Atlas of
Intraocular Tumors

Atlas of Intraocular Tumors

Jerry A. Shields, M.D.
Director, Ocular Oncology Service
Wills Eye Hospital
Professor of Ophthalmology
Thomas Jefferson University
Philadelphia, Pennsylvania

Carol L. Shields, M.D.
Surgeon, Ocular Oncology Service
Wills Eye Hospital
Associate Professor of Ophthalmology
Thomas Jefferson University
Philadelphia, Pennsylvania

LIPPINCOTT WILLIAMS & WILKINS
A **Wolters Kluwer** Company

Philadelphia • Baltimore • New York • London
Buenos Aires • Hong Kong • Sydney • Tokyo

Acquisitions Editor: Christine Battle Rullo/Paula Callaghan
Developmental Editor: Delois Patterson
Manufacturing Manager: Dennis Teston
Production Manager: Jodi Borgenicht
Production Editor: Jonathan Geffner
Cover Designer: QT Design
Indexer: Deana Reese Fowler
Compositor: Lippincott Williams & Wilkins Desktop Division

Printed and bound in China

9 8 7 6 5 4 3 2 1

Library of Congress Cataloging-in-Publication Data
Shields, Jerry A.
    Atlas of intraocular tumors / Jerry A. Shields, Carol L. Shields.
       p.   cm.
    Includes bibliographical references and index.
    ISBN 0-7817-1916-X
    1. Eye—Tumors—Atlases.   I. Shields, Carol L.   II. Title.
RC280.E9 S547 1999
616.99′284 dc21   98-33786
                                                          CIP

Care has been taken to confirm the accuracy of the information presented and to describe generally accepted practices. However, the authors and publisher are not responsible for errors or omissions or for any consequences from application of the information in this book and make no warranty, expressed or implied, with respect to the contents of the publication.

The authors and publisher have exerted every effort to ensure that drug selection and dosage set forth in this text are in accordance with current recommendations and practice at the time of publication. However, in view of ongoing research, changes in government regulations, and the constant flow of information relating to drug therapy and drug reactions, the reader is urged to check the package insert for each drug for any change in indications and dosage and for added warnings and precautions. This is particularly important when the recommended agent is a new or infrequently employed drug.

Some drugs and medical devices presented in this publication have Food and Drug Administration (FDA) clearance for limited use in restricted research settings. It is the responsibility of the health care provider to ascertain the FDA status of each drug or device planned for use in their clinical practice.

To our six wonderful children
Jerry, Patrick, Billy Bob, Maggie Mae, John, and Charlotte Nelle,
who have provided us with endless hours of entertainment
during the preparation of this book.

Contents

Part 1. Tumors of the Uveal Tract

Part 2. Tumors of the Retina and Optic Disc

Part 3. Miscellaneous Intraocular Tumors

Foreword

Atlas of Intraocular Tumors is part of a trilogy on ocular tumors; the other two atlases deal with orbital tumors and eyelid and conjunctival tumors. Clearly, there are no two people more qualified to coauthor such books than Drs. Jerry and Carol Shields. Having worked in the same facility with the Shields for over 25 years, I can attest first-hand to their attention to detail and their thorough documentation of the lesions seen in their oncology practice, which attracts patients from all parts of the world.

The authors have organized this atlas in a concise and understandable format. The text appears on the left-hand page and the figures on the facing right-hand page. The Shields' extensive quest for quality is again reflected in the clarity of the figures—all 1,482 of them! As stated in their preface, the conditions range from the most common lesions, such as uveal nevi, to rare lesions, such as adenocarcinoma of the retinal pigment epithelium.

This atlas is a treasure trove of information about intraocular tumors and pseudotumors. It will be not only an invaluable reference for oncologists and pathologists but also a vital resource for residents, fellows, practicing ophthalmologists, and indeed anyone who uses an ophthalmoscope.

William Tasman, M.D.
Ophthalmologist-in-Chief
Wills Eye Hospital
and Professor of Ophthalmology
Thomas Jefferson University
Philadelphia, Pennsylvania

Foreword

It is a pleasure to write this Foreword to *Atlas of Intraocular Tumors*. Drs. Jerry and Carol Shields have devoted their professional lives to the field of ocular oncology. Both have made significant contributions to our knowledge concerning the diagnosis and treatment of intraocular tumors.

In no other internal organ do we have the opportunity to visualize, photograph, measure, and study the physiology of tumors to the degree possible that we have in the eye. This accessibility allows precise documentation of most of the features of these tumors by the authors and many other investigators. This in turn has greatly increased our ability to identify these tumors that are not readily accessible for histopathological diagnosis.

We are grateful to the authors for sharing their extensive clinical experience through this beautifully illustrated atlas that will greatly enhance the diagnostic and therapeutic skills of all who study ocular oncology.

J. Donald M. Gass, M.D.
Professor of Ophthalmology
Vanderbilt University School
of Medicine
Nashville, Tennessee

Preface

For about 25 years, we have pursued a full-time medical and surgical practice of ophthalmic oncology at Wills Eye Hospital of Thomas Jefferson University in Philadelphia. During that time, we have enjoyed the unusual opportunity to document the clinical and histopathologic characteristics of most neoplasms and related conditions that occur in the eyelids, conjunctiva, intraocular structures, and orbit. In addition, we have been able to photographically document our extensive experience in the clinical diagnosis and management of these conditions. We have incorporated this material into comprehensive lectures on ocular tumors and pseudotumors that we frequently share with ophthalmologists and other physicians. A number of clinicians and ophthalmic pathologists have encouraged us to assemble our excellent slide collection into comprehensive color atlases to assist physicians with recognition of the various ocular tumors and related conditions. Consequently, we have produced three volumes, entitled *Atlas of Eyelid and Conjunctival Tumors*, *Atlas of Intraocular Tumors*, and *Atlas of Orbital Tumors*.

This particular atlas covers tumors and pseudotumors that affect the intraocular structures. Some of these conditions are common and relatively harmless and require no treatment. Some benign lesions are not a threat to the patient's systemic health but can cause serious visual impairment and may require treatment. Some malignant tumors may pose a threat to the patient's vision and life. It is important for the ophthalmologist to correctly diagnose such lesions so that appropriate therapeutic measures can be taken. We have designed this atlas to assist the clinician in that regard.

We have attempted to illustrate and discuss the clinical variations, histopathologic characteristics, and management of most intraocular tumors and pseudotumors. Each specific entity is described in a concise review with pertinent references on the left page and six color figures on the adjacent right page, allowing the reader to obtain a complete uninterrupted overview of the subject without having to turn pages to find corresponding figures and references. This atlas is generously illustrated with 1,482 figures that depict the clinical and pathological variations and management of almost all lesions that are know to affect the uveal tract, retina, and other intraocular structures. It includes common lesions as well as some rare and fascinating conditions. It is rich in clinicopathologic correlations and clinical "pearls" based on our daily experience in the management of affected patients. Surgical principles are illustrated with high-quality professional color drawings and photographs of the surgical procedures.

We hope that this unique atlas will benefit residents and fellows in ophthalmology, general ophthalmologists, ophthalmic subspecialists, and other practitioners who may evaluate patients with intraocular tumors.

Jerry A. Shields, M.D.
Carol L. Shields, M.D.

Acknowledgments

A number of individuals have contributed directly or indirectly to the evolution and publication of this atlas. We are indebted to the many physicians in the United States and abroad who have referred to us their patients with ocular tumors and pseudotumors. Their support of our subspecialty service has enabled us to improve our methods of diagnosis and treatment of patients with ocular tumors and to acquire the extensive collection of photographs that are used in this atlas.

We are particularly appreciative of our wonderful staff on the Oncology Service at Wills Eye Hospital of Thomas Jefferson University. Most of the slides used for photographs were organized and labeled in our department by Mary Ann Venditto, Sandra Dailey, Queen Warwick, and Leslie Botti. We are especially grateful to our office manager, Bridget Walsh, for her continued support and enthusiasm. We also thank Kathy Smallenburg, Joann Delisi, Jacqueline Jurinich, Jeanine Ligon, Amia Scott, Christine Serlenga, and Tamicia Warrick for their assistance with patient care. We appreciate the continued support of the physicians and administrators at Wills Eye Hospital and Thomas Jefferson University.

Many of the excellent clinical photographs used in this atlas were taken by Terrance Tomer, Richard Lambert, Joyce Fellman, Robert Curtin, Jack Scully, and Roger Barone. We are deeply grateful to Robert Curtin and Jack Scully for taking numerous photographs in the operating room and for preparing and copying most of the slides used in the atlas.

We are truly indebted to our colleague and friend, Dr. Ralph C. Eagle, Jr. who over the years has spent many hours providing pathology consultations on our surgical cases. He also took many of the numerous gross pathology photographs and photomicrographs of our patients that appear in this atlas. His talent for documenting photographically the fine details of ocular tumors is unparalleled. The numerous clinicopathologic correlations used in this atlas provide the reader with a better understanding of the ocular tumors.

Most of the photographs in this atlas are of patients whom we evaluated and managed personally, and it was not practical to acknowledge the referring physician in all cases. Some of the clinical and histopathologic photographs are from patients who were not evaluated personally by us but were taken from cases contributed by colleagues to the various ocular pathology societies and from articles published in the literature. In those instances, we have always attempted to give credit to the contributing physician.

We are grateful for the support of Christine Rullo, Paula Callaghan, Delois Patterson, Jonathan Geffner, David Dritsas, James Ryan, and their associates at Lippincott Williams & Wilkins for undertaking the publication of this atlas. With the generous help of these individuals and many others, the completion of this comprehensive atlas has been possible.

Atlas of
Intraocular Tumors

PART I

Tumors of the Uveal Tract

CHAPTER 1

Congenital Uveal Lesions

CONGENITAL IRIS STROMAL CYSTS

Most iris cysts are probably acquired pigment epithelium or stromal lesions that can simulate clinically an iris or ciliary body melanoma (1,2). Such acquired iris cysts are discussed in Chapter 3 under differential diagnosis of iris melanoma. Congenital iris stromal cysts usually are diagnosed in early childhood and are not often confused with iris melanoma.

Clinically, congenital iris stromal cyst can occur in any quadrant of the iris. It has a very thin wall, and the lumen usually contains clear fluid. The cyst attenuates the iris stroma, allowing visualization of the iris pigment epithelium at its posterior surface. The cyst usually is noted in the first few months of life, and it frequently enlarges slowly and often encroaches on the pupil, leading to visual impairment (1–7).

Histopathologically, congenital iris stromal cyst is lined with thin, nonkeratinizing stratified epithelium that contains goblet cells. The pathogenesis usually is undetermined, but the lesion seems to be secondary to embryologic displacement of surface conjunctival epithelium into the anterior chamber. Possible displacement of surface cells into the anterior chamber at the time of prenatal amniocentesis has been implicated (5).

The management is controversial (6,7). When the lesion extends to the pupil, we generally employ aspiration with a 30-gauge needle to collapse the cyst. Cryotherapy or cautery then is applied to the base of the lesion near the limbus. If the lesion recurs, the aspiration can be repeated. Laser treatment to the wall of the cyst also has been used, but recurrence is frequent. In cases that do not respond to these measures, surgical removal by iridectomy or iridocyclectomy may be required. Regardless of the treatment employed, the affected child should have a refraction and appropriate amblyopic therapy with patching of the opposite eye often is necessary.

SELECTED REFERENCES

1. Shields JA, Shields CL. *Intraocular tumors. A text and atlas.* Philadelphia: WB Saunders, 1992:78.
2. Shields JA. Primary cysts of the iris. Theses, American Ophthalmologic Society. *Trans Am Ophthalmol Soc* 1981;79:771–809.
3. Naumann G, Green WR. Spontaneous nonpigmented iris cysts. *Arch Ophthalmol* 1967;78:496–500.
4. Waeltermann JM, Hettinger ME, Cibis GW. Congenital cysts of the iris stroma. *Am J Ophthalmol* 1985;100: 549–554.
5. Cross HE, Maumenee AE. Ocular trauma during amniocentesis. *Arch Ophthalmol* 1973;90:303–304.
6. Lois N, Shields CL, Shields JA, et al. Primary iris stromal cysts: a report of 17 cases. *Ophthalmology* 1998;105:1317–1322.
7. Shields JA, Shields CL, Lois N, Mercado G. Iris cysts in children: classification, incidence and management. The 1998 Torrence A. Makley Jr. Lecture. *Br J Ophthalmol (in press)*.

Congenital Iris Stromal Cysts

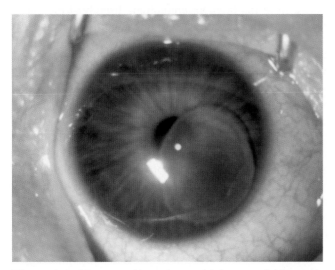

Figure 1-1. Iris stromal cyst located inferonasally in an 8-week-old girl.

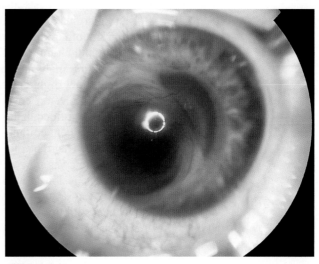

Figure 1-2. Iris stromal cyst located inferotemporally in a 7-week-old child.

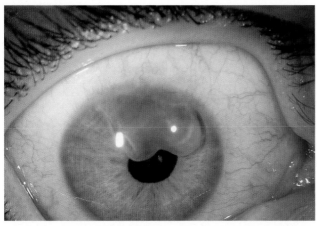

Figure 1-3. Superior iris stromal cyst in a 10-week-old child. The lesion recurred after aspirations and required surgical removal.

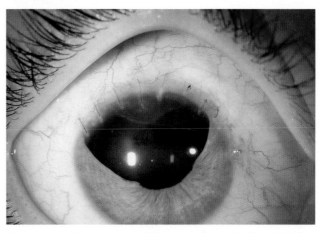

Figure 1-4. Appearance of the eye shown in Fig. 1-3 after surgical removal of the cyst. Note that a sector iridectomy was necessary.

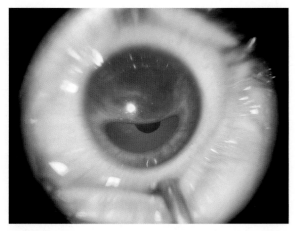

Figure 1-5. Bilobed superior iris stromal cyst in an 8-week-old child. Iridectomy eventually was required.

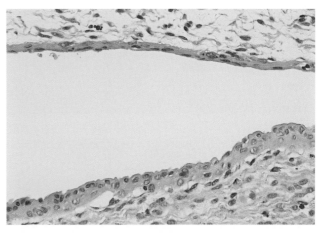

Figure 1-6. Histopathology of the lesion shown in Fig. 1-5. Note that the cyst is lined with nonkeratinizing stratified epithelium and surrounded by iris stromal tissue. No goblet cells are seen in this field (hematoxylin–eosin, original magnification × 15).

CONGENITAL IRIS PIGMENT EPITHELIAL CYSTS

Congenital cysts also can arise from iris pigment epithelium, usually at the pupillary margin. When the lesion is solitary, it is usually a sporadic condition that appears as a smooth, rounded mass that may resemble a melanoma or adenoma of the iris pigment epithelium (1,2). The dense pigment lining the lesions usually prevents transillumination of light. These lesions generally are stationary for many years and only rarely show slight enlargement. No treatment is necessary except for the rare occasion where the lesion covers the entire pupil. The cyst may collapse spontaneously and appear as a flocculent pigmented lesion (2–7).

Iris pigment epithelial cyst at the pupillary margin occasionally can be multiple and bilateral. That type of cyst occasionally can be inherited in an autosomal dominant pattern. The cysts may collapse spontaneously and reform, producing a circumferential irregular lesion around the pupil (iris flocculi). Even when they are extensive, they rarely cause visual impairment, and most lesions remain stable throughout the patient's lifetime (2–4). Although there are usually no systemic associations, one family has been reported with iris flocculi and dissecting aortic aneurysm (6).

SELECTED REFERENCES

1. Shields CL, Shields JA, Cook GR, Von Fricken MA, Augsburger JJ. Differentiation of adenoma of the iris pigment epithelium from iris cyst and melanoma. *Am J Ophthalmol* 1985;100:678–681.
2. Shields JA, Shields CL. *Intraocular tumors. A text and atlas.* Philadelphia: WB Saunders, 1992:78.
3. Shields JA. Primary cysts of the iris. Theses, American Ophthalmological Society. *Trans Am Ophthalmol Soc* 1981;79:771–809.
4. Shields JA, Kline MW, Augsburger JJ. Primary iris cysts. Review of the literature and report of 62 cases. *Br J Ophthalmol* 1984;68:152–166.
5. Lois N, Shields CL,Shields JA, Mercado G. Primary cysts of the iris pigment epithelium: clinical features and natural course in 234 patients. *Ophthalmology* 1998;105:1879–1885.
6. Lewis RA, Merin LM. Iris flocculi and familial aortic dissection. *Arch Ophthalmol* 1995;113:130–131.
7. Shields JA, Shields CL, Lois N, Mercado G. Iris cysts in children: classification, incidence and management. The 1998 Torrence A. Makley Jr. Lecture. *Br J Ophthalmol (in press).*

Congenital Iris Pigment Epithelial Cysts

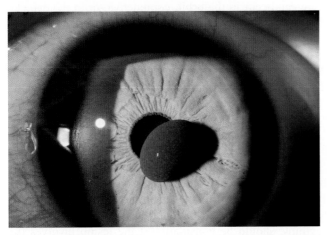

Figure 1-7. Large pupillary margin cyst in a 38-year-old man. The lesion had been present and relatively stable since early childhood.

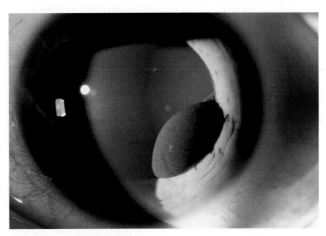

Figure 1-8. Lesion shown in Fig. 1-7 after pupillary dilation. Note that the lesion has now been pulled more into the pupillary aperture.

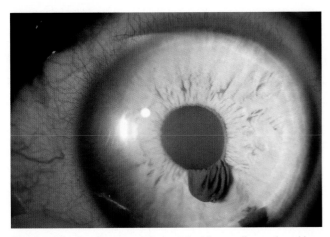

Figure 1-9. Pupillary margin cyst that has collapsed and has a flocculent appearance in a 25-year-old man.

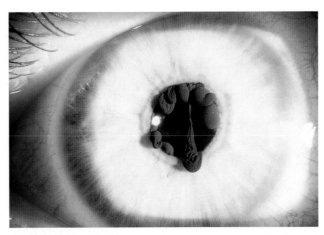

Figure 1-10. Left eye of an 18-year-old man with bilateral multiple pupillary margin cysts (iris flocculi). The lesions were noticed shortly after birth and had not changed.

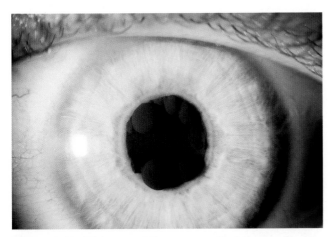

Figure 1-11. Right eye of the same patient depicted in Fig. 1-10 showing a similar appearance to the left eye.

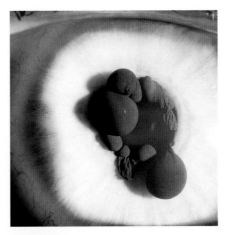

Figure 1-12. Right eye of the same patient 9 years later. Note that the configuration of the lesions had changed, with some lesions having collapsed and others having enlarged. The left eye had undergone similar changes.

INTRAOCULAR LACRIMAL GLAND CHORISTOMA

Ectopic lacrimal gland tissue can occur in the orbit, conjunctiva, or in the eye (1). Intraocular lacrimal gland choristoma is rare, and most such lesions have occurred in the iris. Several theories as to the pathogenesis of intraocular lacrimal gland choristoma have been proposed and are discussed in recent articles on the subject (2,3). Clinically, the lesion generally appears in early infancy as a fleshy reddish-pink mass of the iris and ciliary body (1–5). It appears almost identical to the orbital lacrimal gland as visualized at the time of orbital surgery. Clear cysts appear within the lesion early in the clinical course. These have been likened to lacrimal gland cysts (dacryops).

With regard to the natural course of intraocular lacrimal gland choristoma, the main mass does not tend to grow significantly, but the cysts within the lesion can enlarge progressively and cause iris atrophy, secondary glaucoma, and cataract. Although it is tempting to only follow this benign lesion in young children, we believe that the appearance of a progressively enlarging cyst within the lesion should prompt early surgical removal of the mass in order to prevent glaucoma and visual impairment. Iridocyclectomy, rather than iridectomy, should be considered, if the lesion involves the peripheral iris with extension into the ciliary body (2).

SELECTED REFERENCES

1. Green WR, Zimmerman LE. Ectopic lacrimal gland tissue. Report of eight cases with orbital involvement. *Arch Ophthalmol* 1967;78:318–327.
2. Shields JA, Eagle RC Jr, Shields CL, De Potter P, Poliak JG. Natural course and histopathologic findings of lacrimal gland choristoma of the iris and ciliary body. *Am J Ophthalmol* 1995;119:219–224.
3. Conway VH, Brownstein S, Chisholm IA. Lacrimal gland choristoma of the ciliary body. *Ophthalmology* 1985;92;449–453.
4. Morgan G, Mishin A. Ectopic intraocular lacrimal gland tissue. *Br J Ophthalmol* 1972;56:690–694.
5. O'Donnell BA, Martin FJ, Kan AE, Filipic M. Intraocular lacrimal gland choristoma. *Aust N Z J Ophthalmol* 1990;18:211–213.

Intraocular Lacrimal Gland Choristoma

From Shields JA, Eagle RC Jr, Shields CL, De Potter P, Poliak JG. Natural course and histopathologic findings of lacrimal gland choristoma of the iris and ciliary body. *Am J Ophthalmol* 1995;119:219–224.

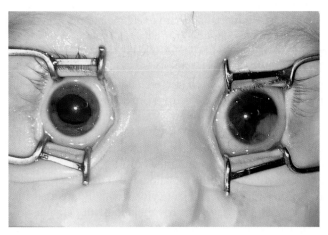

Figure 1-13. Appearance of the iris mass in the left eye of a 7-week-old girl showing a pink mass in the left iris.

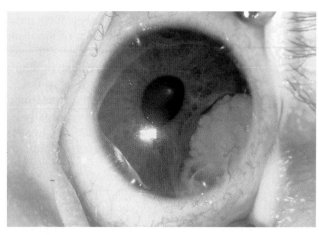

Figure 1-14. Closer view of the lesion shown in Fig. 1-13 more clearly demonstrating a reddish-pink mass with a clear cyst within the lesion inferiorly. The lesion was followed without treatment.

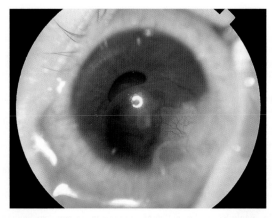

Figure 1-15. Clinical appearance of the mass when the infant was 19 months old. A vascularized corneal pannus now overlies the mass. The inferior cyst is unchanged, but a new cyst is emanating from the mass and filling almost half of the anterior chamber inferotemporally. The lesion was removed by a sector iridectomy.

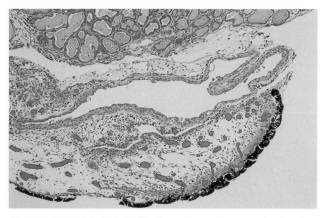

Figure 1-16. Low-magnification photomicrograph showing glandular mass *(above)* and irregular, partially collapsed cyst *(below)* (hematoxylin–eosin, original magnification × 10).

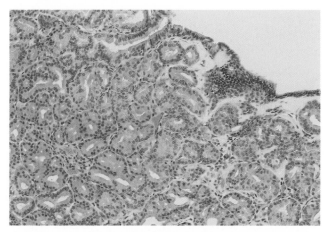

Figure 1-17. Photomicrograph showing glandular acini resembling normal lacrimal gland (hematoxylin–eosin, original magnification × 100).

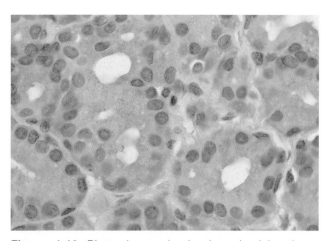

Figure 1-18. Photomicrograph showing glandular tissue identical to normal lacrimal gland (hematoxylin–eosin, original magnification × 200).

CONGENITAL OCULAR MELANOCYTOSIS

Congenital ocular melanocytosis is divided into ocular melanocytosis and oculodermal melanocytosis, or nevus of Ota (1,2). They are identical, except that the latter has periocular cutaneous pigmentation. Both predispose to uveal melanoma, as well as melanoma of the ipsilateral orbit, meninges, and central nervous system (1–6). Several bilaterally affected patients have developed bilateral uveal melanoma (6,7). The most evident finding is unilateral (occasionally bilateral) hyperpigmentation of the sclera and uveal tract. The scleral pigmentation is characterized by flat gray to brown areas of pigmentation. The uveal pigment may have diffuse or sector distribution. The affected iris usually is darker than the iris of the fellow eye. The background fundus pigmentation is greater than in the opposite eye. There is overlying degeneration of the retinal pigment epithelium and numerous drusen. A higher incidence of melanocytoma of the optic nerve in affected eyes has been recognized (1,2).

Histologically, there are dense, heavily pigmented melanocytes in the affected uveal tract. The melanoma that can occur with ocular melanocytosis usually arises in the choroid and/or ciliary body in patients of any age (8). Iris melanoma in patients with ocular melanocytosis is rare (9), and the authors are not aware of a melanoma arising from the affected episcleral pigmentation. Because of the increased incidence of melanoma, affected patients should be examined carefully every 6 to 12 months for their entire life, looking for evidence of uveal, orbital, or brain melanoma.

SELECTED REFERENCES

1. Zimmerman LE. Melanocytes, melanocytic nevi and melanocytomas. The Jonas S. Friedenwald Memorial Lecture. *Invest Ophthalmol* 1965;4:11–41.
2. Shields JA, Shields CL. *Intraocular tumors. A text and atlas.* Philadelphia: WB Saunders, 1992:46–50.
3. Gonder JR, Shields JA, Albert DM, Augsburger JJ, Lavin PT. Uveal malignant melanoma associated with ocular and oculodermal melanocytosis. *Ophthalmology* 1982;89:953–960.
4. Singh AD, De Potter P, Fijal BA, Shields CL, Shields JA, Elston RC. Lifetime prevalence of uveal melanoma in Caucasian patients with ocular (dermal) melanocytosis. *Ophthalmology* 1998;105:195–198.
5. Kiratli H, Bilgig S, Satilmis M. Ocular melanocytosis associated with intracranial melanoma. *Br J Ophthalmol* 1996;80:1025.
6. Gonder JR, Shields JA, Shakin JL, Albert DM. Bilateral ocular melanocytosis and malignant melanoma of the choroid. *Br J Ophthalmol* 1981;65:843–845.
7. Singh AD, Shields CL, Shields JA, De Potter P, Cater JR. Bilateral primary uveal melanoma: bad luck or bad genes? *Ophthalmology* 1996;103:256–262.
8. Gunduz K, Shields JA, Shields CL, Eagle RC Jr. Choroidal melanoma in a 14-year-old patient with ocular melanocytosis. *Arch Ophthalmol* 1998;116:1112–1114.
9. Cu-Unjieng AB, Shields CL, Shields JA, Eagle RC Jr. Iris melanoma in congenital ocular melanocytosis. *Cornea* 1995;14:206–209.

Congenital Ocular Melanocytosis—External Features

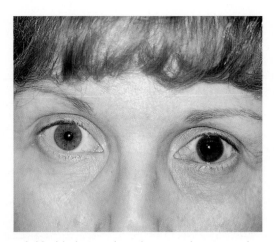

Figure 1-19. Iris heterochromia secondary to ocular melanocytosis in the left eye of a 48-year-old woman. Note that the left iris is darker.

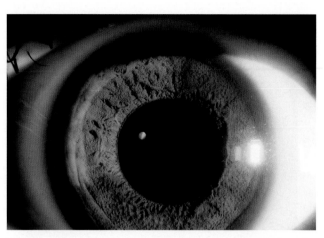

Figure 1-20. Closer view of affected iris in congenital ocular melanocytosis. Note that most of the iris is dark brown and has numerous small nodules. There is a subtle sector of sparing of the iris nasally (to the left).

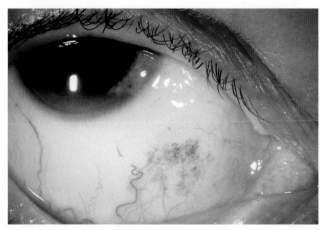

Figure 1-21. Scleral involvement with melanocytosis inferonasally in a 40-year-old man.

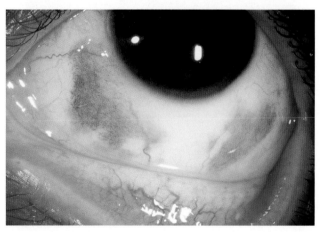

Figure 1-22. Inferior scleral melanocytosis in a 56-year-old woman.

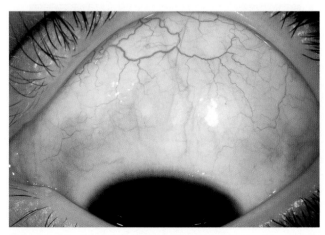

Figure 1-23. Superior scleral melanocytosis in a 40-year-old man.

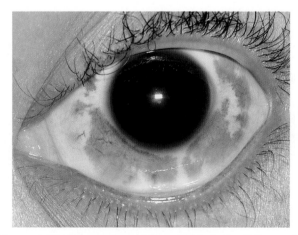

Figure 1-24. More severe melanocytosis in the left eye of a 30-year-old woman. Note that the scleral pigment has a gray color.

Congenital Ocular Melanocytosis—Fundus Features

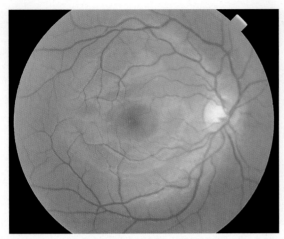

Figure 1-25. Fundus photograph of the unaffected right eye of the patient shown in Fig. 1-24. The background fundus color is normal.

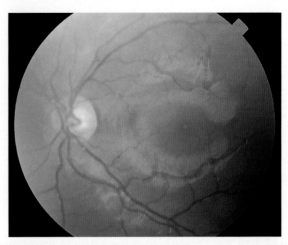

Figure 1-26. Fundus photograph of the affected left eye of the patient shown in Fig. 1-24. The background fundus color is darker than the right eye.

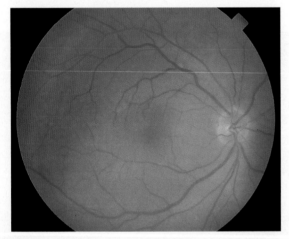

Figure 1-27. Fundus photograph of sector melanocytosis superotemporally in the right eye of a 67-year-old patient. Note that the foveal area is normal and the pigment begins superotemporal to the foveal region.

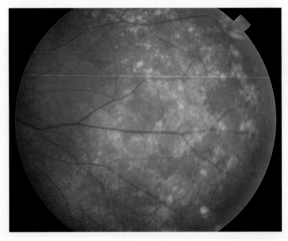

Figure 1-28. Typical peripheral retinal pigment epithelial alterations and drusen in a 48-year-old person with ocular melanocytosis. The extent of these pigment epithelial changes increases with age.

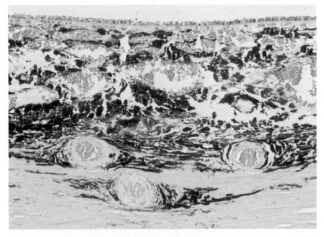

Figure 1-29. Histopathology of the choroid in a patient with ocular melanocytosis. Note the dense pigmentation secondary to increased numbers of choroidal melanocytes (hematoxylin–eosin, original magnification × 40).

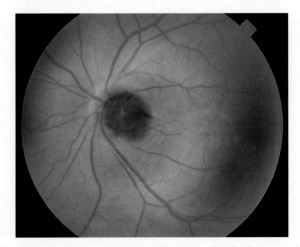

Figure 1-30. Melanocytoma of the optic disc in the opposite eye of the patient shown in Fig. 1-21. There is a slight increased incidence of melanocytoma of the optic disc in patients with ocular melanocytosis. Note the juxtapapillary choroidal component of the lesion.

Oculodermal Melanocytosis (Nevus of Ota)

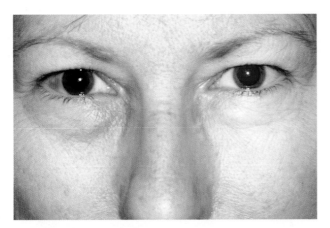

Figure 1-31. Subtle oculodermal melanocytosis of the right eye in a 50-year-old woman.

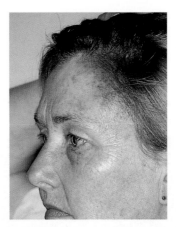

Figure 1-32. Temporal cutaneous melanocytosis in a 51-year-old woman. Pigmentation at the temporal hairline is a frequent finding in patients with oculodermal melanocytosis.

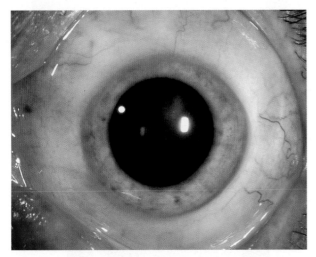

Figure 1-33. Scleral melanocytosis in the patient shown in Fig. 1-32.

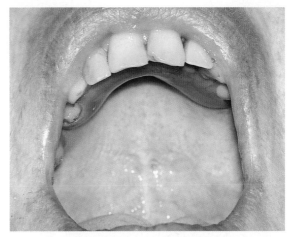

Figure 1-34. Subtle, diffuse pigmentation in the palate of the patient shown in Fig. 1-32. Associated palatine pigmentation is a subtle, often overlooked finding in patients with oculodermal melanocytosis.

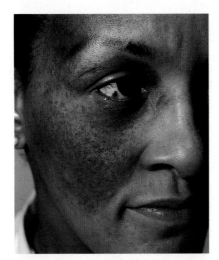

Figure 1-35. Oculodermal melanocytosis on the right side in a 36-year-old African-American patient. Oculodermal melanocytosis may be more difficult to diagnose with dark-skinned individuals. However, like Caucasians, affected black patients also have a higher incidence of melanoma in the pigmented areas.

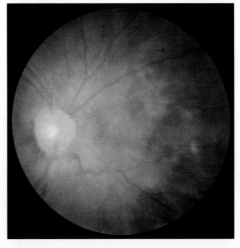

Figure 1-36. Fundus of the right eye in the patient shown in Fig. 1-35. Note the marked pigment epithelial alterations secondary to the thickened, hyperpigmented choroid.

Uveal and Intracranial Melanoma Associated with Congenital Ocular Melanocytosis

There appears to be an increased incidence of both uveal melanoma and intracranial melanoma in patients with ocular and oculodermal melanocytosis.

Fig. 40 from Gunduz K, Shields JA, Shields CL, Eagle RC Jr. Choroidal melanoma in a 14-year-old patient with ocular melanocytosis. *Arch Ophthalmol* 1998;116:1112–1114.

Figs. 1-41 and 1-42 courtesy of Dr. Hayyam Kiratli. From Kiratli H, Bilgig S, Satilmis M. Ocular melanocytosis associated with intracranial melanoma. *Br J Ophthalmol* 1996;80:1025.

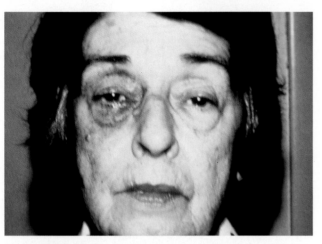

Figure 1-37. Right oculodermal melanocytosis in a 65-year-old woman.

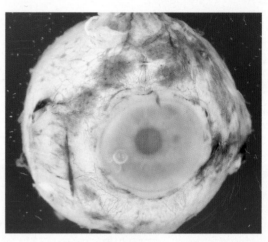

Figure 1-38. Gross appearance of melanoma-containing eye showing the scleral and episcleral pigmentation.

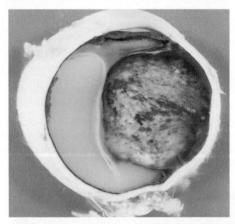

Figure 1-39. Sectioned eye with melanocytosis and melanoma showing large, dome-shaped mass, characteristic of choroidal melanoma, and a secondary retinal detachment.

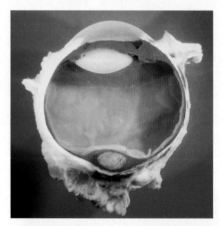

Figure 1-40. Section of eye enucleated for macular melanoma in a 14-year-old boy with marked ocular melanocytosis. Note the ovoid pigmented tumor in the posterior pole.

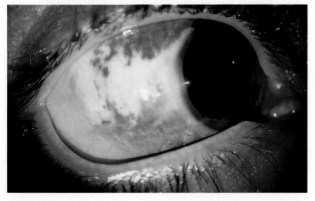

Figure 1-41. Prominent ocular melanocytosis found in the right eye of a 33-year-old woman who presented with a right facial palsy.

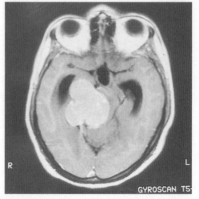

Figure 1-42. Axial magnetic resonance imaging of the brain in the patient shown in Fig. 1-41 showing the large intracranial mass. The lesion was excised and proved to be melanoma.

Bilateral Choroidal Melanoma Associated with Bilateral Ocular Melanocytosis

We have seen several patients with bilateral ocular melanocytosis who eventually developed bilateral uveal melanoma. Patients with bilateral melanocytosis require meticulous periodic ocular examinations to detect melanoma at an early stage.

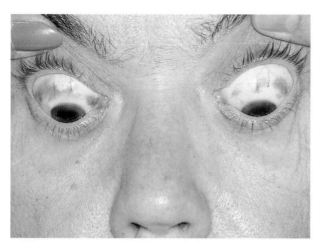

Figure 1-43. Bilateral episcleral pigmentation characteristic of ocular melanocytosis in a 54-year-old man. The lesions had been present since birth.

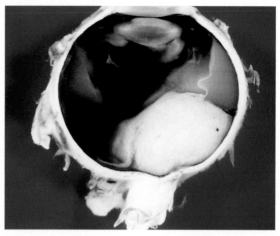

Figure 1-44. Gross section of enucleated left eye showing large, mostly amelanotic choroidal melanoma.

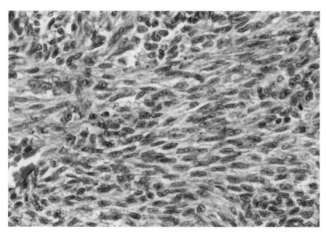

Figure 1-45. Photomicrograph showing spindle-cell–type melanoma of the left eye (hematoxylin–eosin, original magnification × 200).

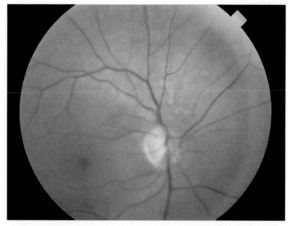

Figure 1-46. Small pigmented fundus lesion with orange pigment appearing in the right eye 8 years after enucleation of the left eye. The patient declined treatment.

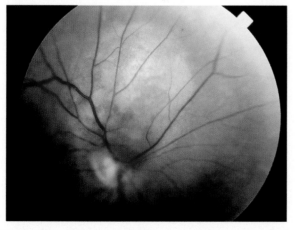

Figure 1-47. Right eye 1 year later showing enlargement of the tumor. The patient still declined treatment.

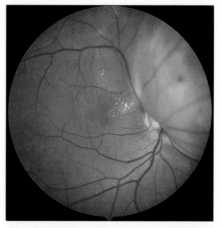

Figure 1-48. Fundus photograph of the right eye 2 years later showing edge of large choroidal melanoma superonasal to the optic disc. The patient was treated with radiotherapy, but ultimately lost all vision in the eye.

CHAPTER 2

Melanocytic Tumors
of the Iris Stroma

IRIS NEVUS

The common iris nevus is covered elsewhere in the literature (1). In contrast to a simple iris freckle, a nevus effaces the architecture of the iris stroma. Iris freckle probably has no malignant potential, whereas an iris nevus may rarely give rise to a malignant melanoma. Iris nevus, like other melanocytic uveal tumors, shows a predilection for Caucasians and becomes apparent during puberty or young adulthood.

Iris nevus can vary in size, shape, and pigmentation. Most are located in the inferior half of the iris. It was once believed that an irregular pupil, angle involvement, secondary cataract, secondary cyst, tapioca configuration, and adjacent transcleral extension were signs of malignant transformation of an iris nevus. It now is realized that many iris nevi can produce such secondary changes and still be benign (1). A variant of iris nevus is melanocytoma, which is a deeply pigmented lesion that can readily undergo necrosis, pigment dispersion, and secondary glaucoma (2,3). Another variant is the diffuse iris nevus (Cogan–Reese syndrome), a condition that may fall in the spectrum of the iridocorneal endothelial syndrome, discussed in Chapter 3. Histopathologically, iris nevus is similar to choroidal nevus discussed later. The cells can range from slender spindle cells to rounded cells similar to those seen in melanocytoma of the optic nerve. Iris nevus may be difficult to differentiate microscopically from a low-grade melanoma (3).

Concerning management, the affected patient should be informed that the chances of malignant transformation are relatively low (1–5). Baseline photographs followed by careful slit lamp biomicroscopy every 6 to 12 months is recommended to detect evidence of growth. Standard angiography and ultrasonography are of little help in diagnosis and management. However, ultrasound biomicroscopy occasionally can be useful to determine the extent of iris and ciliary body involvement. If photographic evidence of growth is documented, local resection of the tumor should be considered. Diffuse or nonresectable iris lesions that have demonstrated growth may require enucleation or plaque radiotherapy (6).

SELECTED REFERENCES

1. Shields JA, Shields CL. *Intraocular tumors. A text and atlas.* Philadelphia: WB Saunders, 1992:62–69.
2. Shields JA, Annesley WH, Spaeth GL. Necrotic melanocytoma of iris with secondary glaucoma. *Am J Ophthalmol* 1977;84:826–829.
3. Fineman M, Eagle RC Jr, Shields JA, Shields CL, De Potter P. Melanocytomalytic glaucoma in eyes with necrotic iris melanocytoma. *Ophthalmology* 1998;105:492–496.
4. Jakobiec FA, Silbert G. Are most iris "melanomas" really nevi? *Arch Ophthalmol* 1981;99:2117–2132.
5. Territo C, Shields CL, Shields JA, Augsburger JJ, Schroeder RP. Natural course of melanocytic tumors of the iris. *Ophthalmology* 1988;95:1251–1255.
6. Shields CL, Shields JA, De Potter P, Singh AD, Hernandez JC, Brady LW. Treatment of nonresectable malignant iris tumors with custom designed plaque radiotherapy. *Br J Ophthalmol* 1995;79:306–312.

Iris Freckle and Nevus

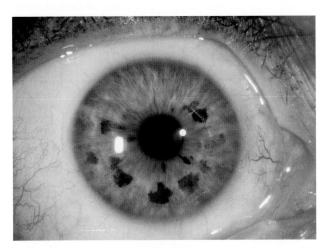

Figure 2-1. Multiple iris freckles in a 46-year-old woman. The freckle does not efface or alter the normal iris architecture.

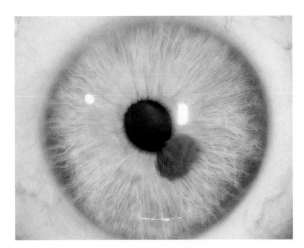

Figure 2-2. Iris nevus adjacent to the pupil in a 69-year-old woman.

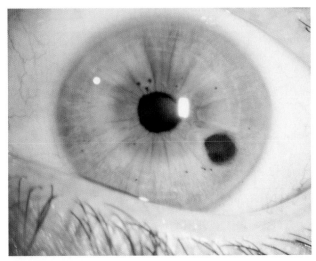

Figure 2-3. Iris nevus in the midportion of the iris in a 40-year-old woman.

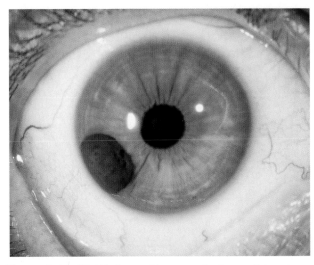

Figure 2-4. Slightly larger iris nevus in the peripheral portion of the iris.

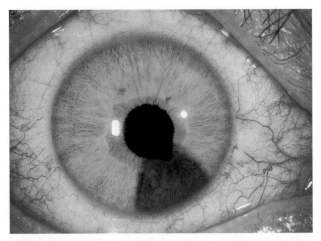

Figure 2-5. Sector inferior iris nevus in a 39-year-old man. Most such sector nevi are noted at birth or shortly thereafter and may represent a localized variant of ocular melanocytosis.

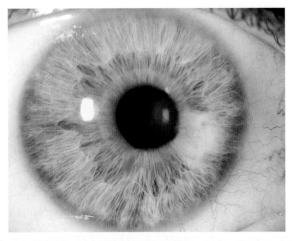

Figure 2-6. Amelanotic iris nevus. The amelanotic form can resemble a leiomyoma, metastasis, lymphoma, and other nonpigmented iris lesions.

Effects of Iris Nevus on Adjacent Structures

Iris nevi can distort the adjacent pupil, involve the anterior chamber angle, produce a secondary cataract and secondary cyst, and even demonstrate transcleral involvement. Such findings can occur with a nevus and do not necessarily indicate that the lesion is malignant. The pupillary changes are probably due to contractile cells like myofibroblasts near the surface of the tumor.

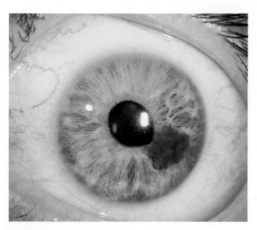

Figure 2-7. Peaking of the pupil secondary to an iris nevus in a 32-year-old man.

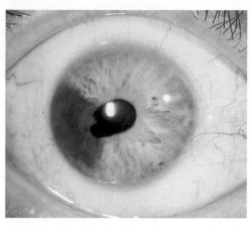

Figure 2-8. Ectropion of the pupillary margin secondary to an iris nevus in a 48-year-old man.

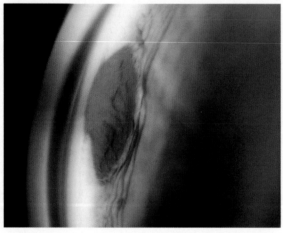

Figure 2-9. Gonioscopic view showing a peripheral iris nevus that affects the angle structures and stops abruptly at Schwalbe's line.

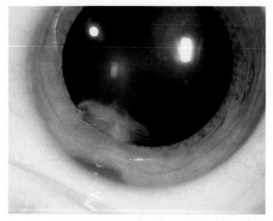

Figure 2-10. Sector cortical cataract secondary to a peripheral iris nevus. Such a cataract can occur with an iris nevus, but transillumination, gonioscopy, and ultrasound biomicroscopy can be used to exclude involvement of the ciliary body.

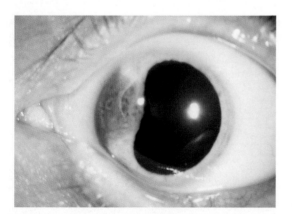

Figure 2-11. Slit lamp view of an iris nevus with a large cyst of the iris pigment epithelium posterior to an iris nevus. Such a cyst should not be misinterpreted as a ciliary body malignant melanoma.

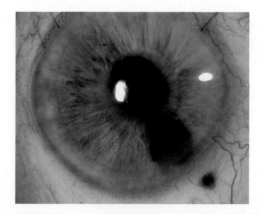

Figure 2-12. Iris nevus with transcleral involvement. Such a finding does not necessarily mean that the tumor has invaded through the sclera. It may be a transcleral component of a congenital nevus and not necessarily extraocular extension of malignant melanoma.

Iris Melanocytoma

Iris melanocytoma is a deeply pigmented variant of iris nevus. It has a tendency to undergo spontaneous necrosis, pigment dispersion, and glaucoma (melanocytomalytic glaucoma). It can rarely transform into malignant melanoma.

Figs. 2-15 through 2-18 from Shields JA, Annesley WH, Spaeth GL. Necrotic melanocytoma of iris with secondary glaucoma. *Am J Ophthalmol* 1977;84:826–829.

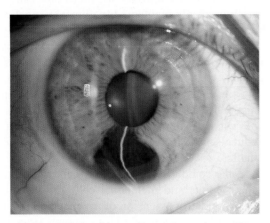

Figure 2-13. Inferior iris melanocytoma in a 40-year-old woman. The lesion was producing seeding into the angle and secondary glaucoma.

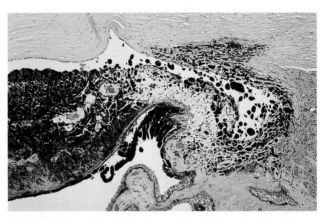

Figure 2-14. Photomicrograph of the lesion shown in Fig. 2-13 after removal by iridocyclectomy. Note the deeply pigmented melanocytes in the iris, trabecular meshwork, and the base of the ciliary body (hematoxylin–eosin, original magnification × 10).

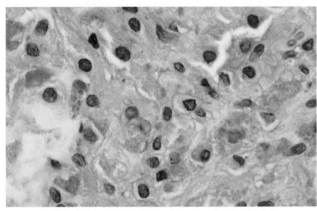

Figure 2-15. Photomicrograph of the lesion shown in Fig. 2-13. The bleached section shows plump round cells with relative uniform nuclei (hematoxylin–eosin, original magnification × 250).

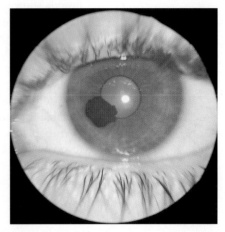

Figure 2-16. Iris melanocytoma in a 23-year-old man as seen in 1972.

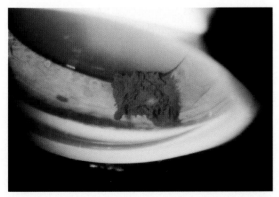

Figure 2-17. Gonioscopic view of the lesion shown in Fig. 2-16, 3 years later. The lesion has produced satellite seeds, pigment deposition into the anterior chamber angle, and secondary glaucoma. Although enucleation was considered, it was elected to remove the lesion by iridectomy.

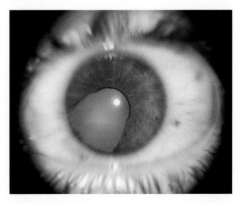

Figure 2-18. Appearance after removal of the main tumor. The satellites and angle pigmentation subsequently resolved and the glaucoma disappeared. The patient continues to do well more than 20 years later.

IRIS MELANOMA

Iris melanoma is a malignant melanocytic tumor that arises in the iris stroma. The clinical features, pathology, diagnostic approaches, management, and prognosis are covered in detail in a comprehensive textbook (1). Clinically, iris melanoma can be circumscribed or diffuse and can range from deeply pigmented to clinically amelanotic. It occurs almost exclusively in white patients.

Circumscribed iris melanoma appears as a variably pigmented, reasonably well-defined mass in the iris stroma and has a definite predilection to occur in the inferior portions of the iris, with more than 80% located below the horizontal meridian. The less common diffuse melanoma has a tendency to produce a classic clinical picture of acquired hyperchromic heterochromia and secondary glaucoma (1,2). Either the circumscribed or diffuse type sometimes can have an irregular tapioca-like surface (tapioca melanoma) (3). Either can produce secondary glaucoma by a variety of mechanisms (4). Histopathologically, smaller iris melanomas have been composed of low-grade melanoma cells, usually of the spindle A or spindle B cell types, but the larger, less cohesive ones may contain epithelioid melanoma cells (5,6). Recently, ultrasound biomicroscopy has been used to detect extension of iris melanoma into the deep iris and ciliary body and in the differentiation of iris melanoma from cystic lesions. In difficult cases, fine-needle aspiration biopsy can be of assistance in the diagnosis of an iris melanoma (7). It should not be used unless the results will influence the therapeutic decision.

With regard to management, only about 5% of untreated suspicious melanocytic iris lesions show growth over the first 5 years after detection (1,8). Therefore, the majority of circumscribed melanocytic iris lesions do not require immediate surgical excision. Lesions that are larger or show growth generally require treatment. The management of circumscribed iris melanoma is local excision with iridectomy, iridocyclectomy, or iridocyclogoniectomy (1,9). A tumor that involves more than half of the iris and trabecular meshwork often requires enucleation, provided that the fellow eye has useful vision. In selected cases, plaque radiotherapy has been used to treat unresectable iris melanoma (1,10). Although iris tumors have shown good regression following plaque radiotherapy, we currently believe that this technique should be reserved for selected growing tumors that are unresectable or when the tumor is located in the patient's only useful eye. The management of diffuse iris melanoma is usually enucleation.

SELECTED REFERENCES

1. Shields JA, Shields CL. *Intraocular tumors. A text and atlas.* Philadelphia: WB Saunders, 1992:69–77.
2. Rones B, Zimmerman LE. The production of heterochromia and glaucoma by diffuse malignant melanomas of the iris. *Trans Am Acad Ophthalmol Otolaryngol* 1957;61:447–463.
3. Reese AB, Mund ML, Iwamoto T. Tapioca melanoma of the iris. I. Clinical and light microscopy studies. *Arch Ophthalmol* 1972;74:840–850.
4. Shields CL, Shields JA, Shields MB, Augsburger JJ. Prevalence and mechanisms of secondary intraocular pressure elevation in eyes with intraocular tumors. *Ophthalmology* 1987;94:839–846.
5. Jakobiec FA, Silbert G. Are most iris "melanomas" really nevi? *Arch Ophthalmol* 1981;99:2117–2132.
6. Zimmerman LE. Clinical pathology of iris tumors: The Ward Burdick Award Contribution. *Am J Clin Pathol* 1963;39:214–228.
7. Shields JA, Shields CL, Ehya H, Eagle RC Jr, De Potter P. Fine needle aspiration biopsy of suspected intraocular tumors. The 1992 Urwick Lecture. *Ophthalmology* 1993;100:1677–1684.
8. Territo C, Shields CL, Shields JA, Augsburger JJ, Schroeder RP. Natural course of melanocytic tumors of the iris. *Ophthalmology* 1988;95:1251–1255.
9. Shields JA, Shields CL. Surgical management of iris melanoma. In: Roy FH ed. *Master techniques in ophthalmic surgery.* Media, PA: Williams & Wilkins, 1995:670–674.
10. Shields CL, Shields JA, De Potter P, Singh AD, Hernandez JC, Brady LW. Treatment of nonresectable malignant iris tumors with custom designed plaque radiotherapy. *Br J Ophthalmol* 1995;79:306–312.

Pigmented Iris Melanoma

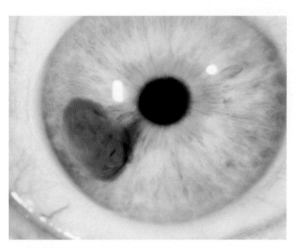

Figure 2-19. Documented growing melanoma in the mid-portion of the iris in a 40-year-old woman.

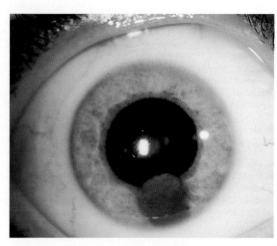

Figure 2-20. Abruptly elevated melanoma in the inferior portion of the iris in a 36-year-old woman.

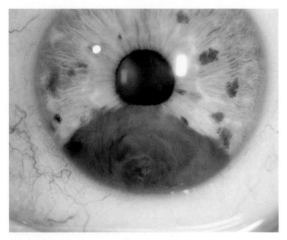

Figure 2-21. Melanoma occupying most of the inferior iris in a 53-year-old woman.

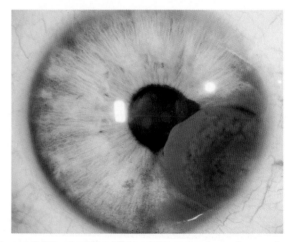

Figure 2-22. Large melanoma causing irregular pupil and touching corneal endothelium in a 61-year-old man.

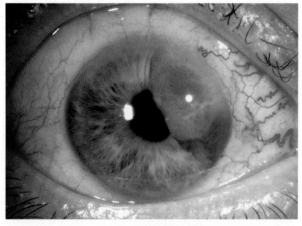

Figure 2-23. Large, mildly pigmented melanoma in the iris superonasally. The atypical superior lesion should raise suspicion that the iris tumor has extended forward from the ciliary body. In this case, the lesion appeared to be primarily in the iris.

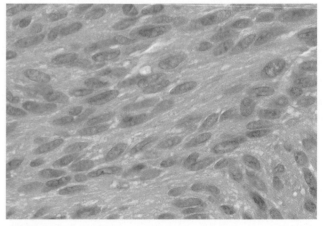

Figure 2-24. Histopathology of iris melanoma showing low-grade spindle-melanoma cells (hematoxylin–eosin, original magnification × 200).

Clinically Amelanotic Iris Melanoma

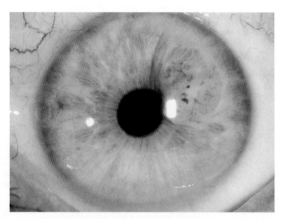

Figure 2-25. Amelanotic iris melanoma near the pupil in a 63-year-old man.

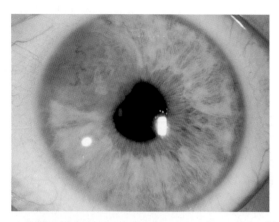

Figure 2-26. Melanoma occupying a quadrant of the iris in a 35-year-old woman.

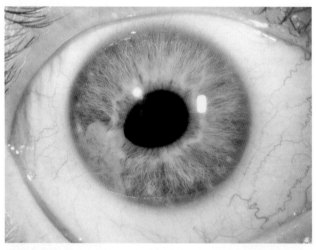

Figure 2-27. Irregular melanoma in the inferotemporal portion of the iris, producing an irregular pupil in a 35-year-old woman in 1979. The lesion was followed without treatment.

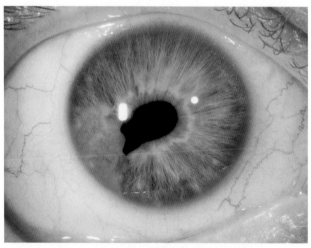

Figure 2-28. Same lesion shown in Fig. 2-27, 9 years later. Note that the tumor has grown slightly and the pupil is more irregular It was removed by iridocyclectomy.

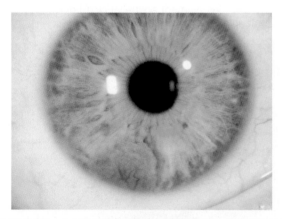

Figure 2-29. Amelanotic tapioca melanoma of the iris. Inferior lesion in a 20-year-old woman. There were numerous tapioca-like nodules scattered in the angle. Fine needle biopsy confirmed diagnosis of melanoma.

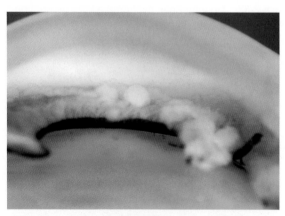

Figure 2-30. Gross photograph of the anterior segment of sectioned eye shown in Fig. 2-29 following enucleation. Note the globular white nodules on the iris and in the angle.

Atypical Clinical Variations of Iris Melanoma

In some instances, iris melanoma can have atypical clinical features, such as a multinodular growth pattern, seeding into the trabecular meshwork, secondary spontaneous hyphema, secondary cyst formation, and band keratopathy.

Figs. 2-35 and 2-36 from Shah PG, Shields CL, Shields JA, DiMarco C. Band keratopathy secondary to an iris melanoma. *Cornea* 1991;10:67–69.

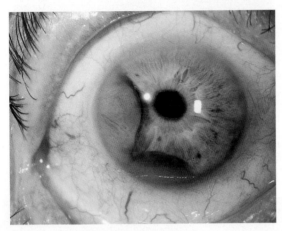

Figure 2-31. Bilobed ring melanoma of the peripheral iris in an 81-year-old man.

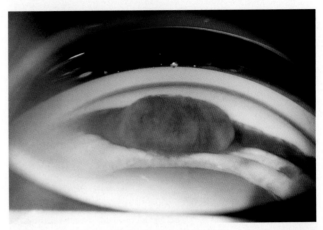

Figure 2-32. Gonioscopic view of a friable, circumscribed iris melanoma with extensive seeding of tumor cells and liberated pigment into the trabecular meshwork in a 66-year-old woman.

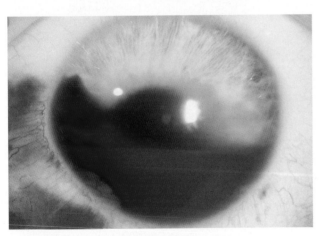

Figure 2-33. Spontaneous hyphema as the presenting feature of an iris melanoma in a 23-year-old man.

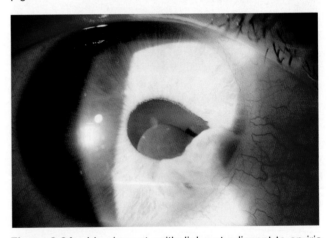

Figure 2-34. Iris pigment epithelial cyst adjacent to an iris melanoma in a 28-year-old woman.

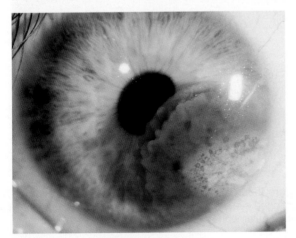

Figure 2-35. Band keratopathy secondary to a large iris melanoma in a 27-year-old man.

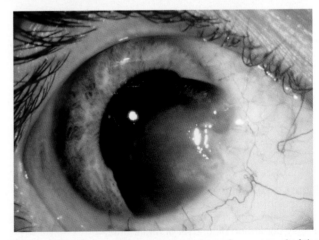

Figure 2-36. Postoperative appearance after removal of the tumor shown in Fig. 2-35 by sector iridocyclectomy. Note that the band keratopathy persists.

Atypical Configurations of Iris Melanoma

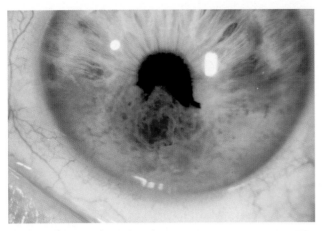

Figure 2-37. Diffuse hemorrhagic tapioca melanoma of the inferior iris in a 53-year-old man.

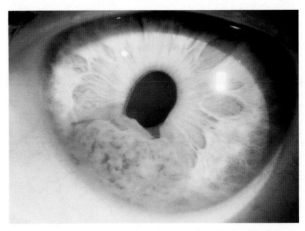

Figure 2-38. Highly vascular amelanotic melanoma with dragging of the pupillary border in a 53-year-old woman.

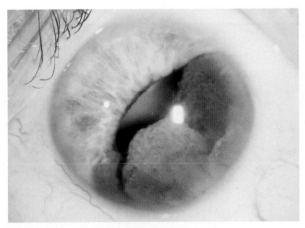

Figure 2-39. Bilobed, partially pigmented melanoma almost covering the pupil in a 59-year-old man.

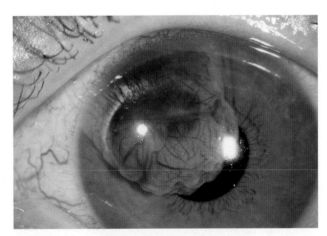

Figure 2-40. Highly pedunculated melanoma in the iris superiorly in a 13-year-old boy. There was some ciliary body involvement and the eye was enucleated. It was not clearly determined whether the tumor originated in the iris or the ciliary body.

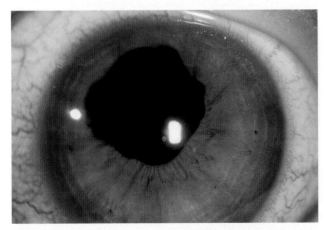

Figure 2-41. Pedunculated, markedly pigmented melanoma arising near the pupillary border and covering the pupil in a 12-year-old girl.

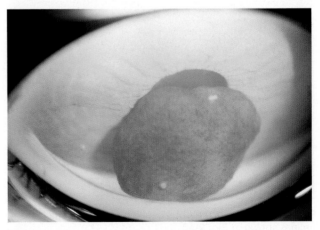

Figure 2-42. Gonioscopic view of the lesion shown in Fig. 2-41. Note the markedly pedunculated shape of the tumor. It proved to be a mixed cell–type melanoma following surgical removal of the tumor.

Diffuse Iris Melanoma

Some diffuse melanomas grow in irregular patches, giving the impression that the tumor is multifocal.

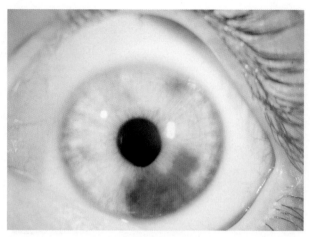

Figure 2-43. Diffuse pigmented lesion in the iris inferiorly in a 10-year-old girl. The lesion was followed conservatively.

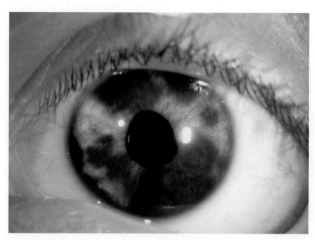

Figure 2-44. Lesion shown in Fig. 2-43, 3 years later. Note that the patchy pigmentation has become more extensive. Secondary glaucoma supervened and histopathology after enucleation revealed a diffuse iris melanoma with involvement of the trabecular meshwork.

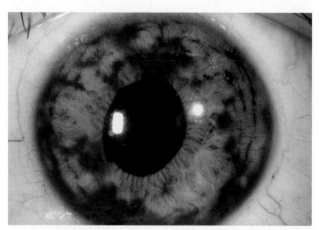

Figure 2-45. Patchy diffuse iris melanoma in an 18-year-old man. Secondary glaucoma supervened and histopathology after enucleation revealed a diffuse iris melanoma with involvement of the trabecular meshwork.

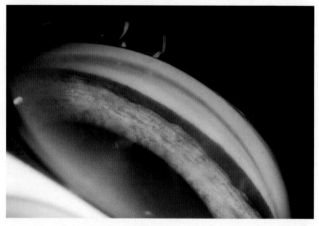

Figure 2-46. Melanoma confined to the region of the trabecular meshwork in a 59-year-old man. Such trabecular melanoma is a rare variant of diffuse iris melanoma.

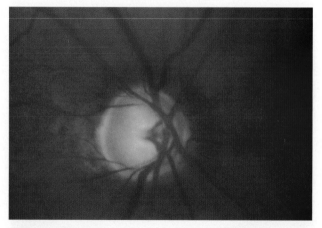

Figure 2-47. Glaucomatous cupping of the optic disc in the patient shown in Fig. 2-46.

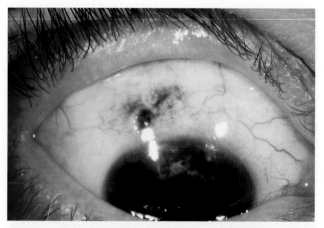

Figure 2-48. Patient with diffuse iris melanoma who had undergone prior filtering surgery for unexplained glaucoma. Note the diffuse iris tumor mostly inferiorly and the pigment within the filtering bleb superiorly. Patients with diffuse iris melanoma are often treated for "idiopathic" glaucoma until the tumor is discovered at a later date.

Diffuse Iris Melanoma—Clinicopathologic Correlation and Follow-up

From Shields JA, Shields CL. Hepatic metastases of diffuse iris melanoma 17 years after enucleation. *Am J Ophthalmol* 1989;106:749–750.

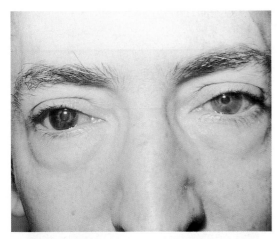

Figure 2-49. Acquired hyperchromic heterochromia in a 52-year-old man. He had an intraocular pressure of 50 mm Hg in the affected right eye.

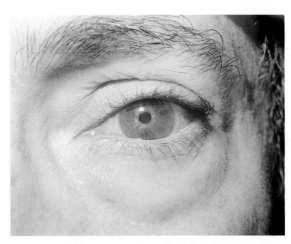

Figure 2-50. Iris of the normal left eye. The color of the iris is blue.

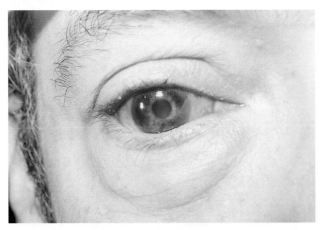

Figure 2-51. Iris of the affected right eye showing diffuse pigmentation. The iris had changed from blue to brown over about 5 years.

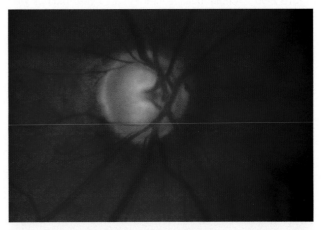

Figure 2-52. Fundus photograph showing glaucomatous cupping of the optic disc in the right eye.

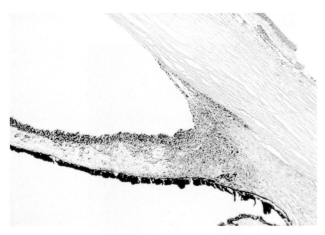

Figure 2-53. Photomicrograph of the anterior segment of the right eye following enucleation. Note the dense pigmentation in the iris and trabecular meshwork (hematoxylin–eosin, original magnification × 15).

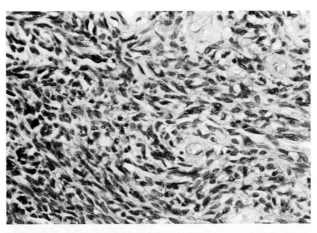

Figure 2-54. Histopathology of the iris tumor showing low-grade spindle cells that comprised the tumor. The patient had no further problems until 17 years later, when he developed hepatic metastasis. There was no local recurrence of tumor in the orbit.

Iris Melanoma in a Patient with Familial Atypical Mole Syndrome (Dysplastic Nevus Syndrome)

The dysplastic nevus syndrome is a familial condition consisting of multiple atypical cutaneous nevi and a high incidence of cutaneous, uveal, and conjunctival melanoma.

From Singh AD, Shields JA, Eagle RC Jr, Shields CL, Marmor M, De Potter P. Iris melanoma in a 10-year-old boy with familial atypical mole-melanoma (FAM-M) syndrome. *Ophthal Pediatr Genet* 1994;15:145–149.

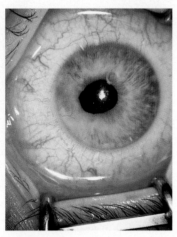

Figure 2-55. Amelanotic iris tumor in a 10-year-old boy who had secondary glaucoma.

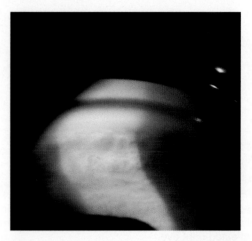

Figure 2-56. Gonioscopic view of the angle showing peculiar amelanotic tissue in the angle. The lesion was removed by iridocyclectomy after subsequent growth was documented.

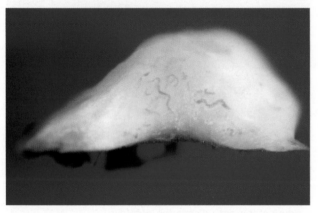

Figure 2-57. Gross appearance of the sectioned specimen showing white vascular tumor.

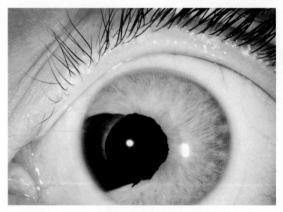

Figure 2-58. Appearance of the anterior segment after successful iridocyclectomy. The glaucoma spontaneously resolved after the tumor was removed and the patient has 20/20 vision 4 years later.

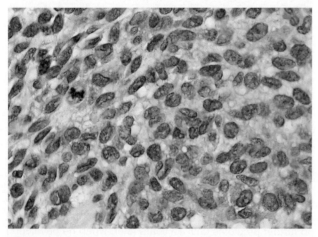

Figure 2-59. Photomicrograph of the tumor showing mixed cell–type melanoma. Note the mitotic figure in the *upper left*.

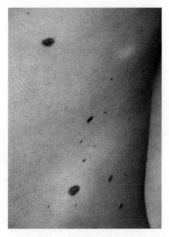

Figure 2-60. Appearance of skin on the patient's back showing several dysplastic nevi.

Iris Melanoma Before and After Surgical Resection by Sector Iridectomy

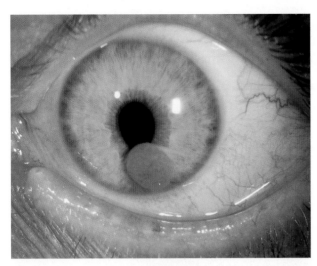

Figure 2-61. Inferior melanoma that had progressively enlarged for 1 year in a 51-year-old woman.

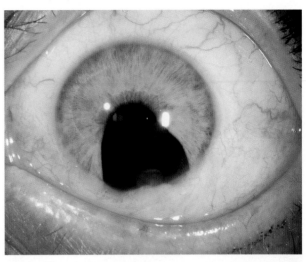

Figure 2-62. Appearance of the eye shown in Fig. 2-61 after surgical removal by sector iridectomy.

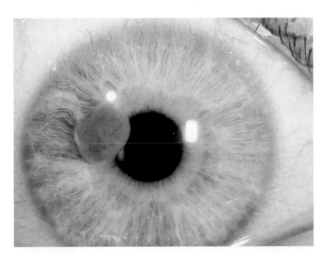

Figure 2-63. Temporal melanoma that had progressively enlarged for 1 year and had produced recurrent hyphemas in a 25-year-old man.

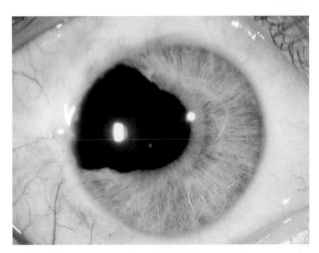

Figure 2-64. Appearance of the eye shown in Fig. 2-63 after surgical removal by sector iridectomy.

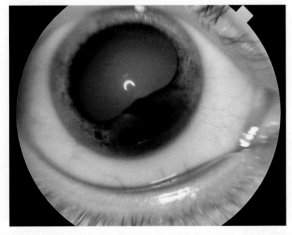

Figure 2-65. Large inferior melanoma in a 10-year-old boy.

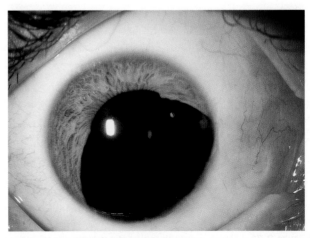

Figure 2-66. Appearance of the eye shown in Fig. 2-65 after surgical removal by iridocyclogoniectomy.

Iris Melanoma Before and After Surgical Resection by Sector Iridectomy and Pupilloplasty

When the tumor is less than 2 clock hours in extent and the iridectomy is small enough, the defect can be partly closed at the time of tumor excision, using a 10-0 non-absorbable suture (Prolene), giving the patient a round pupil rather than a keyhole pupil.

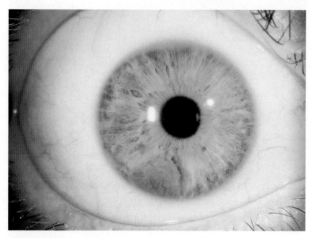

Figure 2-67. Inferior iris melanoma with documented growth in a 20-year-old woman.

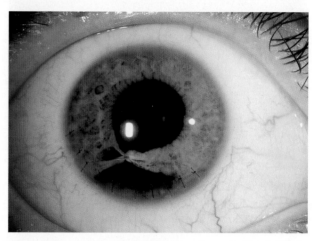

Figure 2-68. Appearance of the eye shown in Fig. 2-67 after surgical removal and pupilloplasty.

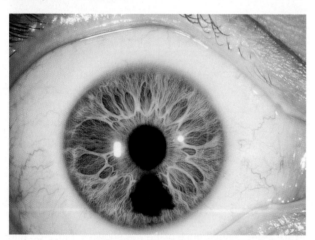

Figure 2-69. Inferior documented growing melanoma in a 27-year-old man. The lesion proved to be a malignant melanoma histopathologically after excision.

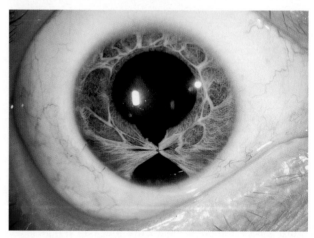

Figure 2-70. Appearance of the eye shown in Fig. 2-69 after surgical removal and pupilloplasty.

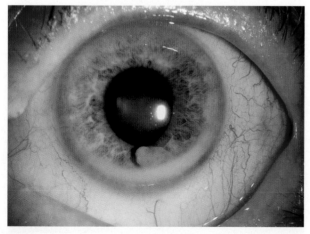

Figure 2-71. Pedunculated amelanotic melanoma with documented growth and recurrent hyphema in a 73-year-old woman.

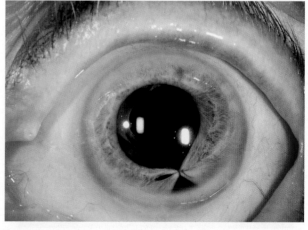

Figure 2-72. Appearance of the eye shown in Fig. 2-71 after surgical removal and pupilloplasty.

Management of Unresectable Iris Melanomas with Plaque Radiotherapy

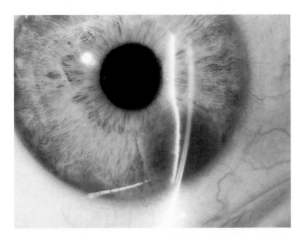

Figure 2-73. Slit lamp view of lightly pigmented tapioca-type melanoma in a 37-year-old man. Angle involvement for more than 180 degrees inferiorly made surgical resection inadvisable.

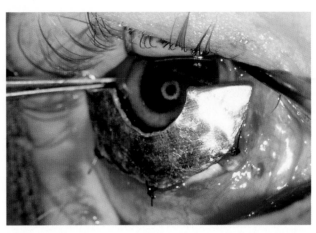

Figure 2-74. Custom-designed plaque placed on the eye of the patient shown in Fig. 2-73.

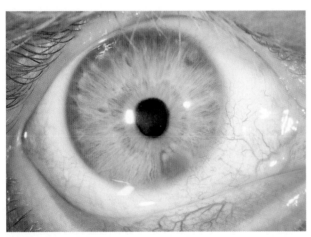

Figure 2-75. Appearance of the tumor shown in Fig. 2-73, 3 years later, showing marked regression of the tumor.

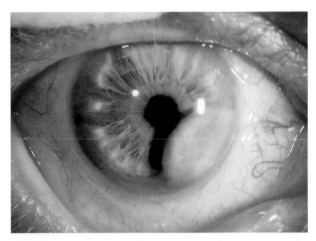

Figure 2-76. Nodular melanoma with extension throughout the inferior half of the iris in a 63-year-old man. His opposite eye was blind from childhood trauma.

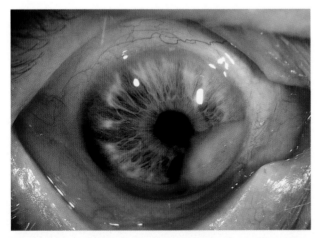

Figure 2-77. Appearance of the eye shown in Fig. 2-76, 4 months after radiotherapy showing decrease in tumor size.

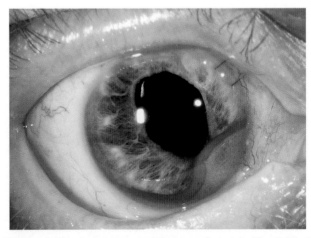

Figure 2-78. Appearance of the eye shown in Fig. 2-76, 2 years after radiotherapy. The tumor had not recurred, and a radiation-induced cataract had been removed and intraocular lens inserted.

CHAPTER 3

Conditions That Simulate
Iris Melanoma

CONDITIONS THAT SIMULATE IRIS MELANOMA

Several conditions can clinically simulate iris melanoma (1–11). Tumors and cysts are discussed elsewhere in this atlas. This section covers selected other nonneoplastic, noncystic conditions that simulate iris melanoma, including iridocorneal endothelial (ICE) syndrome, foreign body, miscellaneous nonneoplastic conditions, and adenoma of the iris pigment epithelium.

The ICE syndrome is an idiopathic condition that usually occurs unilaterally in adult women and is characterized by corneal endothelial guttata, corneal edema, peripheral anterior synechias, iris stromal dehiscence, characteristic iris nodules, and secondary glaucoma. The findings vary from patient to patient and form a spectrum from those with predominant corneal changes (Chandler's syndrome), predominant iris changes (essential iris atrophy), and predominant iris nodules (iris nevus syndrome or Cogan–Reese syndrome). It should be differentiated from diffuse iris melanoma, which would not characteristically show the endothelial changes and iris dehiscence. The clinical and pathologic features of ICE syndrome are discussed in the literature (3–6).

Additional lesions that we have observed to simulate iris melanoma include iris foreign body (1,2,7) granuloma, atypical hemorrhage, retained lens material (8), adenoma of the iris pigment epithelium (1,9), and congenital ectropion iridis. The latter can be idiopathic or associated with neurofibromatosis or the Prader–Willi syndrome (hypotonia, obesity, short stature, hypogonadism, and learning disabilities) (10).

SELECTED REFERENCES

1. Shields JA, Shields CL. *Intraocular tumors. A text and atlas.* Philadelphia: WB Saunders, 1992:77–81.
2. Shields JA, Sanborn GE, Augsburger JJ. The differential diagnosis of malignant melanoma of the iris. A clinical study of 200 patients. *Ophthalmology* 1983;90:716–720.
3. Campbell DG, Shields MB, Smith TR. The corneal endothelium and the spectrum of essential iris atrophy. *Am J Ophthalmol* 1978;86:317–324.
4. Shields MB. Progressive essential iris atrophy, Chandler's syndrome and the iris nevus (Cogan–Reese) Syndrome. A spectrum of disease. *Surv Ophthalmol* 1979;24:3–10.
5. Eagle RC Jr, Font RL, Yanoff M, Fine BS. Proliferative endotheliopathy with iris abnormalities: the iridocorneal endothelial syndrome. *Arch Ophthalmol* 1979;97:2104–2112.
6. Eagle RC Jr, Shields JA. Iridocorneal endothelial syndrome with contralateral guttate endothelial dystrophy. *Ophthalmology* 1987;94:862–870.
7. Eagle RC Jr, Shields JA, Canny CLB, Thompson RL. Intraocular wooden foreign body clinically resembling a pearl cyst. *Arch Ophthalmol* 1977;95:835–836.
8. Olsen TW, Lim JI, Grossniklaus HE. Retained lens material masquerading as a growing, pigmented iris tumor. *Arch Ophthalmol* 1996;114:1154–1155.
9. Shields CL, Shields JA, Cook GR, Von Fricken MA, Augsburger JJ. Differentiation of adenoma of the iris pigment epithelium from iris cyst and melanoma. *Am J Ophthalmol* 1985;100:678–681.
10. Ritch R, Forbes M, Hetherington J Jr, Harrison R, Podos SM. Congenital ectropion uveae with glaucoma. *Ophthalmology* 1984;91:326–331.
11. Ferry AP. Lesions mistaken for malignant melanoma of the iris. *Arch Ophthalmol* 1975;74:9–18.

Iridocorneal Endothelial Syndrome

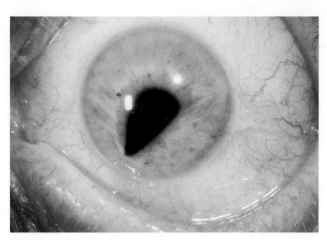

Figure 3-1. Iridocorneal endothelial syndrome in a 70-year-old-woman showing downward displacement of the pupil toward a peripheral anterior synechia. Iris dehiscence had not developed.

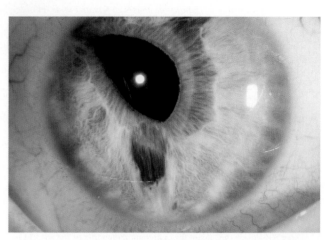

Figure 3-2. Iridocorneal endothelial syndrome in a 45-year-old woman showing upward displacement of the pupil toward a synechia and a secondary dehiscence of the iris stroma inferiorly.

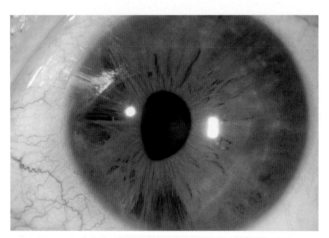

Figure 3-3. Iridocorneal endothelial syndrome in a 40-year-old woman showing irregular pupil and two iris dehiscences.

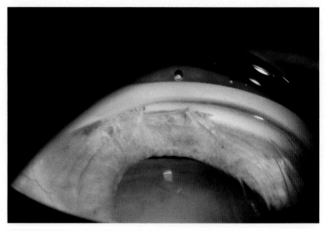

Figure 3-4. Typical peripheral anterior synechia in a 64-year-old woman with iridocorneal endothelial syndrome.

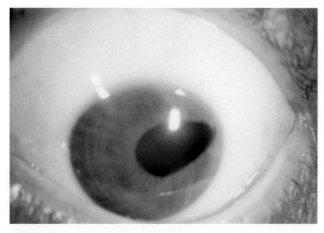

Figure 3-5. Superotemporal displacement of the pupil in a 49-year-old woman with iridocorneal endothelial syndrome. Note that there are no iris dehiscences.

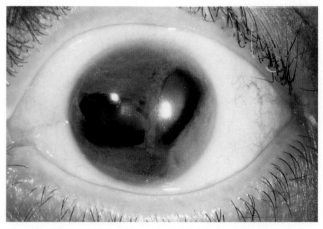

Figure 3-6. Same patient as shown in Fig. 3-5 seen 5 years later. Note that a large iris dehiscence has developed nasally.

Iris Foreign Bodies that Simulate Iris Neoplasms

Occasionally a patient is diagnosed as having an iris melanoma or other iris tumor in which the lesion proves to be a foreign body upon further evaluation. In our experience, such patients often do not recall any prior trauma, in spite of the fact that the foreign body apparently has penetrated the globe anteriorly. Some examples are shown here. The lesion usually can be recognized by its rusty, metallic appearance. If melanoma is a serious diagnostic consideration, ultrasonography or computed tomography might reveal the nature of the lesion.

Fig. 3-12 from Eagle RC Jr, Shields JA, Canny CLB, Thompson RL. Intraocular wooden foreign body clinically resembling a pearl cyst. *Arch Ophthalmol* 1977;95: 835–836.

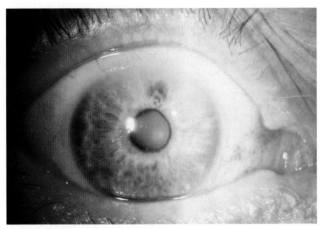

Figure 3-7. Metallic foreign body in the superior iris of a 73-year-old man.

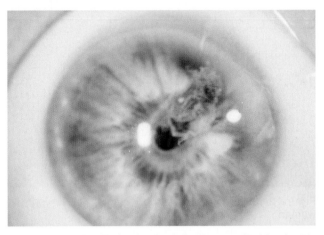

Figure 3-8. Metallic foreign body in the superior iris of a 71-year-old man.

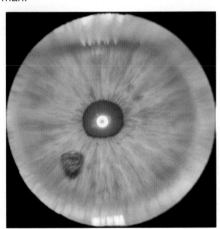

Figure 3-9. Metallic foreign body in the inferior iris of a 19-year-old man.

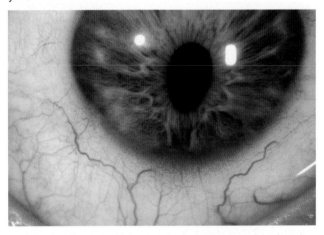

Figure 3-10. Metallic foreign body in the anterior chamber angle inferiorly, causing downward displacement of the pupil.

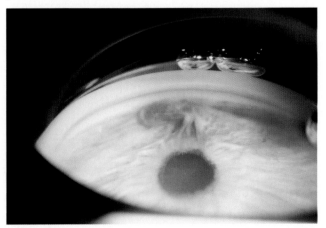

Figure 3-11. Gonioscopic view of the eye shown in Fig. 3-10 showing the metallic foreign body in the iris stoma inferiorly.

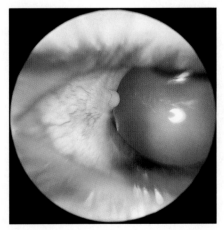

Figure 3-12. Wooden foreign body in the peripheral iris of a young boy, simulating a tumor.

Miscellaneous Nonneoplastic Conditions that Simulate Iris Melanoma

Figs. 3-17 and 3-18 courtesy of Dr. Hans Grossniklaus. From Olsen TW, Lim JI, Grossniklaus HE. Retained lens material masquerading as a growing, pigmented iris tumor. *Arch Ophthalmol* 1996;114:1154–1155.

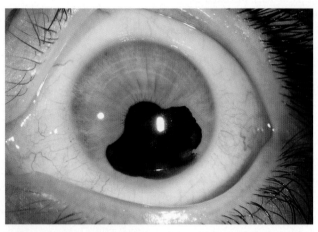

Figure 3-13. Congenital ectropion iridis in a 29-year-old woman.

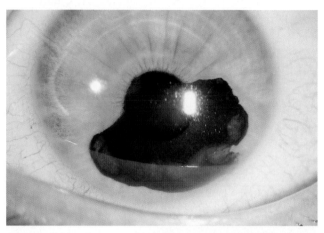

Figure 3-14. Closer view of the lesion shown in Fig. 3-13.

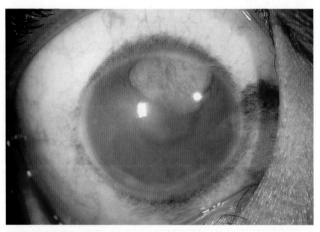

Figure 3-15. Granuloma in the superior iris secondary to sarcoidosis.

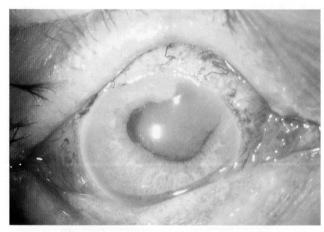

Figure 3-16. Atypical globular hemorrhage in the anterior chamber, presumably arising from a cataract wound.

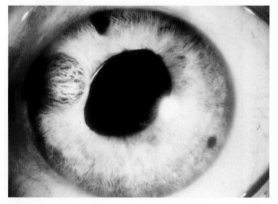

Figure 3-17. Retained lens material in the anterior chamber following cataract surgery.

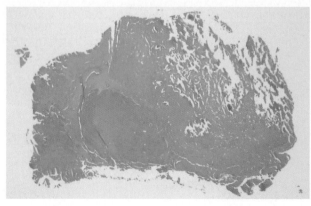

Figure 3-18. Histopathology of the lesion shown in Fig. 3-17 showing typical cataractous lens material.

Adenoma of the Iris Pigment Epithelium

Adenoma of the iris pigment epithelium is discussed in Chapter 19. However, because it is a very important lesion in the differential diagnosis of iris nevus, melanoma, and cyst, it also is covered briefly here. In contrast to nevus and melanoma, it is generally black in color, has more well-defined, abruptly elevated margins, is more likely to occur in the peripheral iris, and does not arise from the iris stroma.

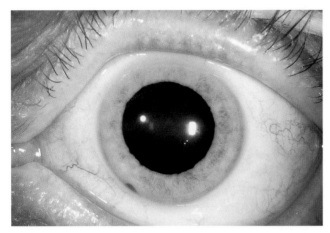

Figure 3-19. Adenoma of the iris pigment epithelium in a 63-year-old woman.

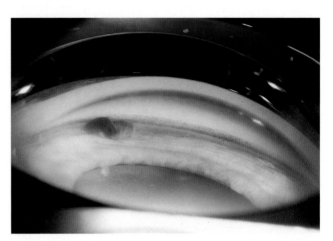

Figure 3-20. Gonioscopic view of the lesion shown in Fig. 3-19.

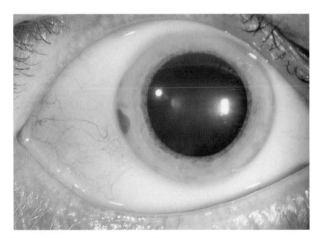

Figure 3-21. Adenoma of the iris pigment epithelium in a 64-year-old woman.

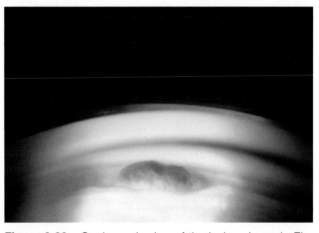

Figure 3-22. Gonioscopic view of the lesion shown in Fig. 3-21.

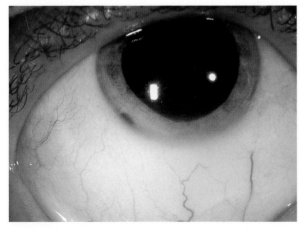

Figure 3-23. Adenoma of the iris pigment epithelium in a 76-year-old man.

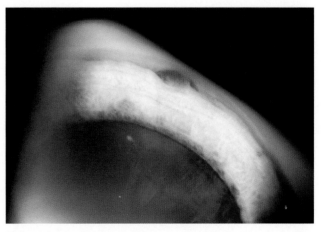

Figure 3-24. Gonioscopic view of the lesion shown in Fig. 3-23.

CHAPTER 4

Acquired Iris Cysts

ACQUIRED IRIS CYSTS

Cystic lesions of the iris can assume any of several clinical variations and can simulate iris melanoma or other iris tumors. The classification, clinical features, pathology, and management of iris cysts are reported (1–5) and are only summarized briefly here.

Iris cysts can be classified as congenital or acquired, primary or secondary, or by their location (pigment epithelial or stromal). Iris pigment epithelial cysts are subclassified into pupillary, midzonal, peripheral (iridociliary), and free floating. Acquired stromal cyst can be idiopathic, or it can occur secondary to surgery or penetrating ocular trauma. Most pupillary margin pigment epithelial cysts and many stromal cysts are congenital and were discussed in Chapter 1.

Iris pigment epithelial cyst: The pupillary margin variant of iris pigment epithelial cyst is usually congenital and was discussed in Chapter 1. The more common peripheral (iridociliary) cyst usually is unilateral and is more common in young adult women. It causes localized anterior bulging of the iris stroma that is detected coincidentally on slit lamp biomicroscopy. With the pupil widely dilated, it sometimes can be visualized directly with slit lamp biomicroscopy and gonioscopy. Ultrasound biomicroscopy can be used to confirm the suspected diagnosis in those that cannot be visualized directly. The midzonal iris cyst can be unilateral or bilateral and solitary or multiple, has a smooth appearance, blocks transmission of light, and, in contrast to iris or ciliary body melanoma, changes shape with dilation of the pupil. Iris pigment epithelial cyst can be dislodged and float freely into the vitreous or anterior chamber (6). Free-floating cysts can become fixed in the anterior chamber angle. Unlike melanoma in the angle, a fixed cyst has sharp abrupt borders, rather than gradual sessile borders.

Iris stromal cyst: Primary iris stromal cysts are so named because they occur in the iris stroma and are not lined with pigment epithelial cells. However, they usually are lined with cells similar to conjunctival epithelium. The pathogenesis is uncertain. Unlike secondary iris stromal cysts, they occur without a history of surgery or trauma (7).

Secondary iris cyst can occur as an epithelial downgrowth or implantation following intraocular surgery or trauma. It usually has a clear lumen but occasionally contain keratin and desquamated epithelium, imparting a yellow color to the lesion (8).

SELECTED REFERENCES

1. Shields JA, Shields CL. *Intraocular tumors. A text and atlas.* Philadelphia: WB Saunders, 1992:78.
2. Shields JA. Primary cysts of the iris. Theses, American Ophthalmological Society. *Trans Am Ophthalmol Soc* 1981;79:771–809.
3. Shields JA, Kline MW, Augsburger JJ. Primary iris cysts. Review of the literature and report of 62 cases. *Br J Ophthalmol* 1984;68:152–166.
4. Lois N, Shields CL, Shields JA, De Potter P, Mercado G. Primary cysts of the iris pigment epithelium: clinical features and natural course in 234 patients. *Ophthalmology* 1998;105:1879–1885.
5. Shields JA, Shields CL, Lois N, Mercado G. Iris cysts in children: classification, incidence and management. The 1998 Torrence A Makley Jr. Lecture. *Br J Ophthalmol (in press)*.
6. Shields JA, Shields CL, De Potter P, Wagner RS, Caputo AR. Free-floating cyst in the anterior chamber of the eye. *J Pediatr Ophthalmol Strabismus* 1996;33:330–331.
7. Lois N, Shields CL, Shields JA, Mercado G. Primary iris stromal cysts: a report of 17 cases. *Ophthalmology* 1998;105:1317–1322.
8. Sanborn GE, Shields JA. Epithelial cyst of the anterior segment following cataract surgery. *Ophthalmologica* 1981;183:221–224.

Peripheral (Iridociliary) Iris Cyst

This is the most common type of iris cyst. It may simulate an iris or ciliary body melanoma. However, an iris melanoma is located in the iris stroma and not posterior to the iris. In addition, the iridociliary cyst transmits light, whereas most melanomas fail to transmit light with transillumination techniques.

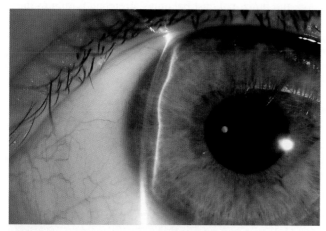

Figure 4-1. Slit lamp view of iridociliary cyst in a 40-year-old woman. Note the anterior displacement of the stroma seen with the slit beam.

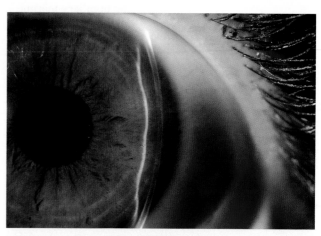

Figure 4-2. Slit lamp view of iridociliary cyst in a 24-year-old woman. Note the anterior displacement of the stroma seen with the slit beam.

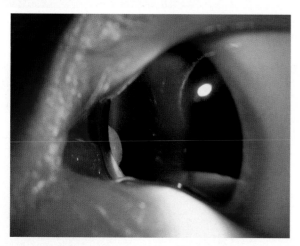

Figure 4-3. Direct view of an iridociliary cyst nasally in a 12-year-old boy. The cyst is best seen by widely dilating the pupil and adjusting the slit lamp beam to the side.

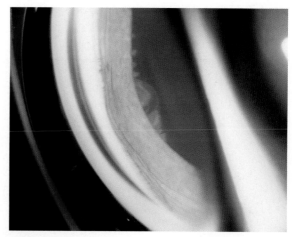

Figure 4-4. Gonioscopic view of iridociliary cyst in a 25-year-old woman. Note that two ciliary processes can be seen behind the transparent cyst, a finding that would not be likely with a melanoma.

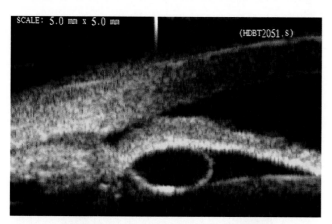

Figure 4-5. Ultrasound biomicroscopy of an iridociliary cyst. This technique can be used to confirm the suspected cystic nature of the lesion. It also has led to the discovery of unexpected iridociliary cysts, indicating that such cysts may be more common than previously believed.

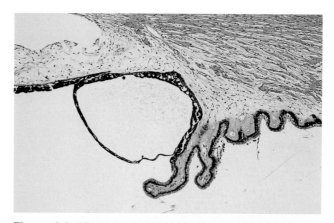

Figure 4-6. Histopathology of iridociliary cyst found on routine sectioning of an eye enucleated for an unrelated choroidal melanoma. Note the round thin-walled cyst in the iridociliary sulcus (hematoxylin–eosin, original magnification × 10).

Midzonal Iris Cyst

A midzonal iris cyst can resemble an iris or ciliary body melanoma. However, a melanoma ordinarily would not arise from the back surface of the iris and overhang the pupillary margin. In addition, the midzonal cyst becomes stretched with pupillary dilation, which would not occur with a melanoma. In contrast to iridociliary cysts, the midzonal cyst tends to block transmission of light.

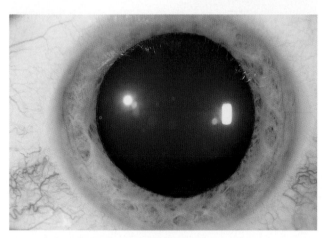

Figure 4-7. Midzonal iris cyst inferiorly in a 40-year-old man.

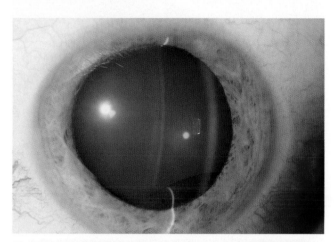

Figure 4-8. Lesion shown in Figure 4-7 as seen with slit lamp beam.

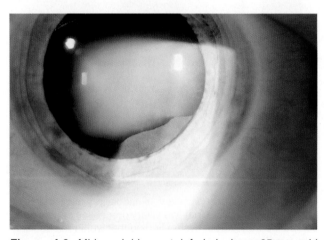

Figure 4-9. Midzonal iris cyst inferiorly in a 65-year-old woman.

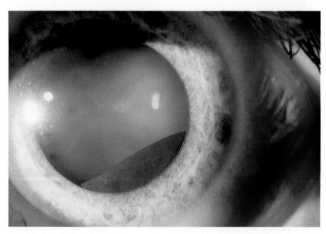

Figure 4-10. Midzonal iris cyst inferiorly in a 42-year-old man.

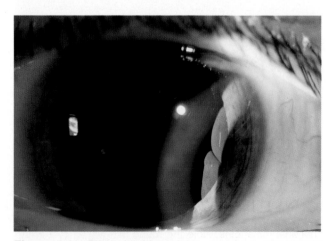

Figure 4-11. Bilobed midzonal iris cyst in a 43-year-old woman.

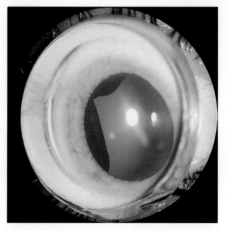

Figure 4-12. Two separate but adjacent midzonal iris cysts in a 40-year-old man.

Free-floating Iris Cyst

A free-floating iris cyst probably was originally attached in the iridociliary sulcus in most cases and became dislodged into the adjacent ocular fluids. The cyst is heavier than aqueous humor, so it sinks to the dependent part of the eye.

From Shields JA, Shields CL, De Potter P, Wagner RS, Caputo AR. Free-floating cyst in the anterior chamber of the eye. *J Pediatr Ophthalmol Strabismus* 1996;33:330–331.

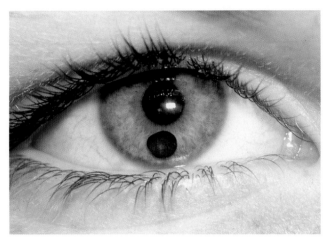

Figure 4-13. Free-floating cyst in the anterior chamber of the right eye in a 12-year-old girl.

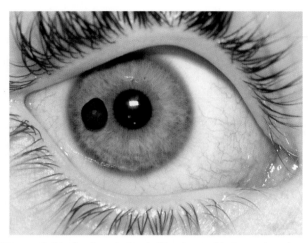

Figure 4-14. Lesion shown in Fig. 4-13 with the patient lying on the right side.

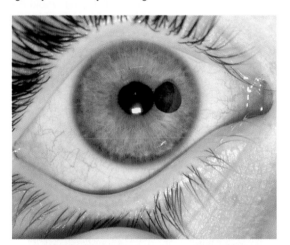

Figure 4-15. Same lesion with the patient lying on the left side.

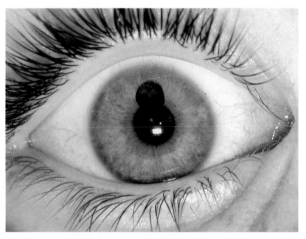

Figure 4-16. Same lesion with the patient bending her head downward.

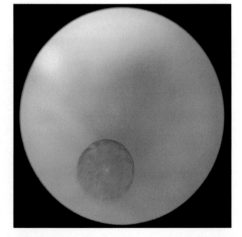

Figure 4-17. Free-floating cyst in the midvitreous cavity. The cyst is in focus but the retina posteriorly is out of focus.

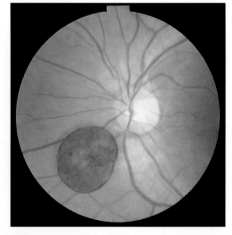

Figure 4-18. Free-floating vitreous cyst near the retinal surface in another patient. The cyst and the retina are in good focus.

Free-floating Cysts with Subsequent Fixation in the Anterior Chamber Angle

Cysts can become dislodged from their pigmented epithelial location, migrate into the anterior chamber, and subsequently become fixed in the anterior chamber angle.

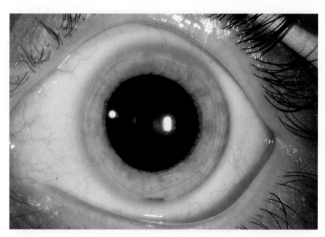

Figure 4-19. Fixed cyst in anterior chamber angle at 6 o'clock position. With this view the lesion can resemble a nevus, melanoma, or adenoma of the pigment epithelium.

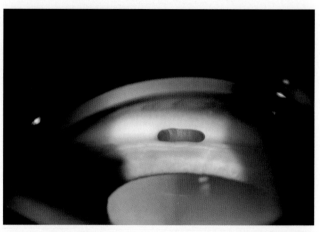

Figure 4-20. Gonioscopic view of the lesion shown in Fig. 4-19. Note the abrupt rounded margins and the location anterior to the iris stroma. A nevus or melanoma would have a more sessile shape and would be located in the iris stroma.

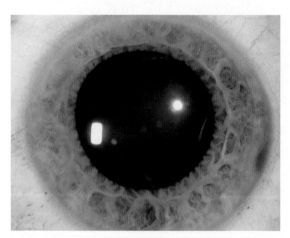

Figure 4-21. Lesion located nasally in the right eye of a 53-year-old woman.

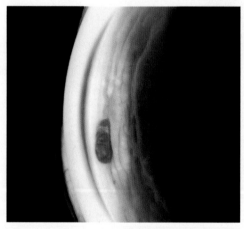

Figure 4-22. Gonioscopic view of the lesion shown in Fig. 4-21 showing similar characteristics to that shown in Fig. 4-20.

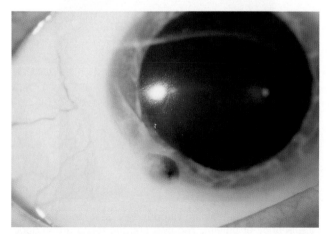

Figure 4-23. Fixed cyst in the anterior chamber inferotemporally. In this case, the lesion has thinned the overlying limbal tissues and appears like a limbal lesion.

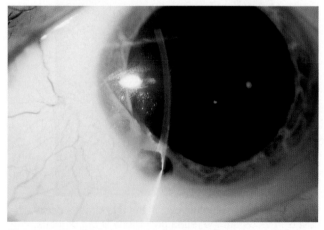

Figure 4-24. Slit lamp view of the lesion shown in Fig. 4-23 depicting the elevation and corneal thinning.

Acquired Spontaneous Iris Stromal Cysts

This peculiar cyst seems to occur spontaneously, usually in adults who have no history of trauma or ocular surgery. In contrast to acquired pigment epithelial cyst, this lesion sometimes can enlarge slowly and cause inflammation, elevated intraocular pressure, and visual loss. In some instances, the cyst has a tendency to enlarge for a period of time, then spontaneously deflate, and then reinflate spontaneously.

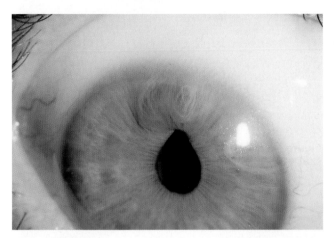

Figure 4-25. Superior iris stromal cyst in a 45-year-old man.

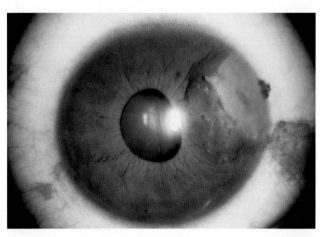

Figure 4-26. Superonasal iris stromal cyst in a 40-year-old woman.

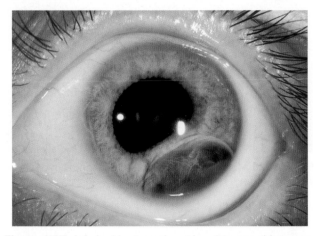

Figure 4-27. Inferior iris stromal cyst in a 34-year-old woman.

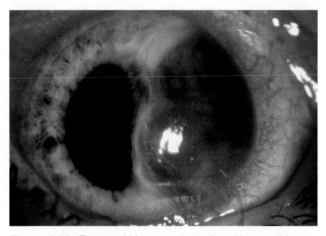

Figure 4-28. Temporal iris stromal cyst in a 32-year-old man.

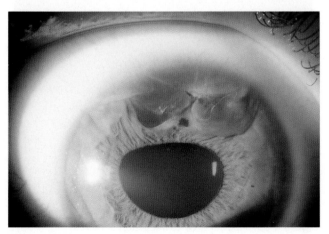

Figure 4-29. Multiloculated iris cyst superiorly in a 24-year-old woman.

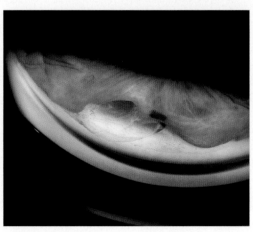

Figure 4-30. Gonioscopic view of the lesion shown in Fig. 4-29 showing the clear cyst.

Natural Course and Treatment of Spontaneous Iris Stromal Cysts

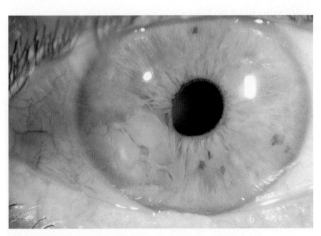

Figure 4-31. Inferonasal iris stromal cyst in a 71-year-old man. Note the turbid appearance to the lumen of the cyst and the subtle "pseudohypopyon" level inferiorly within the cyst.

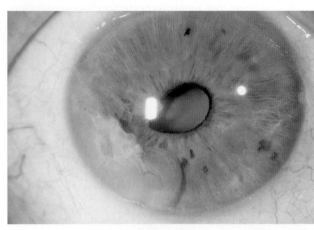

Figure 4-32. Lesion shown in Fig. 4-31, 1 year later, demonstrating slight enlargement and more irregularity of the pupil.

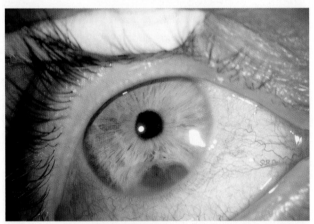

Figure 4-33. Inferonasal iris stromal cyst in a 61-year-old man. The dark color is secondary to complete disappearance of the stroma and exposure of the iris pigment epithelium posterior to the cyst.

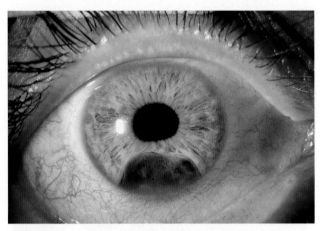

Figure 4-34. Appearance of the lesion 6 months later showing enlargement of the cyst.

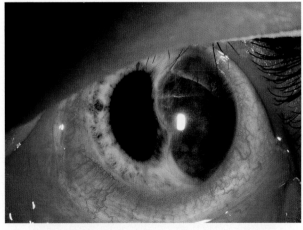

Figure 4-35. Spontaneous iris stromal cyst located temporally in a 36-year-old man.

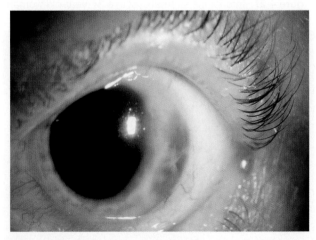

Figure 4-36. Appearance of the lesion shown in Fig. 4-35, 2 months later, showing good result of aspiration of cyst with cryotherapy to its base near the limbus.

Epithelial Downgrowth Stromal Cysts after Trauma and Surgery

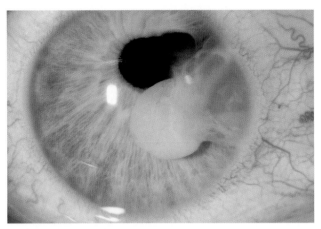

Figure 4-37. Pedunculated epithelial downgrowth cyst at the site of prior perforating limbal trauma in a 52-year-old man.

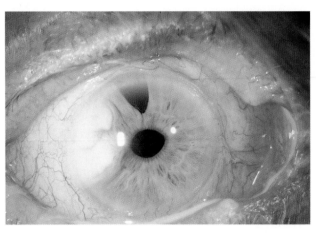

Figure 4-38. Epithelial downgrowth cyst arising at the temporal margin of incision for cataract surgery.

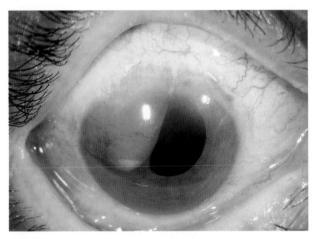

Figure 4-39. Epithelial downgrowth cyst arising at the temporal margin of incision for cataract surgery. Note the "pseudohypopyon" due to epithelial debris in the inferior aspect of the cyst.

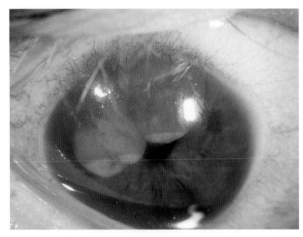

Figure 4-40. Multiloculated epithelial downgrowth cyst arising from incision for prior cataract surgery. Note the "pseudohypopyon" levels in the individual cystic areas.

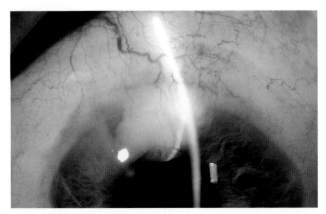

Figure 4-41. Epithelial downgrowth cyst arising from cataract wound in a 52-year-old man. Because of recurrent bouts of intraocular inflammation, the lesion was excised.

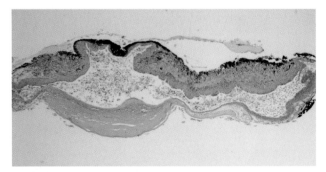

Figure 4-42. Histopathology of the lesion shown in Fig. 4-41 depicting the wall of the cyst lined with stratified squamous epithelium (hematoxylin–eosin, original magnification × 20).

CHAPTER 5

Choroidal Nevus

CHOROIDAL NEVUS

Choroidal nevus is a common intraocular tumor (1–8). It usually becomes apparent in early adulthood as a flat or minimally elevated pigmented or amelanotic lesion with distinct or ill-defined margins. It is usually between 1.5 to 5.0 mm in diameter and usually less than 2 mm in thickness. Overlying drusen are common. Associated orange pigment and subretinal fluid are considered suspicious features for future growth (1). Secondary choroidal neovascularization and detachment of the retinal pigment epithelium are rare. Histopathologically, choroidal nevus is composed of a low-grade proliferation of spindle-shaped, ovoid, or round melanocytes with variable amounts of pigmentation. Fluorescein angiographic features vary from hypofluorescence of smaller, darker lesions, to more hyperfluorescence of larger, less pigmented lesions. Ultrasonography has little diagnostic value, because of the minimal elevation of the lesion; however, it can be used for baseline thickness measurements for elevated lesions.

The frequency with which a choroidal nevus shows growth and evolution into melanoma has been reported (1,8). A typical, stationary choroidal nevus requires no active treatment. Baseline fundus photography and sometimes ultrasonography may be helpful in detecting growth. In cases with symptomatic secondary subretinal fluid, specific methods of laser photocoagulation to bring about resolution of the subretinal fluid have been employed (1). Lesions that show clear evidence of growth generally should be managed like a small melanoma, a subject covered subsequently.

SELECTED REFERENCES

1. Shields JA, Shields CL. *Intraocular tumors. A text and atlas.* Philadelphia: WB Saunders, 1992:85–100.
2. Ganley JP, Comstock GW. Benign nevi and malignant melanomas of the choroid. *Am J Ophthalmol* 1973;76:19–25.
3. Hale PN, Allen RA, Straatsma BR. Benign melanomas (nevi) of the choroid and ciliary body. *Arch Ophthalmol* 1965;74:532–538.
4. Naumann GO, Hellner K, Naumann LR. Pigmented nevi of the choroid. Clinical study of secondary changes in the overlying tissue. *Trans Am Acad Ophthalmol Otolaryngol* 1971;75:110–123.
5. Shields JA, Rodrigues MM, Sarin LK, Tasman WS, Annesley WH. Lipofuscin pigment over benign and malignant choroidal tumors. *Trans Am Acad Ophthalmol Otolaryngol* 1976;81:871–881.
6. Pro M, Shields JA, Tomer TL. Serous detachment of the fovea associated with presumed choroidal nevi. *Arch Ophthalmol* 1979;96:1374–1377.
7. Mims J, Shields JA. Follow-up studies on suspicious choroidal nevi. *Ophthalmology* 1978;85:929–943.
8. Shields CL, Shields JA, Kiratli H, Cater JR, De Potter P. Risk factors for metastasis of small choroidal melanocytic lesions. *Ophthalmology* 1995;102:1351–1361.

Pigmented Choroidal Nevi

The majority of choroidal nevi have some degree of pigmentation and are located in the posterior part of the choroid. More long-standing nevi or slightly elevated nevi can cause overlying drusen.

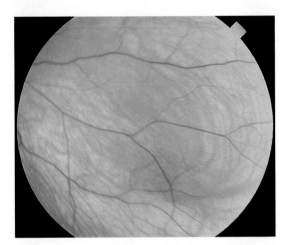

Figure 5-1. Choroidal freckle appearing as a subtle pigmented lesion in the inferior part of the photograph.

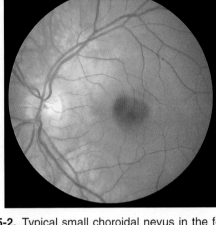

Figure 5-2. Typical small choroidal nevus in the fovea of a 20-year-old man.

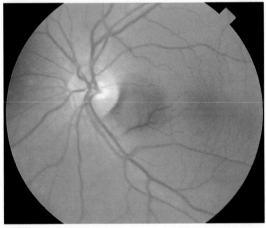

Figure 5-3. Choroidal nevus on the temporal margin of the optic disc in a 39-year-old man.

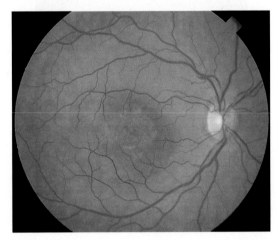

Figure 5-4. Slightly larger choroidal nevus centered in the foveal region. Such lesions eventually can cause visual loss due to photoreceptor degeneration and still be benign.

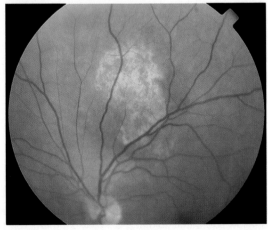

Figure 5-5. Slightly larger, elevated choroidal nevus with surface drusen in a 46-year-old man.

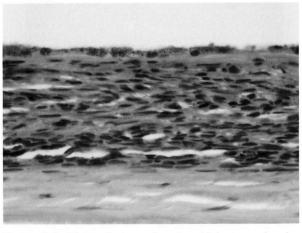

Figure 5-6. Histopathology of a choroidal nevus showing closely compact benign spindle cells (hematoxylin–eosin, original magnification × 15).

Pigment Variations in Choroidal Nevi

An amelanotic choroidal nevus can be ophthalmoscopically similar to a choroidal metastasis, granuloma, or other amelanotic choroidal tumors. Some nevi are partly pigmented and partly nonpigmented. Some have a halo appearance.

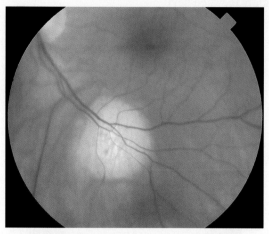

Figure 5-7. Amelanotic choroidal nevus along the inferior vascular arcade in a 46-year-old man.

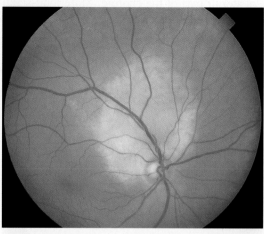

Figure 5-8. Juxtapapillary amelanotic choroidal nevus in a 62-year-old woman.

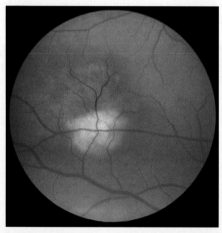

Figure 5-9. Choroidal nevus in which the upper half is pigmented and the lower half is nonpigmented in a 62-year-old man.

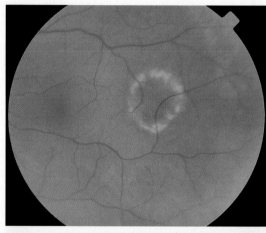

Figure 5-10. Halo choroidal nevus in which the central portion is pigmented and the peripheral ring is amelanotic. Most halo nevi have this configuration. The halo usually is due to balloon cell degeneration in the peripheral portions of the tumor.

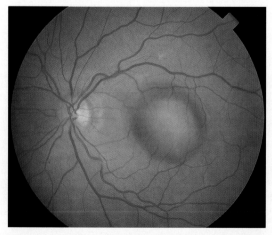

Figure 5-11. Small reverse halo nevus with the pigmented ring in the peripheral portion of the lesion in a 30-year-old woman.

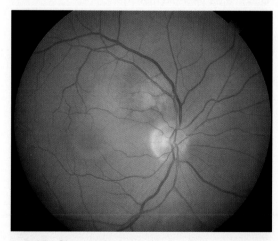

Figure 5-12. Choroidal nevus with overlying orange pigment and shallow subretinal fluid in a 61-year-old man. The presence of orange pigment and subretinal fluid is a sign that the lesion has caused disruption of the retinal pigment epithelium and may be growing slowly.

Choroidal Nevi with Secondary Changes on Adjacent Structures

In addition to the overlying drusen and orange pigment mentioned previously, an elevated choroidal nevus occasionally can induce a secondary serous retinal detachment, detachment of the retinal pigment epithelium, or choroidal neovascularization.

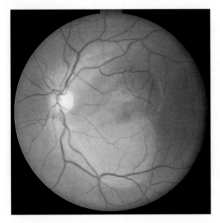

Figure 5-13. Choroidal nevus with secondary serous retinal detachment affecting the foveal region in a 28-year-old man.

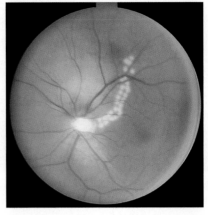

Figure 5-14. Choroidal nevus after delimiting argon laser photocoagulation to induce resorption of the subretinal fluid. A delimiting laser can be used when the margin of the nevus is greater than 1 mm from the foveola.

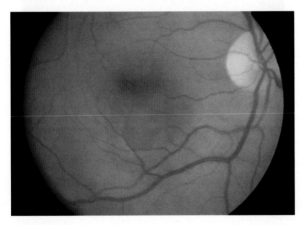

Figure 5-15. Choroidal nevus with overlying detachment of the retinal pigment epithelium. Note the ring of orange pigment that characteristically encircles the base of a pigment epithelial detachment over a choroidal nevus (or melanoma).

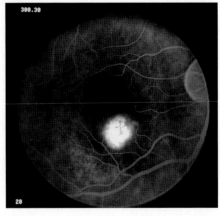

Figure 5-16. Late fluorescein angiogram of the lesion shown in Fig. 5-15 showing characteristic hyperfluorescence of the retinal pigment epithelium detachment.

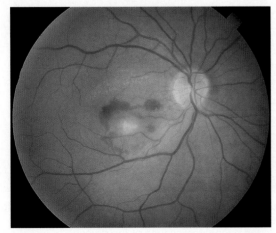

Figure 5-17. Choroidal nevus with overlying subretinal neovascularization in a 68-year-old woman. Note the characteristic crescent-shaped hemorrhage adjacent to the membrane.

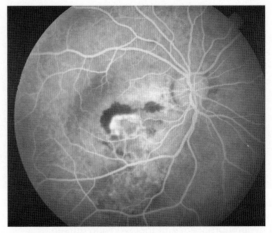

Figure 5-18. Fluorescein angiogram in recirculation phase showing the characteristic pattern of a subretinal neovascular membrane of choroidal origin.

Fluorescein Angiography of Choroidal Nevus

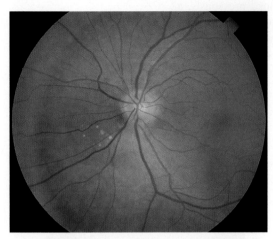

Figure 5-19. Typical choroidal nevus nasal to the optic disc in a 52-year-old woman.

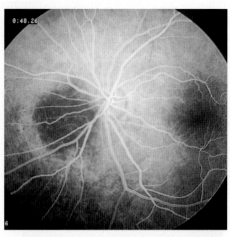

Figure 5-20. Fluorescein angiogram in recirculation phase showing hypofluorescence of the lesion shown in Fig. 5-19.

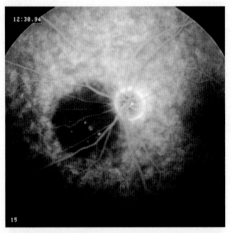

Figure 5-21. Late angiogram showing continued hypofluorescence of the nevus shown in Fig. 5-19.

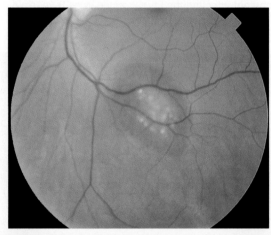

Figure 5-22. Choroidal nevus with overlying drusen in a 44-year-old man.

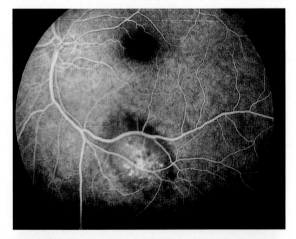

Figure 5-23. Fluorescein angiogram in recirculation phase showing hypofluorescence of the lesion shown in Fig. 5-22 and hyperfluorescence of the overlying drusen.

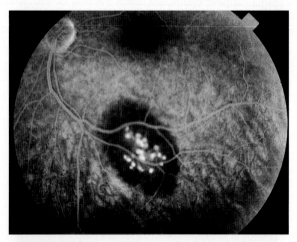

Figure 5-24. Late angiogram of the lesion shown in Fig. 5-22 showing continued hypofluorescence of the nevus and continued hyperfluorescence of the drusen.

Growth of Small Choroidal Nevi into Small Choroidal Melanomas

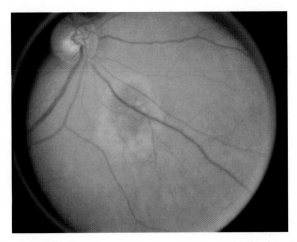

Figure 5-25. Halo nevus inferonasal to the optic disc in a 60-year-old woman.

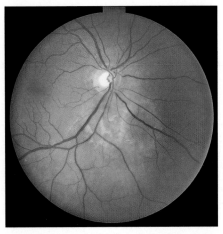

Figure 5-26. Appearance of the lesion shown in Fig. 5-25, 4 years later, showing growth of the lesion temporally and accumulation of overlying orange pigment.

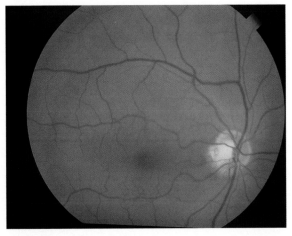

Figure 5-27. Small choroidal nevus in the foveal region in a 65-year-old man.

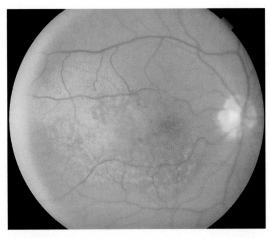

Figure 5-28. Appearance of the lesion shown in Fig. 5-27, when the patient returned 3 years later, showing growth of the lesion and accumulation of orange pigment.

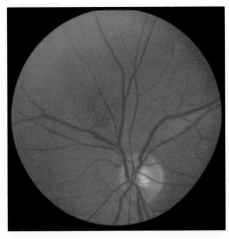

Figure 5-29. Small choroidal nevus superonasal to the optic disc in a 60-year-old man. The lesion had been followed for 10 years without change.

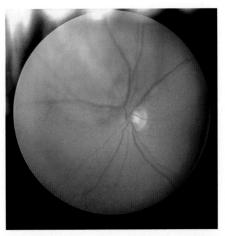

Figure 5-30. Appearance of the lesion shown in Fig. 5-29, 1 year later. The nevus had grown rapidly and evolved into a melanoma. The tumor eventually metastasized in spite of prompt enucleation.

CHAPTER 6

Posterior Uveal
Melanocytoma

POSTERIOR UVEAL MELANOCYTOMA

Melanocytoma is a variant of nevus, located on the optic disc or in the uveal tract (1–5). This congenital, nonhereditary lesion is deeply pigmented and usually located on or adjacent to the optic disc. Unlike uveal melanoma, it does not have a predilection for Caucasians. Of those located at the optic disc, 77% of patients have a feathery margin due to involvement of the nerve fiber layer, 47% have a juxtapapillary choroidal component identical to a choroidal nevus, and 30% have an afferent pupillary defect, even when visual acuity is good (6). Visual fields show enlargement of the blind spot in 90%, sometimes with a nerve fiber bundle defect (6). About 15% show subtle enlargement over the course of several years (5).

Histopathologically, melanocytoma is a deeply pigmented benign tumor (1–3). Bleached preparations reveal the cells to be ovoid with abundant cytoplasm, relatively small nuclei, and few prominent nucleoli. Melanocytoma of the iris (7), ciliary body (8), and choroid (9) have identical histopathologic features. A presumed melanocytoma has been identified in the sensory retina (10).

Fluorescein angiography typically shows hypofluorescence throughout the angiogram, sometimes with hyperfluorescence of secondary disc edema or retinal pigment epithelium atrophy. Rarely, a melanocytoma of the optic disc can evolve into malignant melanoma (11). Therefore, fundus photography and clinical evaluation should be done once or twice a year. Small degrees of growth may not signify malignant change. However, more progressive growth and visual loss should suggest malignant transformation.

SELECTED REFERENCES

1. Zimmerman LE, Garron LK. Melanocytoma of the optic disc. *Int Ophthalmol Clin* 1962;2:431–440.
2. Zimmerman LE. Melanocytes, melanocytic nevi, and melanocytomas: the Jonas S. Friedenwald Memorial Lecture. *Invest Ophthalmol* 1965;4:11–40.
3. Shields JA, Shields CL. *Intraocular tumors. A text and atlas.* Philadelphia: WB Saunders, 1992:101–115.
4. Shields JA. Melanocytoma of the optic nerve head. A review. *Int Ophthalmol* 1978;1:31–37.
5. Joffe L, Shields JA, Osher RH, Gass JDM. Clinical and follow-up studies of melanocytomas of the optic disc. *Ophthalmology* 1979;86:1067–1078.
6. Osher RH, Shields JA, Layman PR. Pupillary and visual field evaluation in patients with melanocytoma of the optic disc. *Ophthalmology* 1979;97:1096–1099.
7. Shields JA, Annesley WH, Spaeth GL. Necrotic melanocytoma of iris with secondary glaucoma. *Am J Ophthalmol* 1977;84:826–829.
8. Shields JA, Augsburger JJ, Bernardino V, Eller AW, Kulczycki E. Melanocytoma of the ciliary body and iris. *Am J Ophthalmol* 1980;89:632–635.
9. Shields JA, Font RL. Melanocytoma of the choroid clinically simulating a malignant melanoma. *Arch Ophthalmol* 1972;87:396–400.
10. Jurgens I, Roca G, Sedo S. Pujol O, Berniell JA, Quintana M. Presumed melanocytoma of the macula. *Arch Ophthalmol* 1994;112:305-306.
11. Shields JA, Shields CL, Eagle RC, Lieb WE, Stern S. Malignant melanoma associated with melanocytoma of the optic disc. *Ophthalmology* 1990;97:225–230.

Melanocytomas Confined to the Optic Disc Region

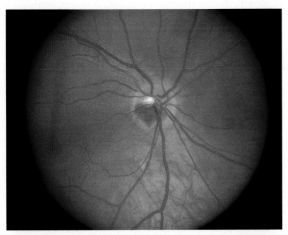

Figure 6-1. Small melanocytoma of the optic disc in a 22-year-old man.

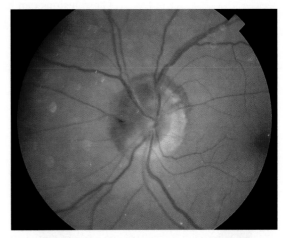

Figure 6-2. Melanocytoma of the optic disc in a 60-year-old woman.

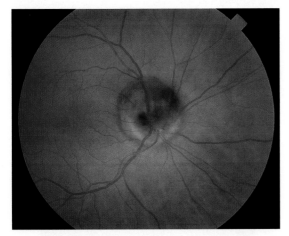

Figure 6-3. Melanocytoma of the optic disc in a 34-year-old man.

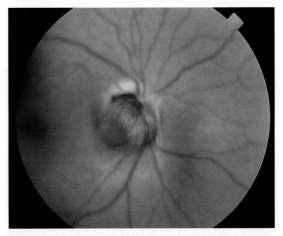

Figure 6-4. Melanocytoma of the optic disc in a 47-year-old woman.

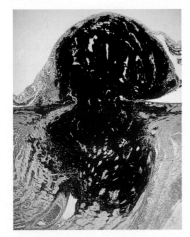

Figure 6-5. Low-magnification photomicrograph of a melanocytoma of the optic disc showing the deeply pigmented lesion causing elevation of the optic nerve and extending into the retrolaminar portion of the optic nerve (hematoxylin–eosin, original magnfication × 20). (Courtesy of Dr. Lorenz Zimmerman and the Armed Forces Institute of Pathology, Washington, DC.)

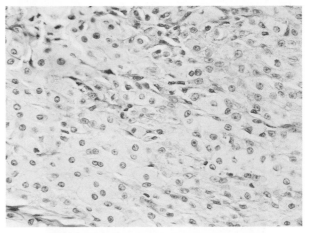

Figure 6-6. Bleached preparation of a melanocytoma showing round cells with abundant cytoplasm and uniform nuclei (hematoxylin–eosin, original magnification × 100).

Melanocytomas of the Optic Disc with Retinal Nerve Fiber Layer Involvement

These lesions can have a feathery or fibrillated margin because of the anatomic arrangement of the juxtapapillary nerve fibers.

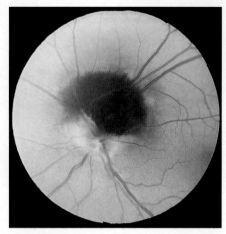

Figure 6-7. Melanocytoma over the superior portion of the optic disc in a 40-year-old woman as seen in 1977. This lesion was followed from about 1960 through 1996, and it showed no appreciable change.

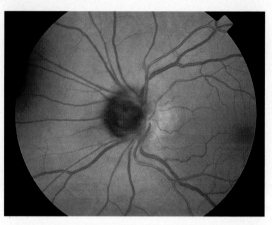

Figure 6-8. Melanocytoma over the nasal portion of the optic disc in a 40-year-old woman.

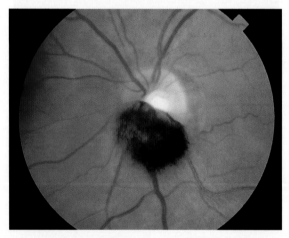

Figure 6-9. Melanocytoma over the inferior portion of the optic disc in a 51-year-old man.

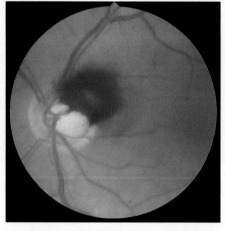

Figure 6-10. Melanocytoma over the superotemporal portion of the optic disc in a 30-year-old man.

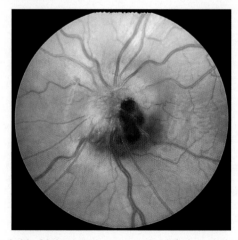

Figure 6-11. Melanocytoma over the inferior portion of the optic disc in a 16-year-old boy as shown in 1977.

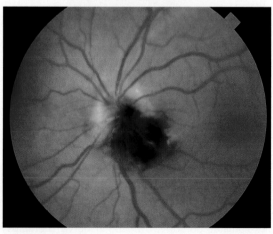

Figure 6-12. Appearance of the lesion shown in Fig. 6-11 as seen in 1993 showing no appreciable change in the lesion over a 16-year period.

Melanocytomas of the Optic Disc with a Juxtapapillary Choroidal Component

These lesions are juxtapapillary melanocytic nevi in which a portion of the lesion involves the lamina choroidalis and appears clinically on the surface of the disc. In many cases, the epipapillary component is more pigmented and the choroidal portion appears less pigmented because the overlying retinal pigment epithelium does not allow its dark color to show.

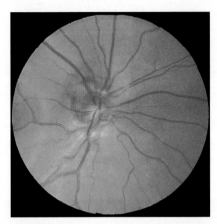

Figure 6-13. Melanocytoma of the juxtapapillary choroid with minimal optic disc involvement in a 12-year-old girl.

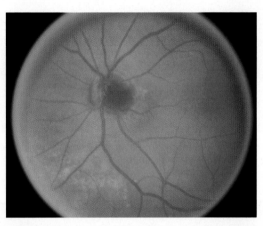

Figure 6-14. Melanocytoma on the temporal aspect of the optic disc in a 60-year-old man.

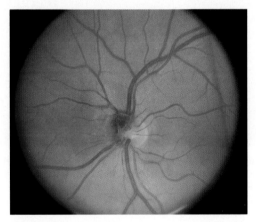

Figure 6-15. Melanocytoma on the nasal aspect of the optic disc in a 30-year-old man.

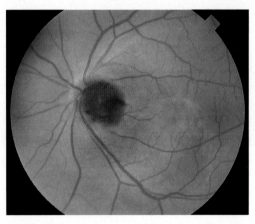

Figure 6-16. Melanocytoma over the temporal portion of the optic disc in a 60-year-old man.

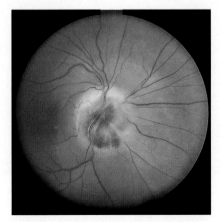

Figure 6-17. Melanocytoma over the inferotemporal portion of the optic disc in a 19-year-old woman.

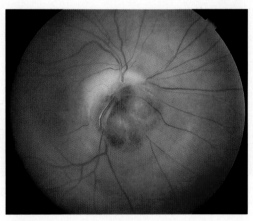

Figure 6-18. Appearance of the lesion shown in Fig. 6-17 after 12 years. It has shown only questionable enlargement.

Fluorescein Angiography of Melanocytoma of the Optic Disc

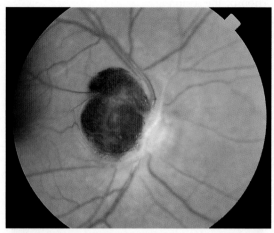

Figure 6-19. Melanocytoma over the temporal portion of the optic disc in a 28-year-old man.

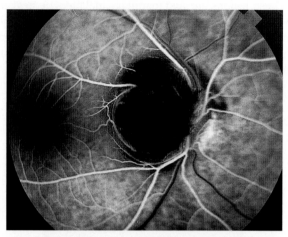

Figure 6-20. Fluorescein angiogram in early laminar venous phase showing hypofluorescence of the lesion.

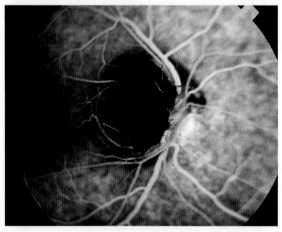

Figure 6-21. Fluorescein angiogram in full venous phase showing continued hypofluorescence of the lesion.

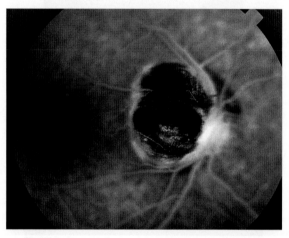

Figure 6-22. Fluorescein angiogram in late phase showing continued hypofluorescence of the lesion with only mild focal staining.

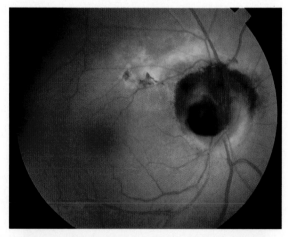

Figure 6-23. Melanocytoma of the optic disc with adjacent atrophy of the retinal pigment epithelium.

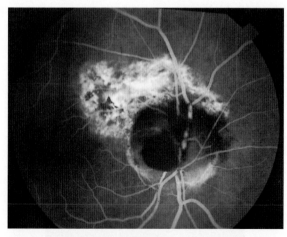

Figure 6-24. Fluorescein angiogram of the lesion shown in Fig. 6-23 in recirculation phase showing hypofluorescence of the melanocytoma and transmission hyperfluorescence through the pigment epithelial defects.

Associations and Variations of Melanocytomas

Melanocytoma seems to occur more frequently in patients with ocular melanocytosis and congenital hypertrophy of the retinal pigment epithelium. A rare case of probable melanocytoma of the retina also has been recognized.

Figs. 6-29 and 6-30 courtesy of Dr. Manuel Quintana. From Jurgens I, Roca G, Sedo S, Pujol O, Berniell JA, Quintana M. Presumed melanocytoma of the macula. *Arch Ophthalmol* 1994;112:305–306.

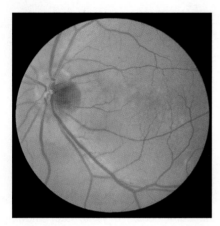

Figure 6-25. Melanocytoma of the optic disc and juxtapapillary choroid in a 43-year-old man.

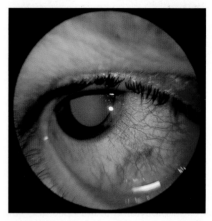

Figure 6-26. Ocular melanocytosis of the opposite eye in the patient shown in Fig. 6-25.

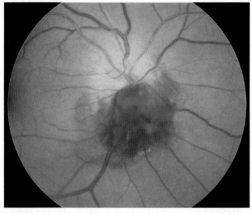

Figure 6-27. Melanocytoma of the optic disc in a 45-year-old African-American patient.

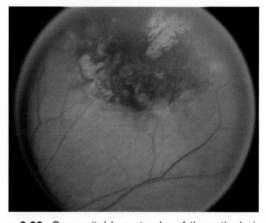

Figure 6-28. Congenital hypertrophy of the retinal pigment epithelium in the same eye shown in Fig. 6-27.

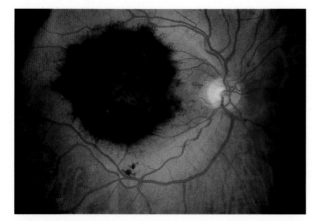

Figure 6-29. Presumed melanocytoma of the sensory retina in the macular region.

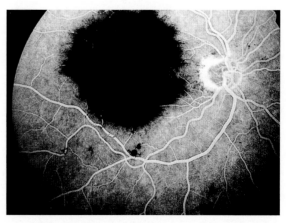

Figure 6-30. Fluorescein angiogram of the lesion shown in Fig. 6-29 showing hypofluorescence of the lesion.

Malignant Melanoma Apparently Arising from Melanocytoma Involving the Optic Disc

Well-documented cases of malignant transformation of melanocytoma of the optic disc are rare. A case is cited.

From Shields JA, Shields CL, Eagle RC, Lieb WE, Stern S. Malignant melanoma associated with melanocytoma of the optic disc. *Ophthalmology* 1990;97:225–230.

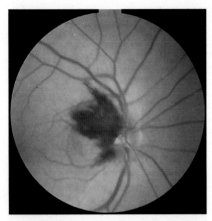

Figure 6-31. Melanocytoma of the optic disc, juxtapapillary choroid, and retinal nerve fiber layer in a 54-year-old man.

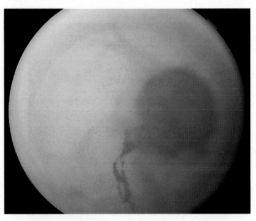

Figure 6-32. Same lesion 6 years later showing marked growth and vitreal seeding.

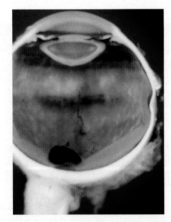

Figure 6-33. Section of enucleated eye showing pigmented tumor in posterior pole of the eye.

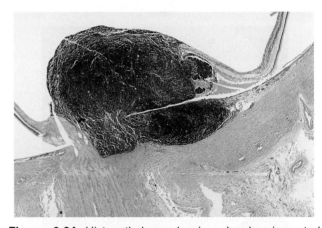

Figure 6-34. Histopathology showing deeply pigmented lesion of choroid, epipapillary region, and sensory retina (hematoxylin–eosin, original magnification × 10).

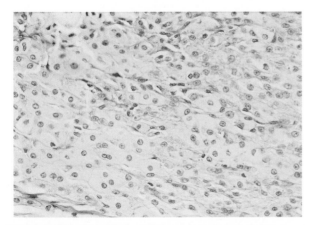

Figure 6-35. Bleached sections of an area of the tumor showing cells compatible with melanocytoma (hematoxylin–eosin, original magnification × 150).

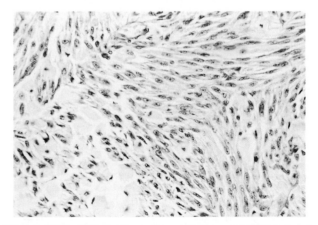

Figure 6-36. Bleached sections of an area of the tumor showing cells compatible with low-grade, spindle-cell melanoma (hematoxylin–eosin, original magnification × 150).

Melanocytomas of the Ciliary Body

Melanocytoma in the ciliary body can attain a large size and still be cytologically benign. Two cases are illustrated.

Figs. 6-37 through 6-40 from Shields JA, Augsburger JJ, Bernardino V, Eller AW, Kulczycki E. Melanocytoma of the ciliary body and iris. *Am J Ophthalmol* 1980;89: 632–635.

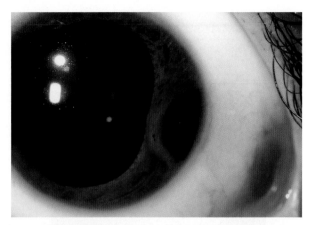

Figure 6-37. Melanocytoma of the ciliary body with iris extension in a 29-year-old woman as seen in 1979. At that time, melanoma was suspected and the patient elected to have enucleation. Today we recommend local resection for tumors such as this.

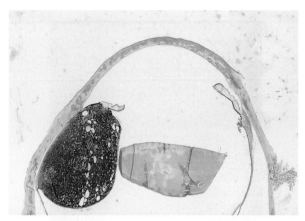

Figure 6-38. Low-magnification photomicrograph of the enucleated eye shown in Fig. 6-37 showing the well-defined ciliary mass with extension through the iris root (hematoxylin–eosin, original magnification × 3).

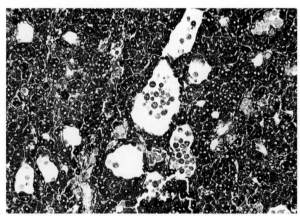

Figure 6-39. Photomicrograph of the lesion shown in Fig. 6-37 showing deeply pigmented tumor cells with pseudocysts with macrophages containing liberated pigment (hematoxylin–eosin, original magnification × 50).

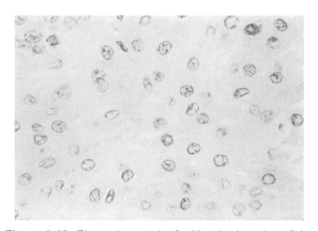

Figure 6-40. Photomicrograph of a bleached section of the lesion shown in Fig. 6-37. Note the typical melanocytoma cells (hematoxylin–eosin, original magnification × 200).

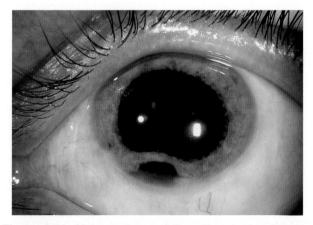

Figure 6-41. Melanocytoma of the ciliary body with secondary iris invasion in a 48-year-old man. The lesion was removed successfully by iridocyclectomy.

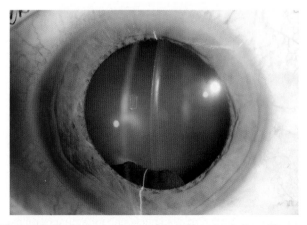

Figure 6-42. Melanocytoma of the ciliary body in a 49-year-old man. The lesion was removed successfully by iridocyclectomy.

Melanocytomas of the Choroid

Figs. 6-43 through 6-46 from Shields JA, Font RL. Melanocytoma of the choroid clinically simulating a malignant melanoma. *Arch Ophthalmol* 1972;87:396–400.

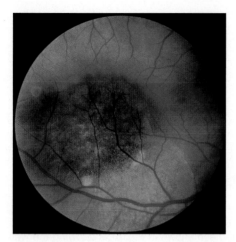

Figure 6-43. Melanocytoma of the choroid temporal to the foveal area.

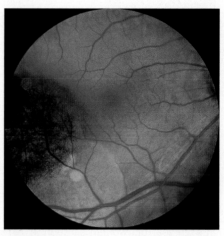

Figure 6-44. Shallow retinal detachment of the fovea secondary to the lesion shown in Fig. 6-43. The patient was seen in 1967 and enucleation was performed because of suspected melanoma. Enucleation probably would not be performed today.

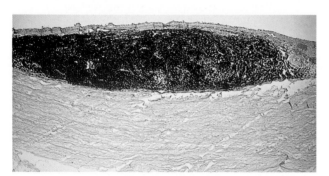

Figure 6-45. Photomicrograph of the lesion shown in Fig. 6-44. Note the deeply pigmented placoid lesion (hematoxylin–eosin, original magnification × 5).

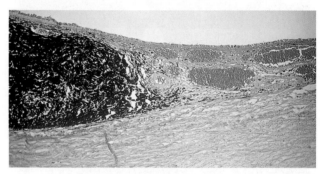

Figure 6-46. Photomicrograph of the lesion shown in Fig. 6-44. Note the distinct margin between the lesion and the adjacent choroid (hematoxylin–eosin, original magnification × 5).

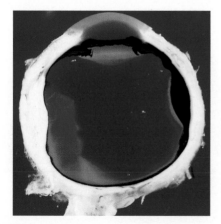

Figure 6-47. Section of eye enucleated for a peripheral pigmented lesion suspected to be a choroidal melanoma. (Courtesy of Dr. Kurt Gitter.)

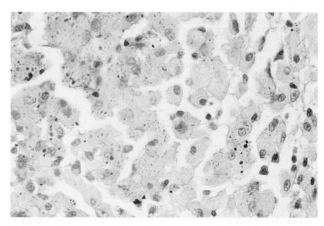

Figure 6-48. Photomicrograph of the lesion shown in Fig. 6-47 depicting the typical melanocytoma cells (hematoxylin–eosin, original magnification × 100). (Courtesy of Dr. Kurt Gitter.)

Melanoma Arising from Giant Diffuse Melanocytoma in a Patient with Oculodermal Melanocytosis

There seems to be a close relationship between uveal melanocytoma and ocular melanocytosis. The two may represent clinical variations of the same histopathologic entity. When this condition gives rise to malignancy, the melanoma often is nonpigmented and of spindle cell type, quite different from the cells of the primary lesion. A case is illustrated.

From Shields JA, Shields CL, Santos C. Melanoma arising from giant diffuse melanocytoma in a patient with oculodermal melanocytosis *(submitted)*.

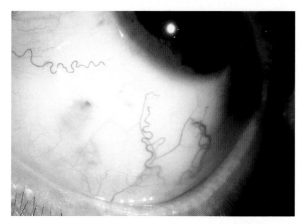

Figure 6-49. Episcleral pigmentation compatible with ocular melanocytosis in a 51-year-old man.

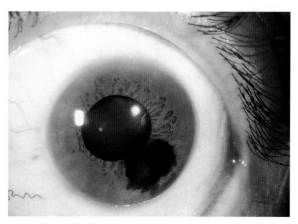

Figure 6-50. Sector pigmented iris lesion in the same eye.

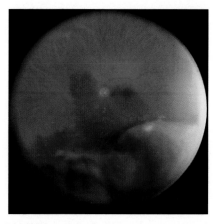

Figure 6-51. Wide-angle fundus photograph showing diffuse elevated mass involving the inferior half of the fundus and surrounding the optic disc.

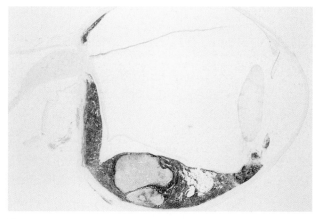

Figure 6-52. Low-magnification photomicrograph depicting diffuse pigmented lesion inferiorly. The deeply pigmented lesion showed areas of transcleral involvement. Note the islands of amelanotic tumor within the pigmented lesion.

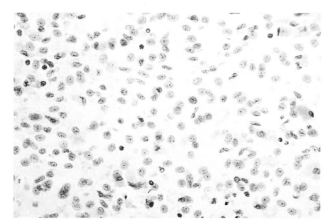

Figure 6-53. Photomicrograph of bleached section from the pigmented area showing typical melanocytoma cells (hematoxylin–eosin, original magnification × 150).

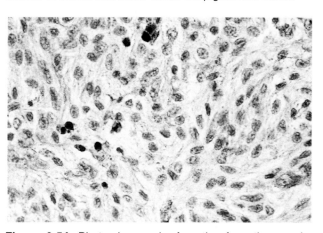

Figure 6-54. Photomicrograph of section from the nonpigmented area showing typical spindle melanoma cells (hematoxylin–eosin, original magnification × 150).

CHAPTER 7

Clinical Features of Posterior Uveal Melanoma

CLINICAL FEATURES OF POSTERIOR UVEAL MELANOMA

Posterior uveal melanoma can assume a variety of clinical features (1–6). In contrast to iris melanoma and most choroidal melanomas, ciliary body melanoma often can attain a larger size before it is recognized clinically. However, it frequently is associated with external ocular signs that suggest the underlying diagnosis. The most important is a dilated episcleral blood vessel (sentinel vessel). A second sign is an epibulbar pigmented lesion characteristic of transcleral extension of the tumor. When the pupil is dilated widely, the ciliary body mass can be visualized in the affected area as a dome-shaped mass. Less frequently, it can assume a diffuse circumferential ring growth pattern (ring melanoma). Ciliary body melanoma can grow to impinge on the lens, causing subluxation and cataract. It can grow posteriorly into the choroid (ciliochoroidal melanoma) and anteriorly into the anterior chamber angle and iris. Localized or diffuse tumors can infiltrate the trabecular meshwork, causing secondary glaucoma (6).

Choroidal melanoma usually presents as a sessile or dome-shaped pigmented mass located deep to the sensory retina. A smaller posterior choroidal melanoma may have surface orange pigment at the level of the retinal pigment epithelium (1–3). A secondary retinal detachment frequently occurs. Occasionally, a choroidal melanoma can be partly or entirely nonpigmented. With continued growth, a choroidal melanoma can rupture Bruch's membrane and assume a mushroom shape. When the tumor is amelanotic, blood vessels in the tumor are visible ophthalmoscopically. Choroidal melanoma also can assume a diffuse growth pattern with only minimal elevation of the tumor (4,5). In some instances, posterior uveal melanoma can cause total cataract, congestive glaucoma, and extraocular extension. Such tumors are generally larger and carry a worse prognosis (6,7).

SELECTED REFERENCES

1. Gass JDM. *Stereoscopic atlas of macular diseases,* vol. 1, 3rd ed. St. Louis: CV Mosby, 1987:190–192.
2. Shields JA, Shields CL. *Intraocular tumors. A text and atlas.* Philadelphia: WB Saunders, 1992:117–136.
3. Char DC. *Clinical ocular oncology*, 2nd ed. Philadelphia: Lippincott–Raven Publishers, 1997:95–98.
4. Font RL, Spaulding AG, Zimmerman LE. Diffuse malignant melanomas of the uveal tract. *Trans Am Acad Ophthalmol Otolaryngol* 1968;72:877–895.
5. Shields CL, Shields JA, De Potter P, Cater J, Tardio D, Barrett J. Diffuse choroidal melanoma: clinical features predictive of metastasis. *Arch Ophthalmol* 1996;114:956–963.
6. Shields CL, Shields JA, Shields MB, Augsburger JJ. Prevalence and mechanisms of secondary intraocular pressure elevation in eyes with intraocular tumors. *Ophthalmology* 1987;94:839–846.
7. Shields JA, Shields CL. Massive orbital extension of posterior uveal melanoma. *J Ophthal Plast Reconstr Surg* 1991;7:238–251.

Sentinel Blood Vessels Associated with Ciliary Body Melanoma

Although dilated episcleral blood vessels usually signify an underlying ciliary body melanoma, they occasionally can be seen with other tumors, such as ciliary body metastasis, leiomyoma, neurilemoma, melanocytoma, and adenoma of the nonpigmented or pigmented ciliary epithelium. On rare occasions, a dilated episcleral vessel is seen as a normal variant with no evidence of a ciliary body mass.

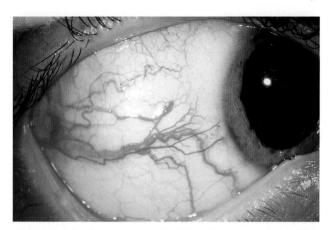

Figure 7-1. Large typical sentinel blood vessels temporally in a 38-year-old man.

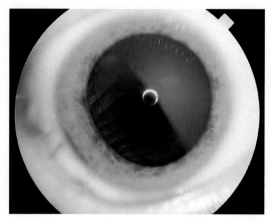

Figure 7-2. Photograph through the dilated pupil of the patient shown in Fig. 7-1 clearly showing the pigmented ciliary body mass.

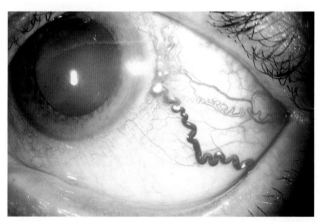

Figure 7-3. Large solitary sentinel vessel over a ciliary body melanoma in a 60-year-old man.

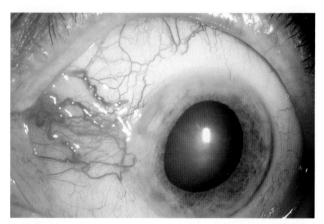

Figure 7-4. Multiple sentinel vessels over a ciliary body melanoma in a 77-year-old man.

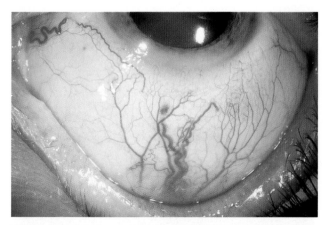

Figure 7-5. Inferior and nasal sentinel vessels over a large ciliary body melanoma in an 84-year-old woman. Note the small focus of the extrascleral extension of the tumor.

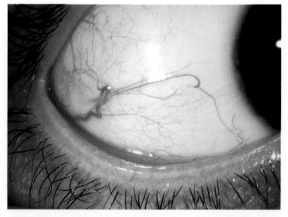

Figure 7-6. Pseudosentinel vessel in a 27-year-old person with an otherwise normal eye. Indirect ophthalmoscopy, gonioscopy, ultrasound biomicroscopy, and transillumination were performed to rule out the possibility of a small occult melanoma.

Transcleral Extension of Ciliary Body Melanoma

Ciliary body melanoma frequently can extend through emissary channels to appear in the episcleral tissues, sometimes forming an extraocular mass. It is more likely to occur with larger, more aggressive tumors, particularly those that grow in a ring pattern. Transcleral extension usually imparts a worse systemic prognosis.

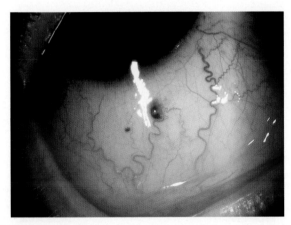

Figure 7-7. Small foci of transcleral extension inferiorly in a 65-year-old man.

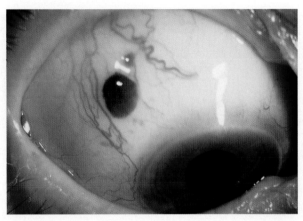

Figure 7-8. More prominent nodules of transcleral extension superiorly in a 77-year-old woman

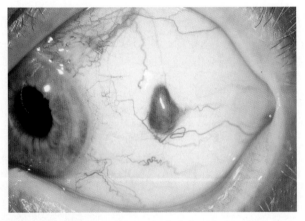

Figure 7-9. Slightly more posteriorly located nodule of transcleral extension in an 83-year-old man.

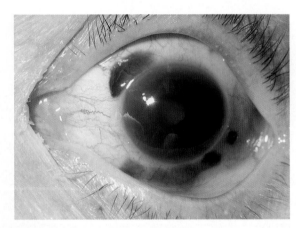

Figure 7-10. Multiple foci of transcleral extension secondary to a ring melanoma of ciliary body in a 70-year-old woman. Ring melanoma with transcleral extension carries a worse prognosis.

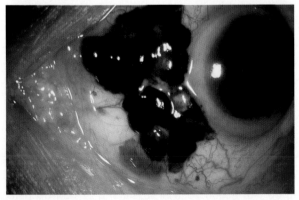

Figure 7-11. Massive transcleral extension and invasion of the overlying conjunctiva in a 58-year-old man with a ciliary body melanoma.

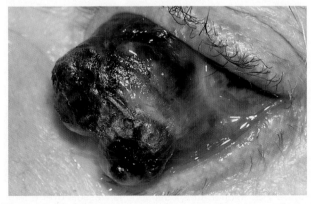

Figure 7-12. Massive extraocular extension of a neglected ciliary body melanoma in an 80-year-old man. He declined treatment for a relatively small ciliary body melanoma detected 3 years earlier.

Iris Extension from Ciliary Body Melanoma

A ciliary body melanoma can grow through the iris root and appear as a mass in the peripheral portion of the iris, simulating a primary iris tumor. Unlike a primary iris melanoma, anterior extension of a ciliary body melanoma tends to pass through the iris root and produce a tumor-induced iridodialysis.

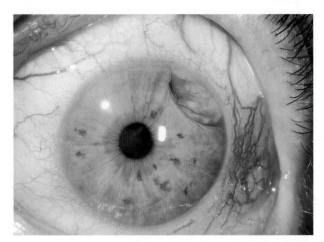

Figure 7-13. Iris extension of a superotemporal ciliary body melanoma in a 70-year-old woman. Note the sentinel vessels.

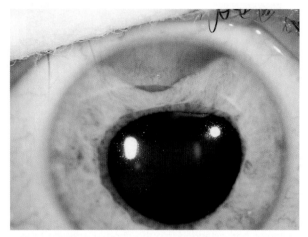

Figure 7-14. Iris extension of a superior ciliary body melanoma in a 52-year-old woman.

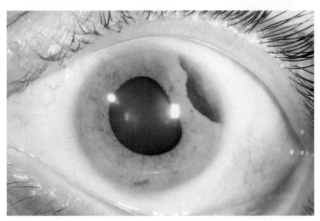

Figure 7-15. Iris extension of a superior ciliary body melanoma in a 37-year-old woman.

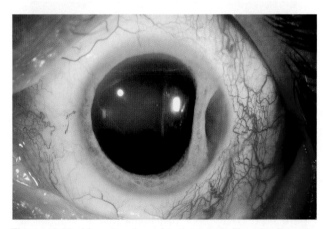

Figure 7-16. Iris extension of a temporal ciliary body melanoma in a 54-year-old man. Note the sentinel vessels and the accordion-like folds in the iris. The ciliary body component of the tumor can be visualized through the dilated pupil.

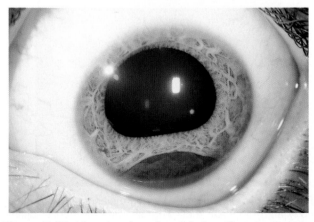

Figure 7-17. Iris extension of an inferior ciliary body melanoma in a 16-year-old girl.

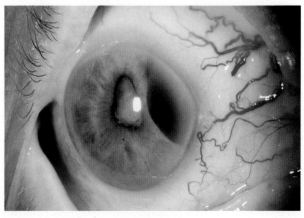

Figure 7-18. Iris extension and secondary cataract in an 85-year-old man with a large temporal ciliary body melanoma. Note the numerous sentinel vessels.

Clinical Appearance of Ciliary Body Melanoma Through Dilated Pupils

Ciliary body melanoma generally appears as a dome-shaped pigmented mass that can encroach on the lens, producing subluxation and cataract. It can extend posteriorly into the choroid (ciliochoroidal melanoma). Occasionally it grows in a ring, rather than a nodular pattern.

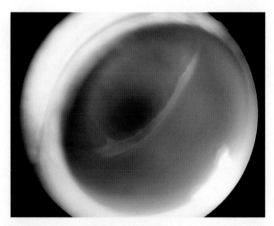

Figure 7-19. Ciliary body melanoma in a 63-year-old man. The tumor has extended into the choroid and lifted the ora serrata, so that it is visible on the dome of the tumor.

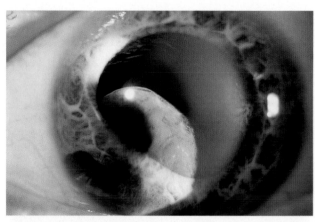

Figure 7-20. Dome-shaped ciliary body melanoma in a 54-year-old man.

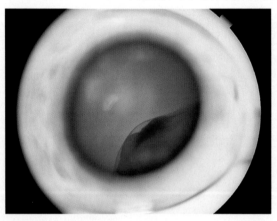

Figure 7-21. Ciliary body melanoma with an irregular surface in a 47-year-old man.

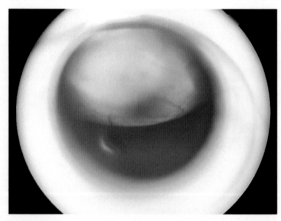

Figure 7-22. Amelanotic ciliary body melanoma in a 39-year-old man. This lesion is atypical, as most amelanotic ciliary body melanomas appear pigmented clinically because of the overlying pigment epithelium of the ciliary body.

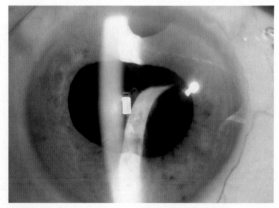

Figure 7-23. Ciliary body melanoma in a 63-year-old man. A unilateral cataract was removed when the melanoma was not suspected. Any patient with an unexplained unilateral cataract should be evaluated for underlying ciliary body melanoma.

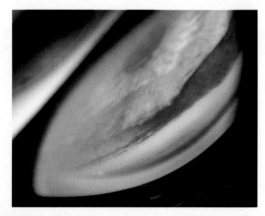

Figure 7-24. Gonioscopy of a ring melanoma of the ciliary body and trabecular meshwork showing the dense, diffuse pigment in the anterior chamber angle. Such tumors can cause intractable secondary glaucoma and often require enucleation of the eye.

Clinicopathologic Correlation of a Ring Melanoma of Ciliary Body with Extraocular Extension and Secondary Glaucoma

In some instances, a ciliary body melanoma can cause cataract and secondary glaucoma, and the patient may be subjected to glaucoma surgery while the melanoma remains unsuspected clinically. A case is illustrated.

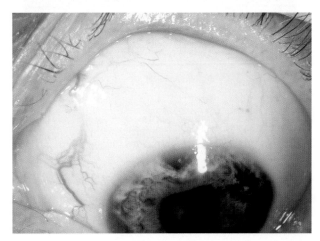

Figure 7-25. Filtering bleb superiorly following trabeculectomy for unexplained unilateral glaucoma in an elderly woman.

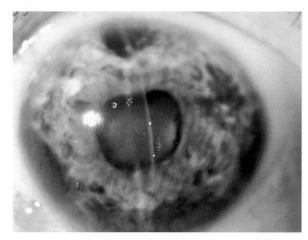

Figure 7-26. Diffuse patches of iris pigmentation. Such pigment dispersion often accompanies ring melanoma of the ciliary body.

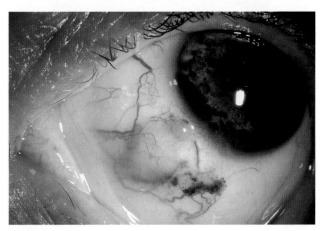

Figure 7-27. Inferonasal amelanotic nodule representing extraocular extension of the tumor.

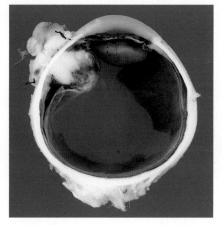

Figure 7-28. Section of enucleated eye showing ciliary body nodule and extraocular mass.

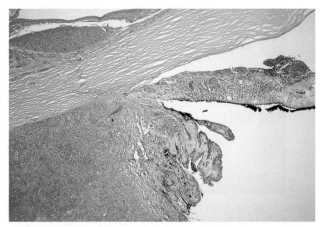

Figure 7-29. Microscopic appearance of the anterior segment showing a ciliary body mass. The tumor extends diffusely around the ciliary body with the one prominent nodule shown in Fig. 7-28 (hematoxylin–eosin, original magnification × 5).

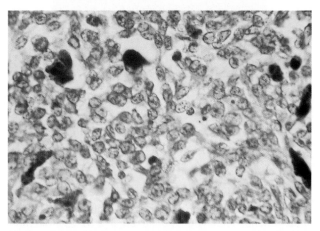

Figure 7-30. Photomicrograph showing mixed cell–type melanoma (hematoxylin–eosin, original magnification × 200).

Pigmented Choroidal Melanoma

The most characteristic feature of choroidal melanoma is an elevated pigmented choroidal mass. Smaller lesions show typical orange pigment on the surface. It typically produces a secondary nonrhegmatogenous retinal detachment.

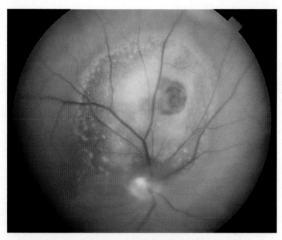

Figure 7-31. Choroidal melanoma superior to the optic disc in a 66-year-old woman. There is a small break through Bruck's membrane on the tumor surface.

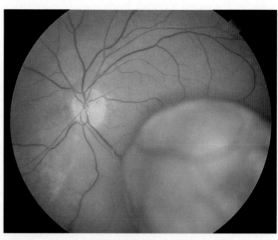

Figure 7-32. Choroidal melanoma in the inferior aspect of the macular region in a 73-year-old man.

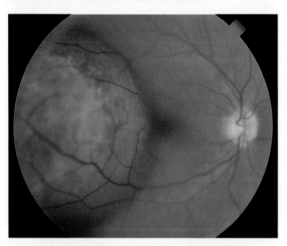

Figure 7-33. Choroidal melanoma temporal to the foveal region in a 38-year-old man.

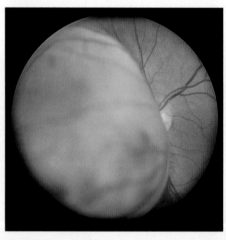

Figure 7-34. Dome-shaped choroidal melanoma overhanging the optic disc in a 40-year-old man.

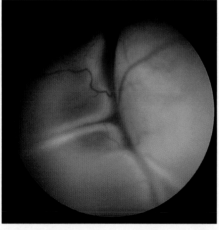

Figure 7-35. Choroidal melanoma (to the *right*) and secondary retinal detachment (to the *left*) in a 51-year-old man.

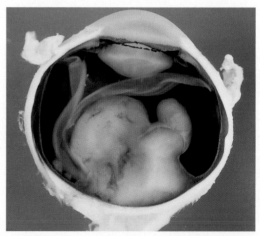

Figure 7-36. Section of enucleated eye shown in Fig. 7-35. Note the large lightly pigmented melanoma with irregular surface due to a break in Bruch's membrane and the overlying retinal detachment extending posterior to the lens.

Partly Pigmented Choroidal Melanoma

On occasion, a choroidal melanoma is partly pigmented and partly nonpigmented. Although the nonpigmented component can suggest another diagnosis, such as choroidal metastasis, any intrinsic pigment in the lesion is a strong suggestion that the lesion is a melanoma.

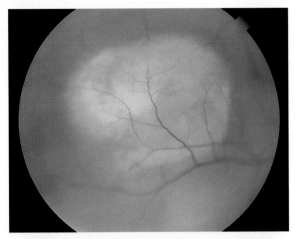

Figure 7-37. Choroidal melanoma in a 43-year-old man showing pigmentation only in the inferior part of the lesion.

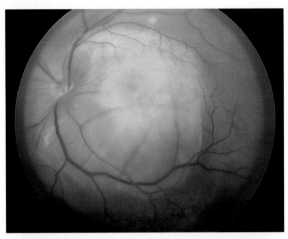

Figure 7-38. Choroidal melanoma in the macular region of a 61-year-old man showing small area of pigmentation in the inferotemporal aspect of the lesion.

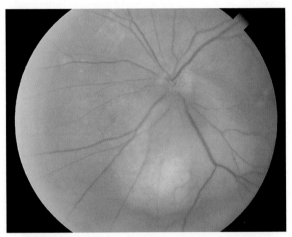

Figure 7-39. Choroidal melanoma adjacent to the optic disc in a 71-year-old woman. In this case, the flat tumor base is pigmented but a more elevated area of vertical growth is amelanotic.

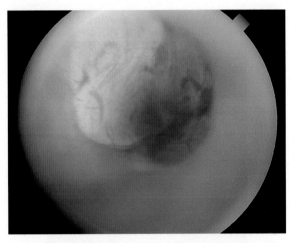

Figure 7-40. Highly elevated choroidal melanoma with pigmented and nonpigmented components in a 72-year-old man.

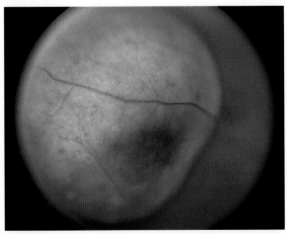

Figure 7-41. Dome-shaped choroidal melanoma with intrinsic pigment in the inferior portion of the lesion in a 54-year-old woman.

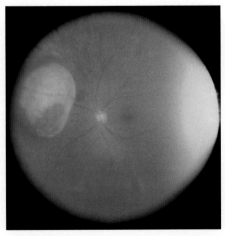

Figure 7-42. Wide-angle photograph of the lesion shown in Fig. 7-41 showing the overall appearance of the mass.

Nonpigmented Choroidal Melanoma

When a melanoma is clinically nonpigmented, the differentiation from choroidal metastasis, hemangioma, lymphoma, osteoma, and other choroidal tumors can be more difficult. However, ophthalmoscopy generally shows well-defined blood vessels in the mass, which suggests melanoma. In addition, melanoma is usually more highly elevated, and drusen and pigment epithelial proliferation are usually more evident over melanoma as compared to metastasis. In the case of nonpigmented melanoma, ancillary studies such as fluorescein angiography and ultrasonography play a greater role in diagnosis.

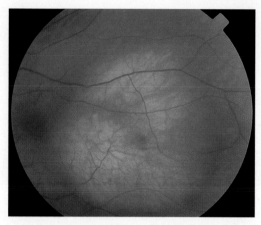

Figure 7-43. Nonpigmented orange-colored melanoma in the macular region in a 34-year-old woman. With close scrutiny, intrinsic vessels can be seen in the tumor.

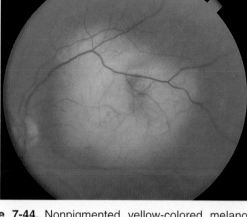

Figure 7-44. Nonpigmented yellow-colored melanoma in the macular region of a 62-year-old woman. Note again the well-defined intrinsic vessels.

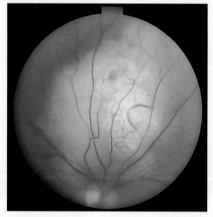

Figure 7-45. Nonpigmented yellow-colored melanoma superior to the optic disc in a 52-year-old woman. Vessels in the tumor are evident.

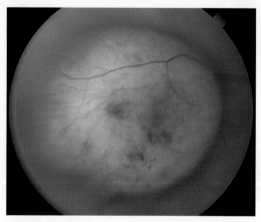

Figure 7-46. Nonpigmented choroidal melanoma in a 52-year-old woman. Note the intrinsic vessels and retinal pigment epithelial proliferation on the surface of the nonpigmented lesion.

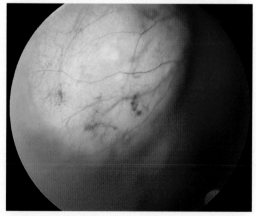

Figure 7-47. Dome-shaped nonpigmented choroidal melanoma in a 40-year-old woman showing both well-defined intrinsic vessels and surface pigment epithelial alterations.

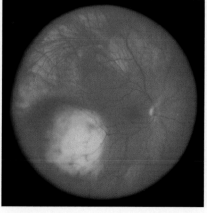

Figure 7-48. Wide-angle photograph of the lesion shown in Fig. 7-47 showing the overall appearance of the mass.

Mushroom-shaped Choroidal Melanoma with Pigmented Dome

When a choroidal melanoma ruptures Bruch's membrane, it grows under the retina as a mushroom-shaped mass. When the apical portion of the tumor is pigmented, prominent intrinsic vessels usually are not evident. When the tumor is adjacent to the optic disc, it may grow around the posterior aspect of Bruch's membrane, rather than rupturing Bruch's membrane, to assume the mushroom shape. When a melanoma breaks through Bruch's membrane, secondary choroidal, subretinal, or vitreal hemorrhage often occurs.

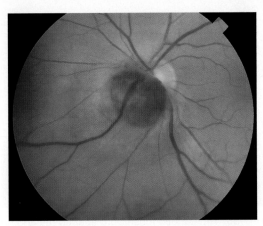

Figure 7-49. Mushroom-shaped choroidal melanoma in a 56-year-old man. In this case, the melanoma apparently grew around the posterior termination of Bruch's membrane.

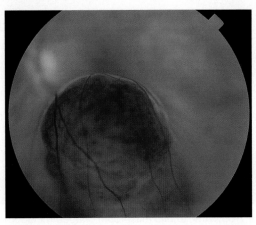

Figure 7-50. Mushroom-shaped choroidal melanoma in a 43-year-old man.

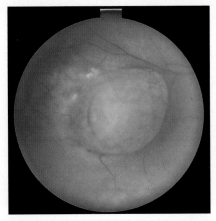

Figure 7-51. Mushroom-shaped choroidal melanoma in a 79-year-old man.

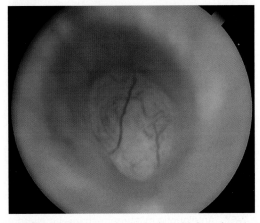

Figure 7-52. Mushroom-shaped choroidal melanoma in a 61-year-old man.

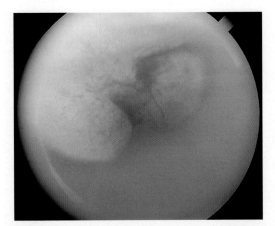

Figure 7-53. Mushroom-shaped choroidal melanoma in a 68-year-old man. Note the small hemorrhage in the area between the base and apex of the lesion.

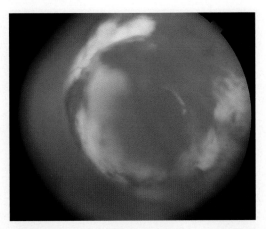

Figure 7-54. Mushroom-shaped choroidal melanoma in a 29-year-old man showing more extensive hemorrhage.

Mushroom-shaped Choroidal Melanoma with Nonpigmented Dome

When the apical portion of the mushroom-shaped melanoma is nonpigmented, prominent intrinsic vessels are usually very evident. Such a finding is highly suggestive, and perhaps pathognomonic, of choroidal melanoma. Note the prominent vessels in each of the illustrated cases.

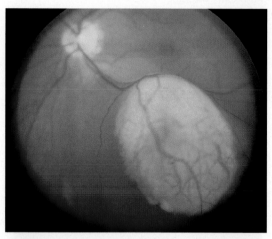

Figure 7-55. Amelanotic mushroom-shaped melanoma in a 55-year-old man.

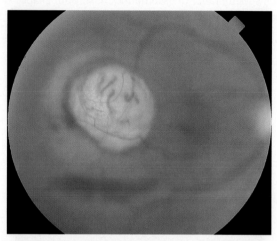

Figure 7-56. Amelanotic mushroom-shaped melanoma in a 63-year-old man. Note the preretinal hemorrhage inferiorly.

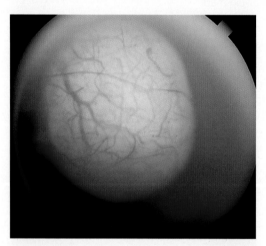

Figure 7-57. Amelanotic mushroom-shaped melanoma in a 69-year-old woman.

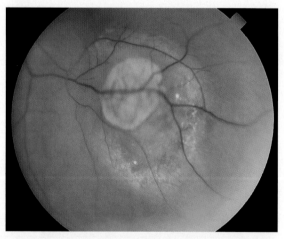

Figure 7-58. Amelanotic mushroom-shaped melanoma in a 49-year-old man.

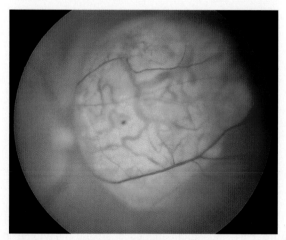

Figure 7-59. Amelanotic mushroom-shaped melanoma in a 45-year-old man.

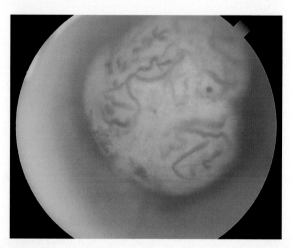

Figure 7-60. Amelanotic mushroom-shaped melanoma in a 68-year-old man.

Wide-angle Photographs of Posterior Uveal Melanoma

Wide-angle photographs allow a better overall view of choroidal melanoma that cannot be visualized by other methods. Wide-angle photographs are helpful in following melanomas that have been treated with radiotherapy.

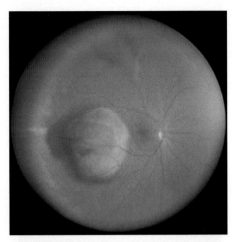

Figure 7-61. Choroidal melanoma temporal to the macular area in a 55-year-old woman.

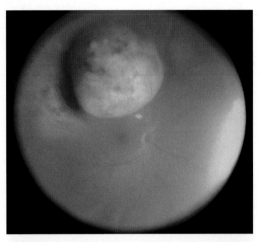

Figure 7-62. Choroidal melanoma located superiorly in a 41-year-old man.

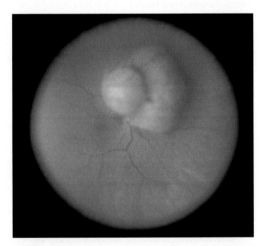

Figure 7-63. Choroidal melanoma with a break through Bruch's membrane in a 55-year-old man.

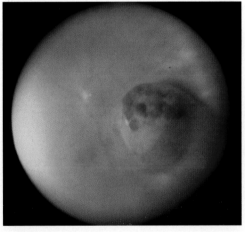

Figure 7-64. Choroidal melanoma with retinal invasion in a 60-year-old woman.

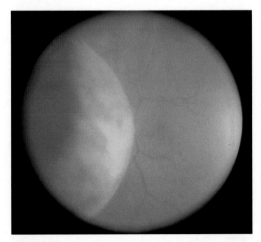

Figure 7-65. Large ciliochoroidal melanoma in a 58-year-old man.

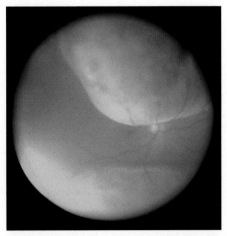

Figure 7-66. Large superior ciliochoroidal melanoma in a 45-year-old man. Note the secondary retinal detachment inferiorly.

Choroidal Melanoma—Effects upon Adjacent Structures

Choroidal melanoma can induce changes in the adjacent structures that should be recognized by the clinician. It can affect the retinal pigment epithelium by causing atrophy and proliferation, or it can produce orange pigment on its surface secondary to aggregation of lipofuscin-laden macrophages. Choroidal melanoma can induce fibrous metaplasia of the retinal pigment epithelium. Juxtapapillary melanoma can invade the optic disc, causing disc hyperemia and edema. In rare instances, choroidal melanoma can induce a circinate exudation around its margins. In some cases, it can induce peripheral choroidal ischemia, which leads to a sectoral paving stone degeneration in the quadrant of the tumor.

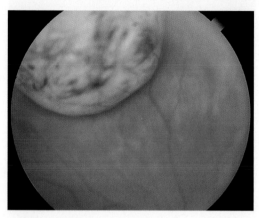

Figure 7-67. Choroidal melanoma with overlying atrophy and proliferation of retinal pigment epithelium in a 40-year-old woman.

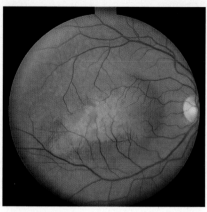

Figure 7-68. Choroidal melanoma with overlying orange pigment in a 54-year-old man.

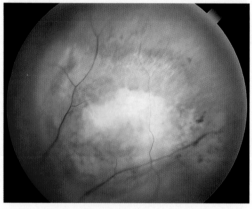

Figure 7-69. Choroidal melanoma with overlying fibrous metaplasia of retinal pigment epithelium in a 41-year-old woman.

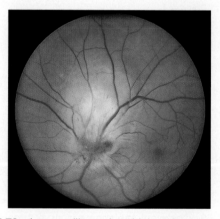

Figure 7-70. Juxtapapillary choroidal melanoma with secondary invasion of the optic disc, causing hyperemia and disc edema.

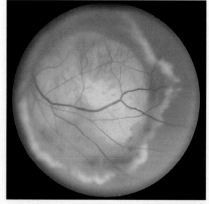

Figure 7-71. Choroidal melanoma with circinate exudation in a 50-year-old man.

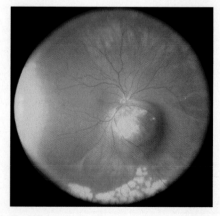

Figure 7-72. Wide-angle photograph of a choroidal melanoma with secondary paving stone degeneration in the quadrant of the lesion inferiorly in a 40-year-old woman.

Choroidal Melanoma with Retinal and Vitreal Invasion

Choroidal melanoma can invade the overlying sensory retina and can break through the retina into the vitreous cavity. Retinal and vitreal invasion is more likely to occur with mushroom-shaped melanoma but can sometimes occur with dome-shaped and diffuse melanomas. The dispersed pigment produces a "pseudoretinitis pigmentosa" appearance ophthalmoscopically and angiographically.

Figs. 7-77 and 7-78 from Eagle RC Jr, Shields JA. Pseudoretinitis pigmentosa secondary to preretinal malignant melanoma cells. *Retina* 1982;2:51–55.

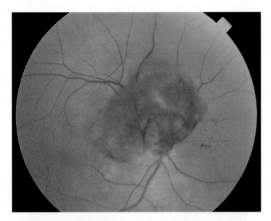

Figure 7-73. Juxtapapillary choroidal melanoma with retinal invasion in a 54-year-old woman.

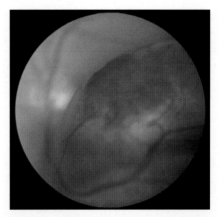

Figure 7-74. Choroidal melanoma in the macular region with retinal invasion in a 41-year-old man. Note the gray-black plaque on the surface of the tumor that obscures the retinal vessels.

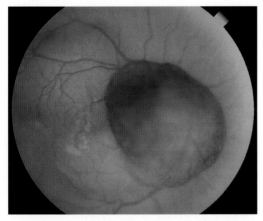

Figure 7-75. Mushroom-shaped choroidal melanoma with retinal invasion in a 73-year-old woman.

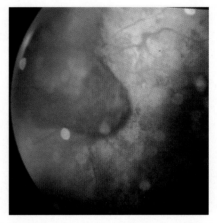

Figure 7-76. Necrotic pedunculated choroidal melanoma with retinal and vitreal invasion in 70-year-old woman.

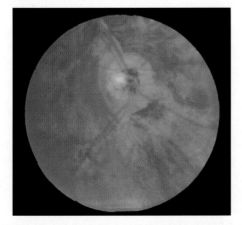

Figure 7-77. Retinal and vitreal invasion of a choroidal melanoma producing a "pseudoretinitis pigmentosa" picture in a 64-year-old woman.

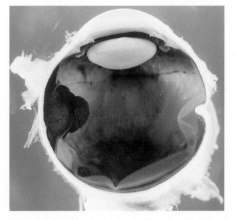

Figure 7-78. Sectioned eye shown in Fig. 7-77. Note the deeply pigmented equatorial mushroom-shaped choroidal melanoma that invaded the retina and vitreous. A line of pigment deposition is evident at the vitreous base.

Retinal Vein Dilation Secondary to Retinal Invasion of Choroidal Melanoma

In some cases of retinal invasion by choroidal melanoma, a retinal vein draining the retinal portion of the tumor becomes dilated and tortuous. Unlike the retinal capillary hemangioma that is associated with a dilated, tortuous artery and vein, only the vein is characteristically abnormal in cases of melanoma. The following clinicopathologic correlation depicts this phenomenon.

From Shields JA, Joffe L, Guibor P. Choroidal melanoma clinically simulating a retinal angioma. *Am J Ophthalmol* 1978;85:67–71.

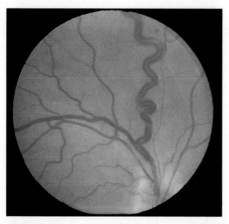

Figure 7-79. Large dilated retinal vein superiorly to the optic disc in a 35-year-old man. Coincidental myelinated retinal nerve fibers are present on the superior margin of the optic disc.

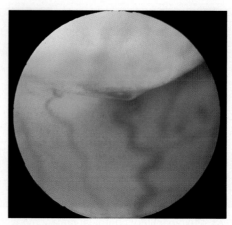

Figure 7-80. Superior fundus showing a large amelanotic mass involving the sensory retina and choroid.

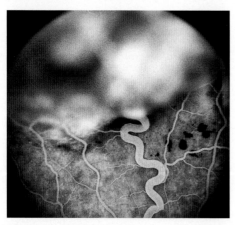

Figure 7-81. Fluorescein angiogram in venous phase showing dilated tortuous retinal vein but no significant dilation of the associated arteries.

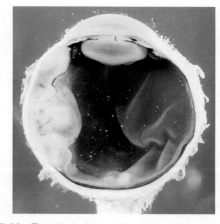

Figure 7-82. Enucleated eye showing amelanotic choroidal mass.

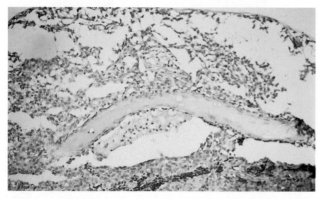

Figure 7-83. Section through tumor-infiltrated retina showing longitudinal section of a large blood vessel (hematoxylin–eosin, original magnification × 15).

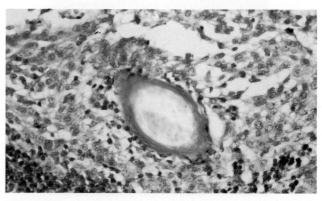

Figure 7-84. Photomicrograph through the retinal portion of the tumor showing a large dilated vessel in cross-section (hematoxylin–eosin, original magnification × 100).

Diffuse Choroidal Melanoma

Choroidal melanoma can grow in a diffuse or flat pattern, rather than the more characteristic nodular or mushroom pattern. As compared to typical choroidal melanoma, diffuse choroidal melanoma generally is more aggressive, has a more malignant cell type, tends to extend extrasclerally, and carries a worse prognosis.

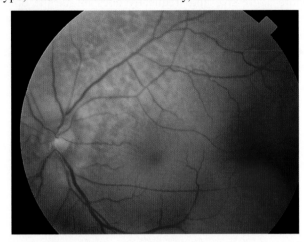

Figure 7-85. Diffuse choroidal melanoma in the posterior pole and superior fundus of a 58-year-old man.

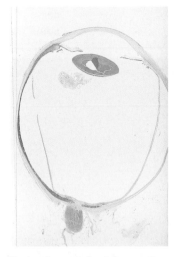

Figure 7-86. Photomicrograph of the section of the enucleated eye shown in Fig. 7-85 through the thickest part of the tumor. Note that the choroid is diffusely thickened to the *left*, which represents the superior fundus.

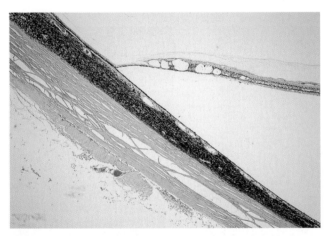

Figure 7-87. Photomicrograph of the eye shown in Fig. 7-85 showing pigmented thickening of the choroid near the ora serrata.

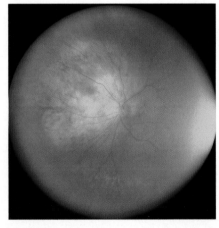

Figure 7-88. Wide-angle fundus photograph of diffuse amelanotic thickening of the choroid nasally in a 55-year-old woman.

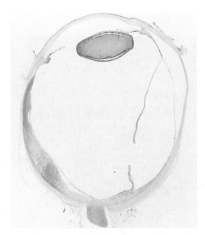

Figure 7-89. Photomicrograph of the section of the enucleated eye shown in Fig. 7-88 through the thickest part of the tumor.

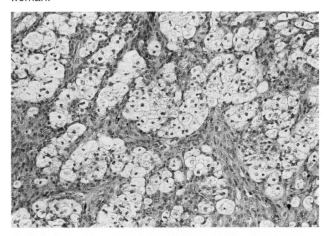

Figure 7-90. Photomicrograph of the tumor shown in Fig. 7-88. Note the large, clear balloon melanoma cells. It was probably these balloon cells that accounted for the yellow color of the lesion.

Diffuse Choroidal Melanoma with Optic Nerve Invasion

Although most typical nodular melanomas have little tendency to invade the optic nerve, diffuse melanoma is more aggressive and frequently does invade the optic nerve. The following is a clinicopathologic correlation of a diffuse choroidal melanoma with optic nerve extension.

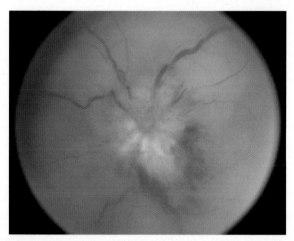

Figure 7-91. Thickening of the optic disc and diffuse choroidal thickening in a 66-year-old man.

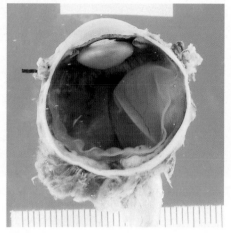

Figure 7-92. Section of enucleated eye showing diffuse amelanotic tumor in the posterior choroid.

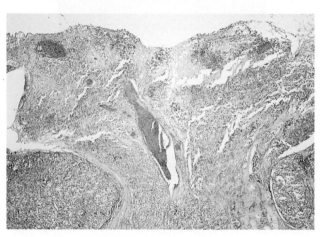

Figure 7-93. Photomicrograph of the optic disc region showing swollen disc with large blood vessels.

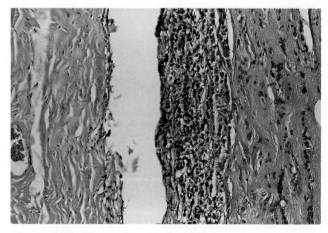

Figure 7-94. Photomicrograph showing melanoma cells in the subarachnoid space (hematoxylin–eosin, original magnification × 40).

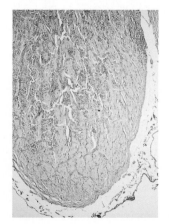

Figure 7-95. Photomicrograph of longitudinal section of the optic nerve showing tumor cell infiltration (hematoxylin–eosin, original magnification × 40).

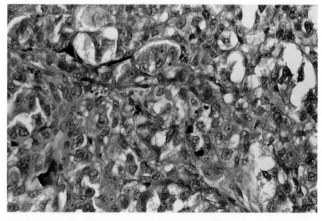

Figure 7-96. Photomicrograph showing mixed cell–type melanoma (hematoxylin–eosin, original magnification × 100).

Advanced Posterior Uveal Melanoma

Most posterior uveal melanomas are diagnosed at a relatively early stage when the tumor is still in the eye and has not produced major complications. In some instances, however, a previously undiagnosed melanoma can cause massive orbital extension.

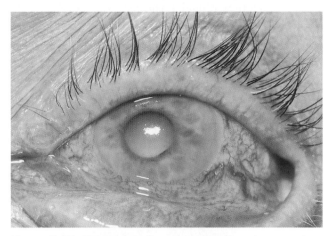

Figure 7-97. Cataract and acute congestive glaucoma in a 70-year-old man with choroidal melanoma.

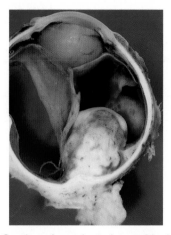

Figure 7-98. Section of enucleated eye with choroidal melanoma, total retinal detachment, and anterior displacement of the cataractous lens causing secondary glaucoma.

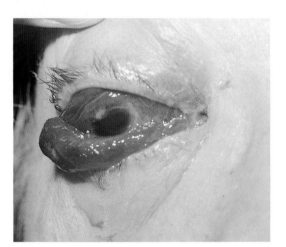

Figure 7-99. Acute glaucoma and conjunctival chemosis simulating endophthalmitis in an 82-year-old woman with choroidal melanoma.

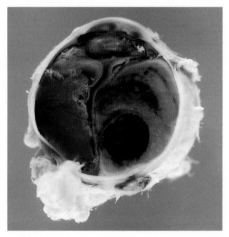

Figure 7-100. Section of enucleated eye of the patient shown in Fig. 7-99, showing necrotic melanoma and subretinal hemorrhage. The necrosis in the tumor probably induced the orbital inflammation simulating panophthalmitis.

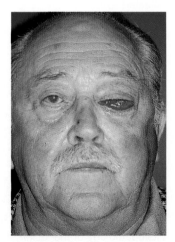

Figure 7-101. Conjunctival chemosis and proptosis secondary to orbital extension of uveal melanoma in a 71-year-old man. Sixteen years earlier, the patient had undergone retinal detachment surgery elsewhere, but no retinal break was detected.

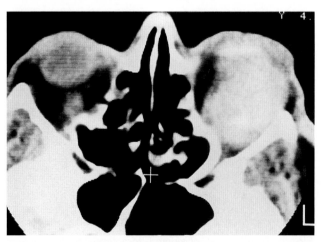

Figure 7-102. Orbital computed tomogram of the patient shown in Fig. 7-101, showing melanoma filling the globe and the orbit. Orbital exenteration was performed.

Extraocular Extension and Orbital Recurrence of Posterior Uveal Melanoma

Uveal melanoma can occur in the posterior orbit by primary transcleral extension or by recurrence after enucleation. If the orbital involvement is small and circumscribed, modified enucleation can be performed by a lateral orbitotomy approach without resorting to orbital exenteration. Sometimes orbital recurrence can develop many years after enucleation. Orbital melanoma also is discussed in *Atlas of Orbital Tumors*.

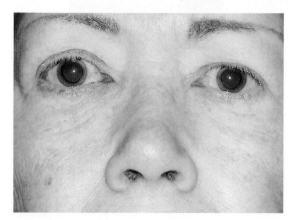

Figure 7-103. Proptosis of the right eye in a 67-year-old woman.

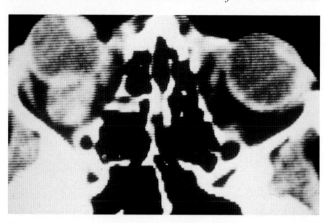

Figure 7-104. Axial computed tomogram showing orbital mass in the patient shown in Fig. 7-103. The relatively flat intraocular portion of the melanoma is very subtle.

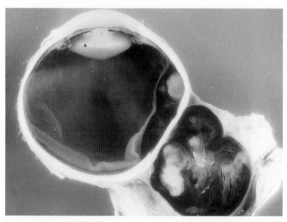

Figure 7-105. Section of eye of the patient shown in Fig. 7-103, removed by a lateral canthotomy approach with about 20 mm of optic nerve showing the large nodule of orbital extension that accounted for the proptosis.

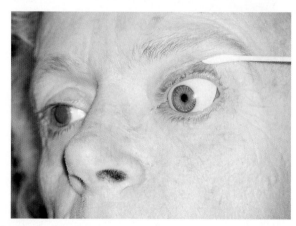

Figure 7-106. Protrusion of prosthesis on the left side of a patient who had enucleation for choroidal melanoma 20 years earlier. In retrospect, a small focus of transcleral extension by spindle melanoma cells was evident histopathologically on the enucleated eye.

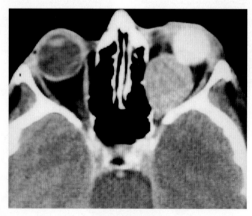

Figure 7-107. Axial computed tomogram of the patient shown in Fig. 7-106 depicting large ovoid mass posterior to the orbital implant.

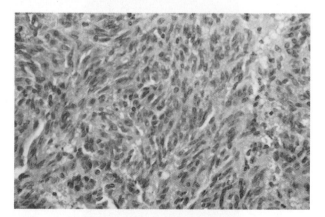

Figure 7-108. Histopathology of the lesion shown in Fig. 7-107, demonstrating low-grade spindle cells.

Spontaneous Necrosis and Regression of Choroidal Melanoma

Uveal melanoma occasionally can undergo spontaneous necrosis and regression for uncertain reasons. Such tumors develop white-yellow areas and pigment dispersion, and they resemble tumors that have been irradiated, except that they lack radiation vasculopathy. Lesions with this appearance should be followed periodically because of a definite tendency to eventually demonstrate regrowth. The cases shown here were all seen after the presumed event, and no photographs were available of the original lesions.

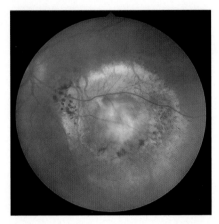

Figure 7-109. Regressed choroidal melanoma with surrounding ring of atrophy of retinal pigment epithelium in a 25-year-old woman.

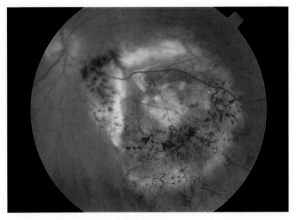

Figure 7-110. Same lesion shown in Fig. 7-109 about 13 years later showing that the lesion is still regressed with no regrowth.

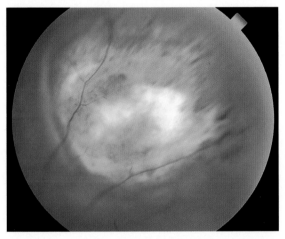

Figure 7-111. Chorodal melanoma with spontaneous necrosis in a 49-year-old woman. The yellow-white areas in the lesion represent fibrous tissue in areas of tumor necrosis.

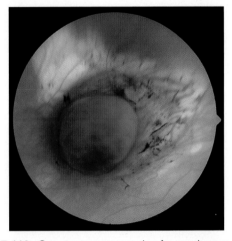

Figure 7-112. Spontaneous necrosis of a mushroom-shaped melanoma in a 67-year-old woman. The base of the tumor is flat and shows extensive pigment epithelial alteration.

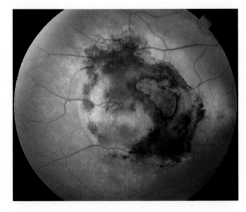

Figure 7-113. Spontaneous regression of a choroidal melanoma in a 25-year-old woman.

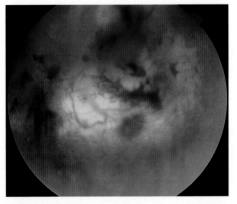

Figure 7-114. Spontaneous regression of a choroidal melanoma in a 45-year-old man. In this case, the tumor appears to be almost completely destroyed. Later, regrowth of the tumor necessitated plaque radiotherapy.

CHAPTER 8

Pathology of Posterior Uveal Melanoma

PATHOLOGY OF POSTERIOR UVEAL MELANOMA

Posterior uveal melanoma can have characteristic features on both gross and microscopic examination (1,2). Observations of growth patterns on grossly sectioned eyes can be helpful to the clinician in understanding the clinical behavior of the tumors. Grossly, a ciliary body melanoma can be dome shaped, mushroom shaped, or diffuse. The mushroom shape occurs from rupture of Bruch's membrane secondary to tumor growth. Melanoma can be deeply pigmented, partly pigmented, or nonpigmented. It can produce a secondary retinal detachment, subluxation of the lens, or secondary cataract. It can invade the anterior chamber, producing secondary glaucoma, or it can extend through the sclera. A diffuse melanoma can assume a ring configuration in the ciliary body region or a flat to slightly elevated appearance in the choroid.

Microscopically, posterior uveal melanoma can be composed of spindle A cells, spindle B cells, and epithelioid cells, or various combinations of spindle and epithelioid cells (mixed-cell melanoma). Areas of necrosis frequently are seen within the tumor. In some instances, extensive necrosis may prevent recognition of the underlying cell type.

SELECTED REFERENCES

1. Shields JA, Shields CL. *Intraocular tumors. A text and atlas.* Philadelphia: WB Saunders, 1992:117–136.
2. McLean IW. Uveal nevi and malignant melanomas. In: Spencer WH, ed. *Ophthalmic pathology. An atlas and textbook.* Philadelphia: WB Saunders, 1996:2121–2217.

Gross Features of Ciliary Body and Ciliochoroidal Melanoma

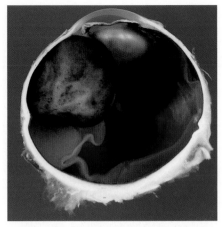

Figure 8-1. Pigmented ciliary body melanoma.

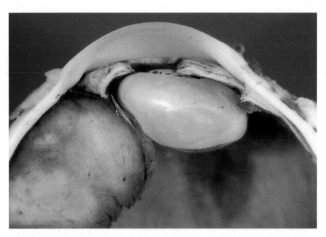

Figure 8-2. Pigmented ciliary body melanoma causing subluxation of the lens and secondary cataract.

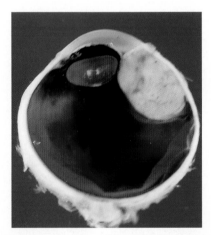

Figure 8-3. Mildly pigmented ciliary body melanoma.

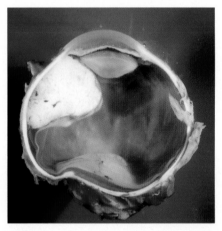

Figure 8-4. Nonpigmented ciliary body melanoma.

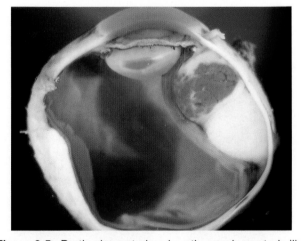

Figure 8-5. Partly pigmented and partly nonpigmented ciliochoroidal melanoma.

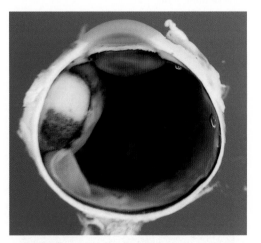

Figure 8-6. Partly pigmented and partly nonpigmented ciliochoroidal melanoma.

Gross Features of Choroidal Melanoma

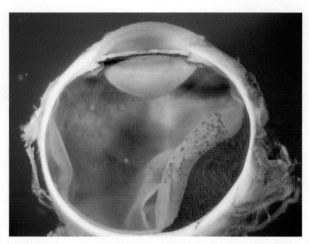

Figure 8-7. Mildly elevated pigmented choroidal melanoma.

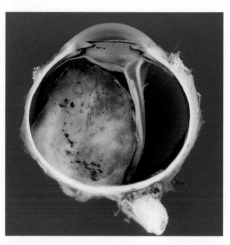

Figure 8-8. Large pigmented choroidal melanoma causing total retinal detachment.

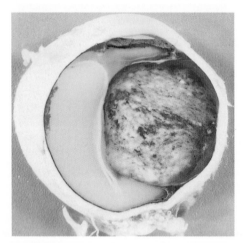

Figure 8-9. Large pigmented choroidal melanoma causing total retinal detachment.

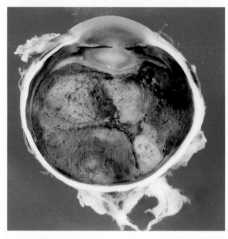

Figure 8-10. Pigmented melanoma filling the entire eye.

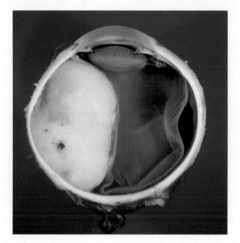

Figure 8-11. Amelanotic dome-shaped choroidal melanoma.

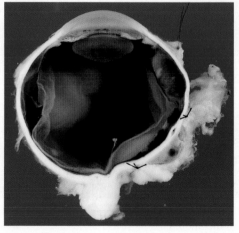

Figure 8-12. Diffuse choroidal melanoma with nodule of extrascleral extension. This was detected with ultrasonography prior to modified enucleation.

Mushroom-shaped Choroidal Melanoma

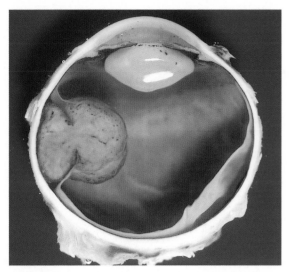

Figure 8-13. Pigmented mushroom-shaped melanoma located near the equator of the globe.

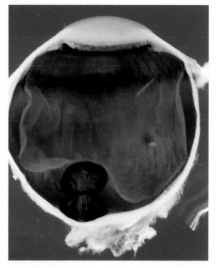

Figure 8-14. Pigmented mushroom-shaped melanoma located in the posterior choroid.

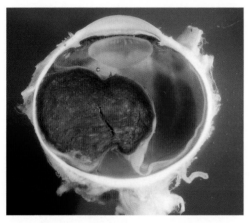

Figure 8-15. Larger, equatorial mushroom-shaped melanoma with total retinal detachment.

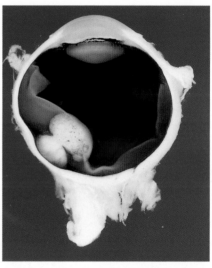

Figure 8-16. Mushroom-shaped nonpigmented melanoma.

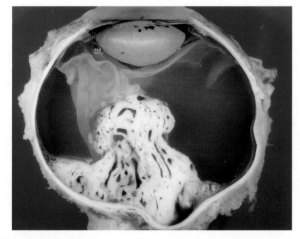

Figure 8-17. Mushroom-shaped nonpigmented melanoma with marked vascularity.

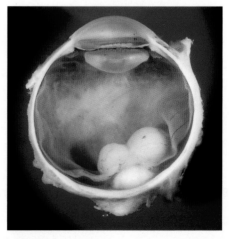

Figure 8-18. Nonpigmented melanoma with two breaks through Bruch's membrane.

Low-magnification Photomicrographs of Choroidal Melanoma

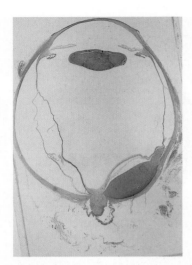

Figure 8-19. Slightly elevated posterior choroidal melanoma.

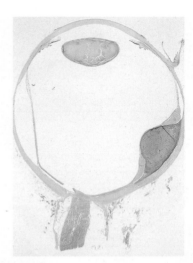

Figure 8-20. Dome-shaped postequatorial choroidal melanoma, with a small break through Bruch's membrane.

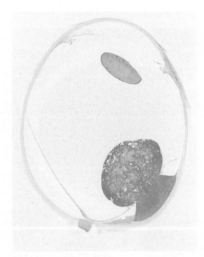

Figure 8-21. Mushroom-shaped choroidal melanoma.

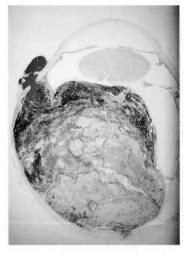

Figure 8-22. Large necrotic choroidal melanoma.

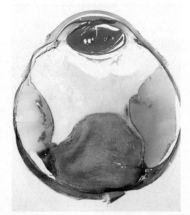

Figure 8-23. Posterior choroidal melanoma with secondary retinal detachment and anterior displacement of the lens-iris diaphragm, which caused secondary glaucoma.

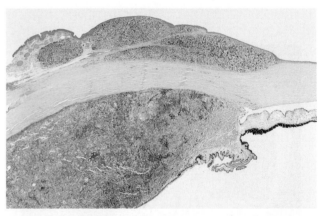

Figure 8-24. Extrascleral extension of ciliary body melanoma.

Cell Types of Uveal Melanoma

The cell type of uveal melanoma generally is defined in terms of the Callender classification. It applies to iris, ciliary body, and choroidal melanoma. A modification of the Callender classification is used in some pathology laboratories.

Figs. 8-25 through 8-30 are photomicrographs taken by Dr. Ralph C. Eagle Jr.

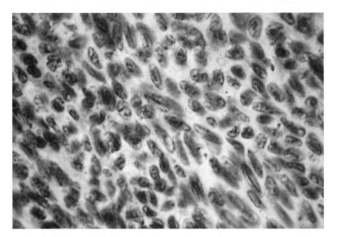

Figure 8-25. Spindle A melanoma (hematoxylin–eosin, original magnification × 200).

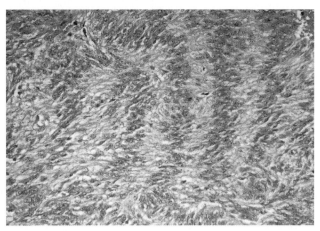

Figure 8-26. Fascicular melanoma. This is a spindle cell melanoma that assumes a fascicular growth pattern, similar to that seen with schwannoma (hematoxylin–eosin, original magnification × 100).

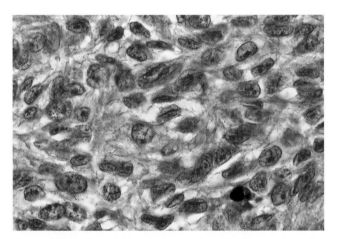

Figure 8-27. Spindle B melanoma (hematoxylin–eosin, original magnification × 200).

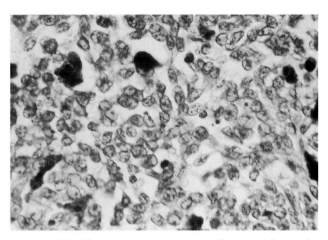

Figure 8-28. Mixed cell–type melanoma (hematoxylin–eosin, original magnification × 200).

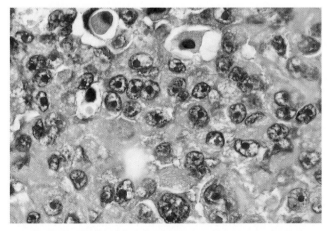

Figure 8-29. Epithelioid cell–type melanoma (hematoxylin–eosin, original magnification × 200).

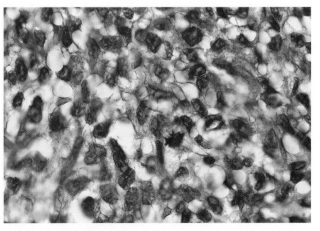

Figure 8-30. Epithelioid cell–type melanoma (hematoxylin–eosin, original magnification × 200).

CHAPTER 9

Diagnostic Approaches to Posterior Uveal Melanoma

DIAGNOSTIC APPROACHES TO POSTERIOR UVEAL MELANOMA

In most instances, the diagnosis of posterior uveal melanoma can be made by recognition of its classic features using slit lamp biomicroscopy or indirect ophthalmoscopy. However, the diagnosis can be supported or confirmed by the judicious use of ancillary studies such as fluorescein angiography, indocyanine green angiography, ultrasonography, computed tomography, magnetic resonance imaging, radioactive phosphorus uptake test, and fine-needle aspiration biopsy. In cases that are typical ophthalmoscopically, these ancillary studies assume a more vital role in diagnosis. These techniques are discussed in detail in the literature (1–6).

With fluorescein angiography, a typical choroidal melanoma shows mottled hyperfluorescence in the vascular filling phases and diffuse late staining of the mass and its overlying subretinal fluid. A larger amelanotic melanoma, particularly one that has broken through Bruch's membrane, may show more clearly the characteristic double circulation in which both the retinal vessels and the choroidal vessels in the tumor are readily evident. Indocyanine green angiography shows characteristic features of uveal melanoma that can be of diagnostic help in difficult cases (2).

With A-scan ultrasonography, choroidal melanoma typically shows medium to low internal reflectivity, and with B scan it shows a choroidal mass pattern with acoustic hollowness and choroidal excavation. Ultrasonography can delineate small nodules of extraocular extension of the tumor (1). It is particularly helpful in eyes with opaque media. Computed tomography and magnetic resonance imaging can be used to visualize uveal melanoma and to completely delineate larger areas of orbital extension (3).

The radioactive phosphorus uptake test can be used to make the diagnosis in difficult cases (4). Although this accurate and reliable test was used extensively in the past, it is used less often today because of the advent and perfection of techniques of fine-needle biopsy. Fine-needle aspiration biopsy can be used to make the diagnosis of choroidal melanoma in difficult cases that defy clinical diagnosis using less invasive measures (5). The most commonly employed technique is a transpars plana, transvitreal approach using a 25-gauge needle. The technique is detailed in the literature (1,5).

SELECTED REFERENCES

1. Shields JA, Shields CL. *Intraocular tumors. A text and atlas.* Philadelphia: WB Saunders, 1992:155–169.
2. Shields CL, Shields JA, De Potter P. Patterns of indocyanine green angiography of choroidal tumors. *Br J Ophthalmol* 1995;79:237–245.
3. De Potter P, Shields JA, Shields CL. Disorders of the globe. Tumors of the uvea. In: De Potter P, Shields JA, Shields CL, eds. *MRI of the eye and orbit.* Philadelphia: JB Lippincott Co., 1995:56–92.
4. Shields JA. Accuracy and limitation of the P-32 test in the diagnosis of ocular tumors. An analysis of 500 cases. *Ophthalmology* 1978;85:950–966.
5. Shields JA, Shields CL, Ehya H, Eagle RC Jr, De Potter P. Fine needle aspiration biopsy of suspected intraocular tumors. The 1992 Urwick Lecture. *Ophthalmology* 1993;100:1677–1684.
6. Shields JA, McDonald PR, Leonard BC, Canny CLB. The diagnosis of uveal melanomas in eyes with opaque media. *Am J Ophthalmol* 1977;82:95–105.

Fluorescein Angiography of Dome-shaped Melanoma

A case of a 29-year-old man is shown.

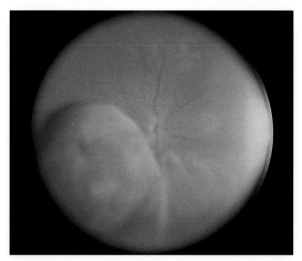

Figure 9-1. Wide-angle photograph of choroidal melanoma inferotemporally in the right eye.

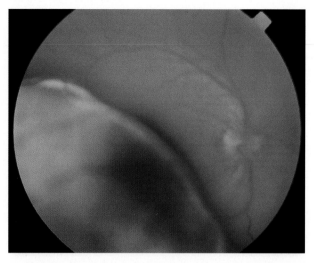

Figure 9-2. Standard fundus photograph of the same lesion.

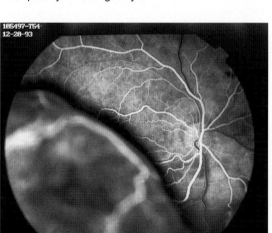

Figure 9-3. Angiogram in late arterial phase, with focus on the optic disc, showing filling of retinal arteries over the tumor and early hyperfluorescence of the tumor.

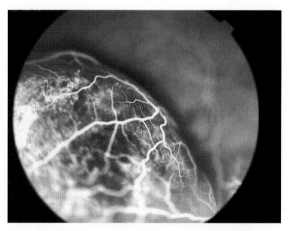

Figure 9-4. Venous phase showing further hyperfluorescence of the mass.

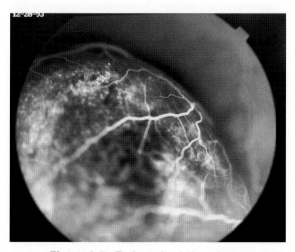

Figure 9-5. Early recirculation phase.

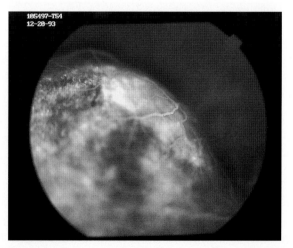

Figure 9-6. Late angiogram showing continued hyperfluorescence of the mass.

Fluorescein Angiography of Mushroom-shaped Melanoma

The prominent blood vessels seen in amelanotic mushroom-shaped choroidal melanoma can impart a "pseudoangiomatous" appearance to the lesion.

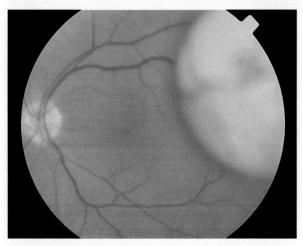

Figure 9-7. Clinical appearance of amelanotic mass temporal to the foveal region.

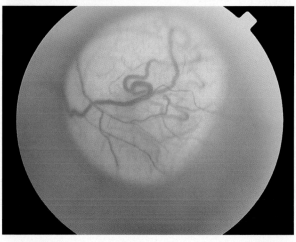

Figure 9-8. Clinical appearance of the dome of the mushroom-shaped mass showing prominent retinal and tumoral blood vessels.

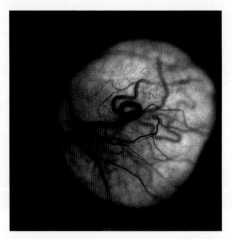

Figure 9-9. Red-free photograph highlighting the prominent blood vessels.

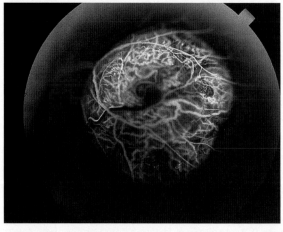

Figure 9-10. Angiogram in early laminar venous phase showing retinal and tumoral blood vessels.

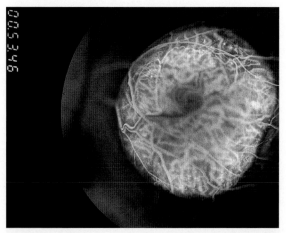

Figure 9-11. Angiogram in early recirculation phase showing continued hyperfluorescence of the vessels in the mass. Note that there is still some laminar flow in the overlying retinal vein.

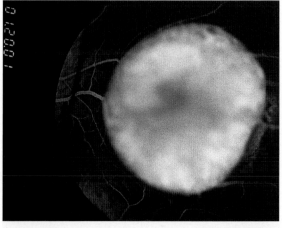

Figure 9-12. Late angiogram showing intense hyperfluorescence of the mass due to leakage from blood vessels in the tumor.

Fluorescein Angiography of Choroidal Melanoma with Overlying Neovascular Membrane of Choroidal Origin

Choroidal neovascularization over a choroidal nevus or melanoma is rare. It has a clinical and angiographic appearance similar to that seen in age-related macular degeneration.

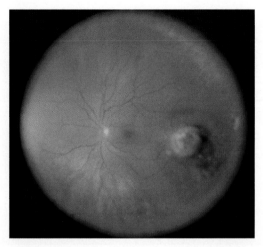

Figure 9-13. Wide-angle fundus photograph of mushroom-shaped melanoma inferotemporally in the left eye of a 40-year-old man.

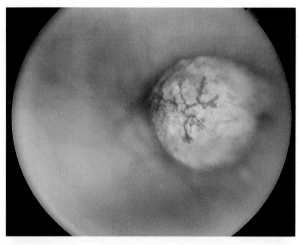

Figure 9-14. Standard fundus photograph showing arborizing blood vessels on the surface of the tumor.

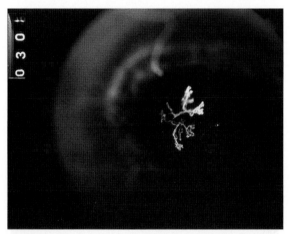

Figure 9-15. Arterial phase showing well-defined hyperfluorescence of the overlying neovascular membrane. Note that no retinal vessels feed the neovascular structure, suggesting that it is of choroidal origin from within the tumor.

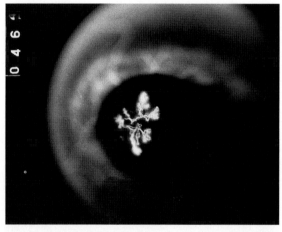

Figure 9-16. Late venous phase showing early leakage from the neovascular membrane.

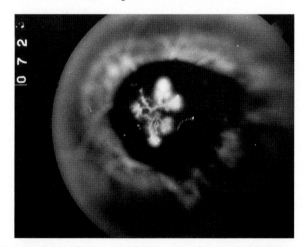

Figure 9-17. Early recirculation phase showing continued leakage.

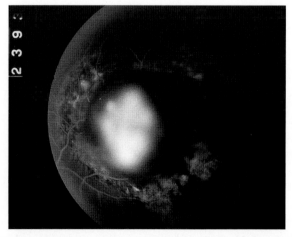

Figure 9-18. Late recirculation phase showing ill-defined hyperfluorescence secondary to leakage of the neovascular membrane.

Indocyanine Green Angiography of Choroidal Melanoma

Indocyanine green angiography shows characteristic, but not pathognomonic, features in cases of choroidal melanoma.

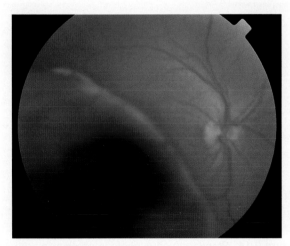

Figure 9-19. Clinical photograph of choroidal melanoma inferotemporally in the right eye of a 29-year-old man.

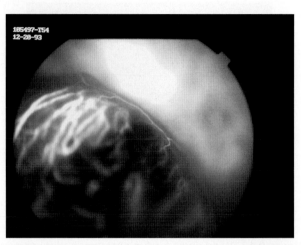

Figure 9-20. Early indocyanine green angiogram of the tumor shown in Fig. 9-19, showing prominent overlying retinal vessels and minimal leakage from tumor vessels.

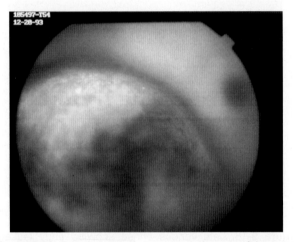

Figure 9-21. Late indocyanine green angiogram of the tumor shown in Fig. 9-19, showing moderate hyperfluorescence of the mass.

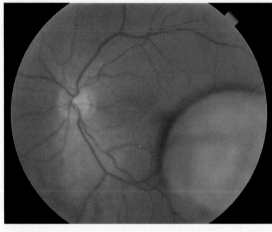

Figure 9-22. Clinical photograph of choroidal melanoma inferotemporal to the fovea in a 51-year-old man.

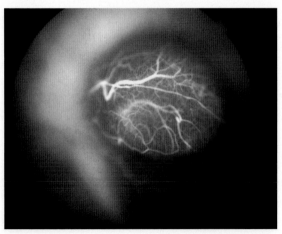

Figure 9-23. Early indocyanine green angiogram of the tumor shown in Fig. 9-22, showing prominent overlying retinal vessels and minimal leakage from tumor vessels.

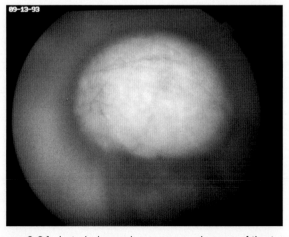

Figure 9-24. Late indocyanine green angiogram of the tumor shown in Fig. 9-22, showing moderate hyperfluorescence of the mass.

Ultrasonography of Posterior Uveal Melanoma

Ultrasonography using A-scan or B-scan is a commonly employed technique that is readily available in many ophthalmologists' offices. It shows characteristic features that can support the diagnosis of choroidal or ciliary body melanoma. In cases with opaque ocular media, such as corneal edema, cataract, or vitreal hemorrhage, it can provide evidence of an underlying melanoma.

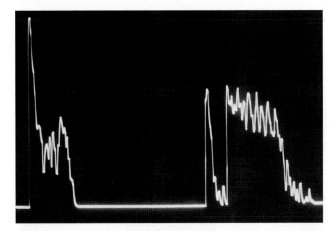

Figure 9-25. A-scan of small choroidal melanoma showing clear vitreous (to the *left*), high initial spike, and low internal reflectivity in the tumor.

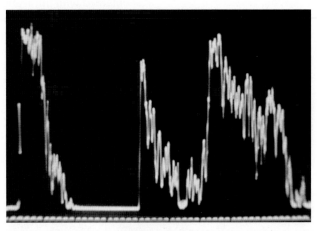

Figure 9-26. A-scan of larger choroidal melanoma showing progressively decreasing amplitude in the tumor (angle kappa).

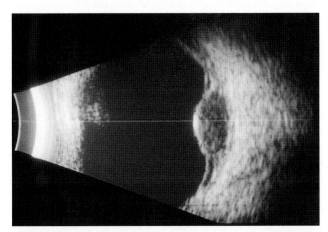

Figure 9-27. B-scan of medium-sized, dome-shaped choroidal melanoma showing characteristic acoustic hollowness and choroidal excavation.

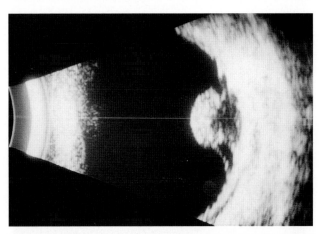

Figure 9-28. B-scan of medium-sized, mushroom-shaped choroidal melanoma showing typical acoustic hollowness and choroidal excavation.

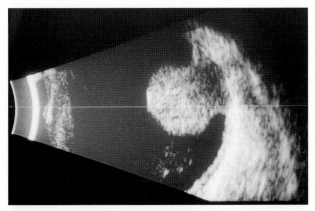

Figure 9-29. B-scan of larger, mushroom-shaped choroidal melanoma. This lesion shows more acoustic solidity near the tumor apex, suggesting congested tumor vessels or tumor necrosis.

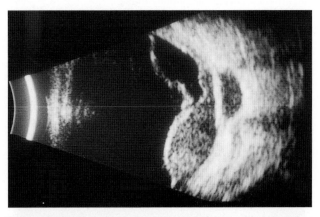

Figure 9-30. B-scan of choroidal melanoma with extrascleral extension. The echolucent area in the orbital fat represents the nodule of extrascleral tumor. Note also the linear echo superior to the solid tumor representing a secondary retinal detachment.

Computed Tomography and Magnetic Resonance Imaging of Posterior Uveal Melanoma

Although computed tomography and magnetic resonance imaging can demonstrate a posterior uveal melanoma, they provide little clinical information that cannot be obtained with ultrasonography. However, in cases with massive orbital extension of the uveal melanoma, these techniques are better than ultrasonography for demonstrating the full extent of the tumor.

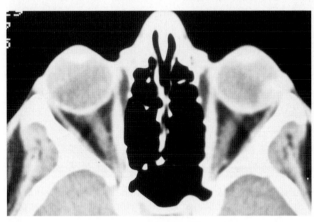

Figure 9-31. Axial computed tomogram of equatorial choroidal melanoma.

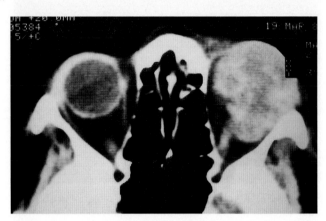

Figure 9-32. Axial computed tomogram of choroidal melanoma with transscleral orbital extension of the tumor.

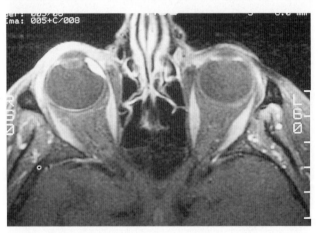

Figure 9-33. Axial magnetic resonance imaging in T1-weighted image with fat suppression and gadolinium enhancement showing ciliary body mass.

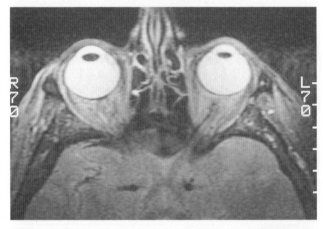

Figure 9-34. Axial magnetic resonance imaging in T2-weighted image showing same mass seen in Fig. 9-33.

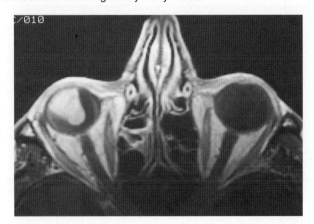

Figure 9-35. Axial magnetic resonance imaging in T1-weighted image with gadolinium enhancement showing a mushroom-shaped ciliary-body melanoma.

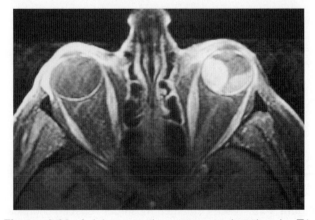

Figure 9-36. Axial magnetic resonance imaging in T1-weighted image with fat suppression and gadolinium enhancement showing a dome-shaped choroidal melanoma (to the *left*) and a secondary retinal detachment (to the *right*).

Radioactive Phosphorus Uptake Test and Fine-needle Aspiration Biopsy

The radioactive phosphorus uptake (P-32) test and fine-needle aspiration biopsy are two highly reliable methods for making the diagnosis in difficult cases where the differential diagnosis is between a melanoma and a simulating lesion.

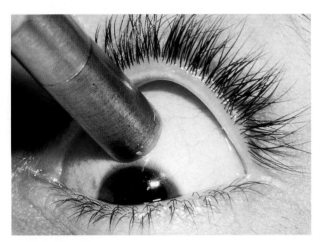

Figure 9-37. Method of nonincisional radioactive phosphorus test for a ciliary body lesion.

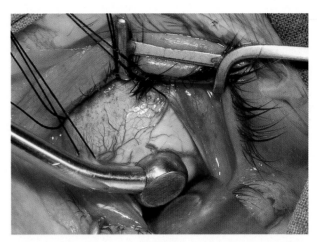

Figure 9-38. Method of incisional radioactive phosphorus test for a posterior choroidal lesion.

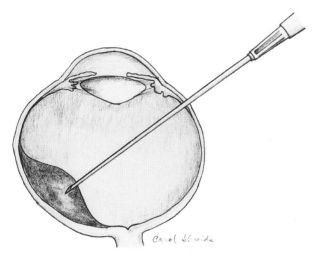

Figure 9-39. Diagram of transpars plana, transvitreal technique of fine-needle aspiration biopsy. Indirect ophthalmoscopy is used to guide the needle.

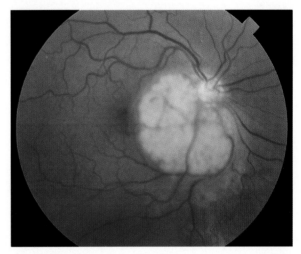

Figure 9-40. Atypical juxtapapillary lesion for which fine-needle aspiration biopsy was employed to make a diagnosis.

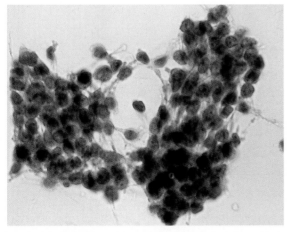

Figure 9-41. Cytology of the lesion shown in Fig.9-40 showing spindle cells compatible with melanoma (Papanicolaou, original magnification × 100).

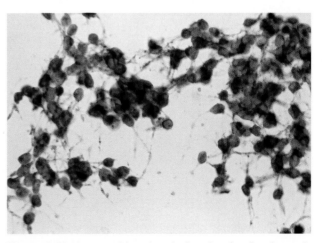

Figure 9-42. Immunohistochemical stain of cells shown in Fig. 9-41 showing positive immunoreactivity for melanoma-specific antigen (HMB-45, original magnification × 100).

CHAPTER 10

Management of Posterior Uveal Melanoma

MANAGEMENT OF POSTERIOR UVEAL MELANOMA

There are several methods of management for posterior uveal melanoma (1–14). The selected management should depend on factors such as the size, location, and activity of the melanoma as well as the status of the opposite eye and the age, general health, and psychological status of the patient. Each patient should undergo a detailed ophthalmic evaluation and the size and extent of the tumor should be carefully documented. The known risk factors for growth and metastasis should be considered (11) and the patient then should be counseled thoroughly as to the therapeutic options (12).

The details of the therapeutic methods are described elsewhere (1–9). Small lesions in which the diagnosis is questionable can be followed with serial fundus photographs and ultrasonography to document growth before undergoing definitive treatment.

Some small and some medium-sized melanomas can be managed with techniques of laser photocoagulation. Photocoagulation for choroidal melanoma initially was performed with the xenon arc photocoagulator, but more recently the argon laser has been employed. The laser can be used primarily for lesions less than 3 mm in thickness that have documented growth or other significant risk factors for growth and metastasis (3). Photocoagulation is used less often today because transpupillary thermotherapy has shown more promise.

Transpupillary thermotherapy recently has replaced laser photocoagulation at some centers for treatment of selected small and medium-sized melanoma. It involves heating the tumor using light in the infrared range by way of a modified diode laser delivery system. It gives the best results in cases of small tumors in which growth is detected at an early stage but it has been used successfully for tumors up to 4 mm in thickness (4–6).

Techniques of radiotherapy using radioactive plaque (7) or charged particles (8,9,) can be used for many medium-sized or large posteriorly located melanomas in which there is a reasonable chance of preserving some vision. Plaque radiotherapy is currently the most commonly employed method of treating uveal melanoma. Extensive experience with plaque brachytherapy has suggested that it offers reasonably good tumor control, can often preserve useful vision, and offers as good a prognosis as enucleation. Plaque radiotherapy requires close cooperation among the ocular oncologist, radiation oncologist, and radiation physicist. It is now recognized that plaque radiotherapy can be employed to treat large melanomas, macular melanoma, ciliary body melanoma, and extraocular extension of melanoma (13–14). Similar results have been obtained with charged particle irradiation (8,9).

A melanoma located in the ciliary body and peripheral choroid can be managed by local removal of the tumor using a method of partial lamellar sclerouvectomy (PLSU) (10). It is a difficult procedure that requires considerable skill and experience, but the results are often very gratifying. Enucleation appears to be the best treatment for larger tumors in which there is little hope for salvaging useful vision or tumors that surround or invade the optic nerve. In the rare instance where a uveal melanoma shows massive orbital extension, primary orbital exenteration is warranted. In some instances, combination therapies, such as plaque radiotherapy followed by supplemental transpupillary thermotherapy or laser photocoagulation, are employed.

SELECTED REFERENCES

1. Gass JDM. Observation of suspected choroidal and ciliary body melanomas for evidence of growth prior to enucleation. *Ophthalmology* 1980;87:523–528.
2. Shields JA, Shields CL. *Intraocular tumors. A text and atlas.* Philadelphia: WB Saunders, 1992:171–205.
3. Shields JA, Glazer LC, Mieler WF, Shields CL. Comparison of xenon arc and argon laser photocoagulation in the treatment of choroidal melanomas. *Am J Ophthalmol* 1990;109:647–655.
4. Oosterhuis JA, Journee-de Korver HG, Kakebeeke-Kemme HM, Bleeker JC. Transpupillary thermotherapy in choroidal melanomas. *Arch Ophthalmol* 1995;113:315–321.
5. Shields CL, Shields JA, De Potter P, Kheterpel S. Transpupillary thermotherapy in the management of choroidal melanoma. *Ophthalmology* 1996;103:1642–1650.
6. Shields CL, Shields JA, De Potter P, Lois N, Edelstein C, Mercado G, Gunduz K. Transpupillary thermotherapy for choroidal melanoma. Tumor control and visual outcome in 100 cases. *Ophthalmology* 1998;105:581–590.
7. Shields JA, Shields CL, De Potter P, Cu-Ujieng A, Hernandez C, Brady LW. Plaque radiotherapy for uveal melanoma. *Int Ophthalmol Clin* 1993;33:129–135.
8. Char DH, Kroll SM, Castro JK. Ten-year follow-up of helium ion therapy of uveal melanoma. *Am J Ophthalmol* 1998;125:81–89.
9. Gragoudas ES. Long-term results after proton irradiation of uveal melanomas. *Graefes Arch Clin Exp Ophthalmol* 1997;235:265–267.
10. Shields JA, Shields CL, Shah P, Sivalingam V. Partial lamellar sclerouvectomy for ciliary body and choroidal tumors. *Ophthalmology* 1991;98:971–983.
11. Shields CL, Shields JA, Kiratli H, Cater JR, De Potter P. Risk factors for metastasis of small choroidal melanocytic lesions. *Ophthalmology* 1995;102:1351–1361.
12. Shields JA. Counseling the patient with a posterior uveal melanoma [Editorial]. *Am J Ophthalmol* 1988;106:88–91.
13. Gunduz K, Shields CL, Shields JA, Cater J, Freire J, Brady LW. Plaque radiotherapy of choroidal melanoma with macular involvement. *Am J Ophthalmol (in press).*
14. Gunduz K, Shields CL, Shields JA, Cater J, Freire J, Brady LW. Plaque radiotherapy of ciliary body melanoma. *Arch Ophthalmol (in press).*

Observation of Choroidal Melanocytic Lesions

A tumor less than 2 mm in thickness with surface drusen and no surface orange pigment or subretinal fluid usually can be followed. Additional relative reasons for observation include a small lesion near the fovea in an eye with good vision, the presence of the lesion in the patient's only useful eye, or if the patient is old or in poor general health. Recent recognition of risk factors for metastasis has prompted earlier treatment of many lesions that previously would have been observed. Examples of lesions are shown that initially would be followed without treatment according to current philosophies.

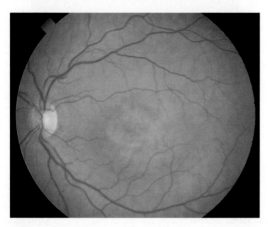

Figure 10-1. Suspicious subfoveal lesion in an asymptomatic 55-year-old woman.

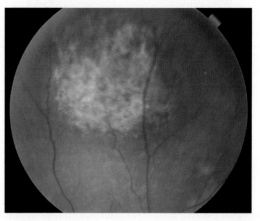

Figure 10-2. Suspicious lesion greater than 2 mm thick with numerous drusen in an asymptomatic 72-year-old woman.

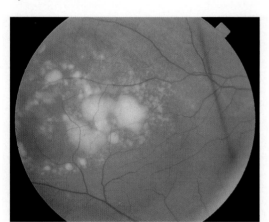

Figure 10-3. Suspicious parafoveal lesion in an asymptomatic 67-year-old woman. The numerous large drusen on the tumor surface suggest that the lesion is relatively dormant.

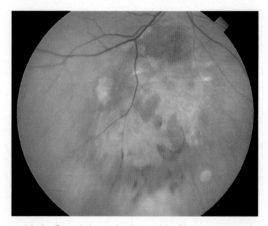

Figure 10-4. Suspicious lesion with fibrous metaplasia of the retinal pigment epithelium in an asymptomatic 75-year-old woman.

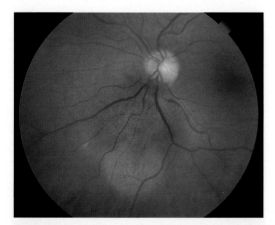

Figure 10-5. Suspicious lesion inferior to the optic disc in an asymptomatic 48-year-old woman. The shallow retinal detachment inferior to the lesion is a bothersome finding, but does not necessarily imply that this small lesion is malignant.

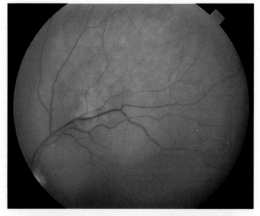

Figure 10-6. Suspicious lesion superotemporal to the optic disc in an asymptomatic 53-year-old woman. Although this lesion has abundant orange pigment on its surface, it is still only 3 mm in diameter and 1 mm in thickness. Careful periodic follow-up to detect early growth is advisable.

Small Melanocytic Choroidal Lesions that Initially were Observed and Eventually Metastasized

There are a few documented cases of small lesions (presumably nevi) that were followed without treatment in patients who later developed metastatic disease. Recognition of risk factors for future metastasis has prompted earlier treatment of many lesions that in the past would have been observed. Small lesions without risk factors should be followed, but once growth is documented, active treatment generally should be considered.

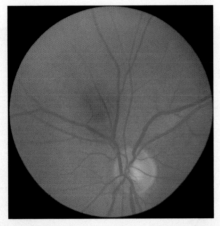

Figure 10-7. Small presumed choroidal nevus superonasal to the optic disc in a 70-year-old man. The lesion had been followed for 10 years and it showed no change.

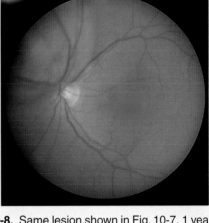

Figure 10-8. Same lesion shown in Fig. 10-7, 1 year later. The lesion had shown pronounced growth. Enucleation was performed but liver metastasis became apparent 5 years later.

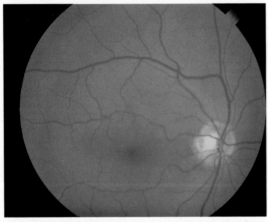

Figure 10-9. Small presumed choroidal nevus temporal to the fovea in a 75-year-old man.

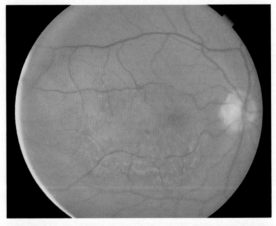

Figure 10-10. Same lesion shown in Fig. 10-9, 3 years later, showing growth and accumulation of orange pigment. Liver metastasis was detected shortly thereafter.

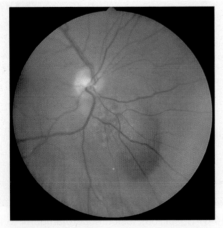

Figure 10-11. Small choroidal melanocytic lesion inferior to the optic disc in a 38-year-old woman seen in 1986. This lesion has risk factors such as proximity to the optic disc, elevation, and orange pigment.

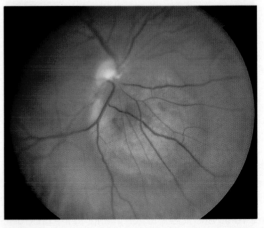

Figure 10-12. Same lesion shown in Fig. 10-11, 1 year later. Growth had occurred and enucleation was performed. The mixed cell–type melanoma demonstrated hepatic metastasis about 8 years later.

Argon Laser Photocoagulation for Choroidal Melanoma

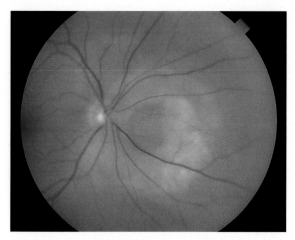

Figure 10-13. Small pigmented choroidal lesion nasal to the optic disc in a 37-year-old woman as seen in January 1992.

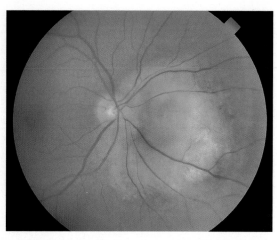

Figure 10-14. Same lesion shown in July 1993 showing slight, but definite, growth.

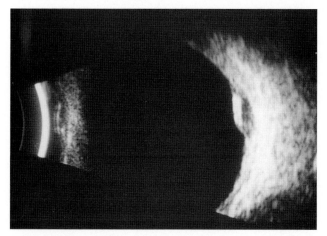

Figure 10-15. B-scan ultrasonogram showing lesion 2.0 mm thick.

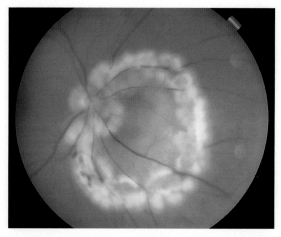

Figure 10-16. Appearance after initial treatment showing surrounding ring of photocoagulation.

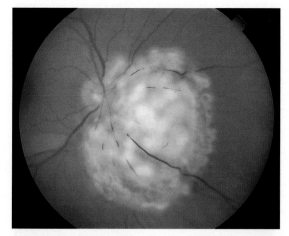

Figure 10-17. Appearance several weeks later showing repeated surrounding treatment and initial surface treatment.

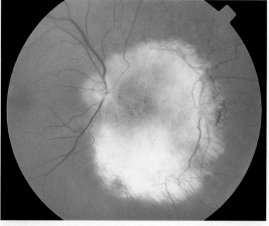

Figure 10-18. Appearance in July 1994 showing complete tumor destruction. The small amount of residual pigment is flat.

Argon Laser Photocoagulation for Small Choroidal Melanoma

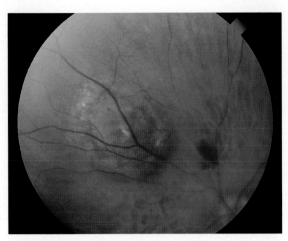

Figure 10-19. Growing pigmented choroidal tumor nasal to the optic disc in a 47-year-old man in June 1994.

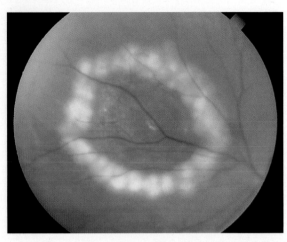

Figure 10-20. Lesion shown in Fig. 10-19 immediately after the initial session of surrounding photocoagulation.

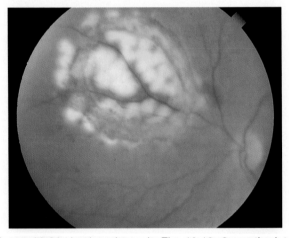

Figure 10-21. Lesion shown in Fig. 10-19, 2 months later, showing surface treatment.

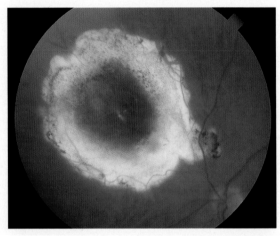

Figure 10-22. Appearance of lesion shown in Fig. 10-19, 2 years later, showing residual, central flat pigment after about six sessions of treatment. No further treatment was given and the residual pigment was unchanged after 3 additional years. Close follow-up is mandatory to detect tumor recurrence.

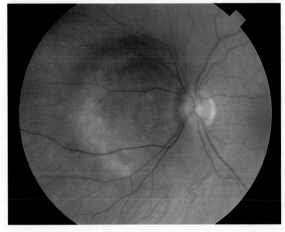

Figure 10-23. Growing choroidal melanoma nasal to the optic disc in a 48-year-old woman.

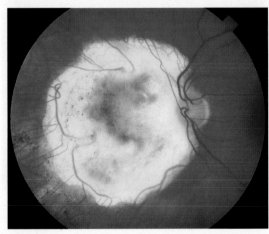

Figure 10-24. Appearance of lesion shown in Fig. 10-23, 2 years after treatment, showing good response to photocoagulation.

Choroidal Pigmented Lesions Amenable to Transpupillary Thermotherapy

Transpupillary thermotherapy is effective for small melanocytic choroidal lesions that are presumed to be melanoma and that show documented growth or risk factors for growth and metastasis. Examples are illustrated.

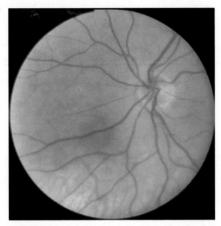

Figure 10-25. Presumed choroidal nevus located nasal to the optic disc in a 50-year-old man in 1986.

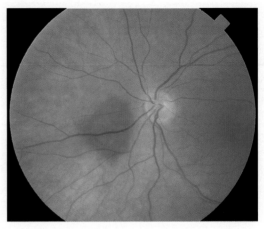

Figure 10-26. Same lesion shown in Fig. 10-25, 10 years later, revealing definite growth. If continued observation is done, the lesion eventually will reach the optic disc, making treatment more difficult and the visual prognosis worse. Such a growing tumor in this location often can be eradicated with thermotherapy without significant visual loss.

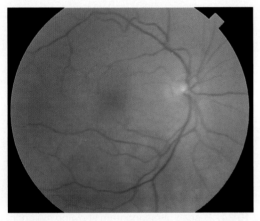

Figure 10-27. Presumed choroidal nevus inferior to the papillomacular bundle in a 60-year-old woman.

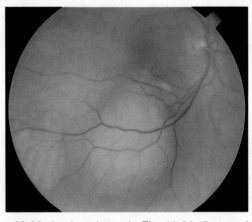

Figure 10-28. Lesion shown in Fig. 10-26, 5 years later. It has grown in diameter, and thickness has increased to 3 mm.

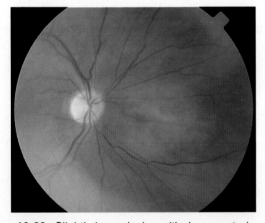

Figure 10-29. Slightly larger lesion with documented growth, located nasal to the optic disc in a 39-year-old woman.

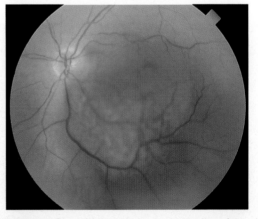

Figure 10-30. Choroidal melanoma extending from inferotemporal margin of the optic disc in a 66-year-old man. Risk factors for metastasis include thickness greater than 2 mm, tumor margin touching the optic disc, and presence of visual symptoms. The orange pigment and subretinal fluid are strong evidence that this lesion will show subsequent growth. Thermotherapy is an ideal treatment in spite of the anticipated central visual loss.

Transpupillary Thermotherapy for Choroidal Melanoma

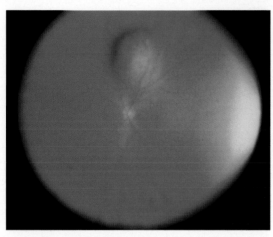

Figure 10-31. Wide-angle photograph of a melanoma superior to the optic disc in a 68-year-old man.

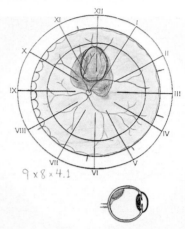

Figure 10-32. Fundus drawing of the same patient showing retinal detachment (shown in blue) extending from the tumor into the foveal region.

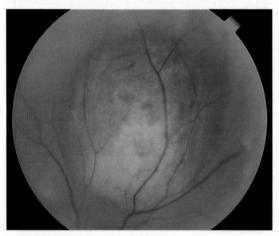

Figure 10-33. Fundus photograph of the lesion with 45-degree camera.

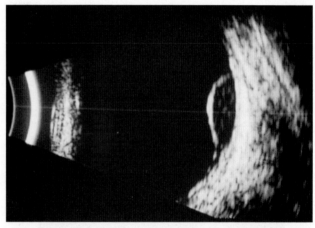

Figure 10-34. B-scan ultrasonogram showing melanoma pattern with lesion thickness of 3.9 mm prior to thermotherapy.

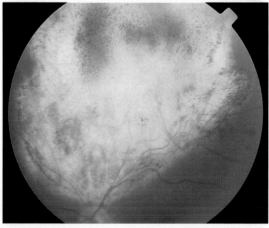

Figure 10-35. Appearance of the lesion after completion of thermotherapy showing disappearance of the tumor.

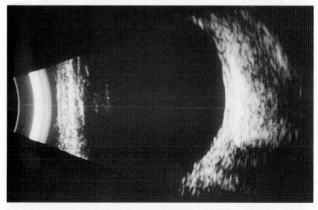

Figure 10-36. B-scan ultrasonogram after treatment showing no residual evidence of tumor. The visual acuity returned to 6/6 after treatment.

Transpupillary Thermotherapy for Choroidal Melanoma

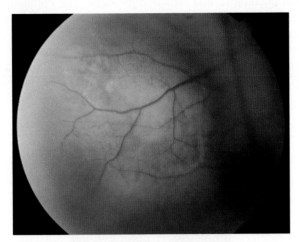

Figure 10-37. Dome-shaped choroidal melanoma temporal to the foveal area in a 33-year-old man.

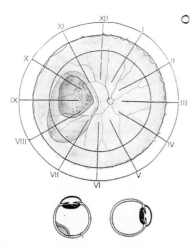

Figure 10-38. Fundus drawing of the same patient showing retinal detachment (shown in blue) extending inferiorly from the tumor.

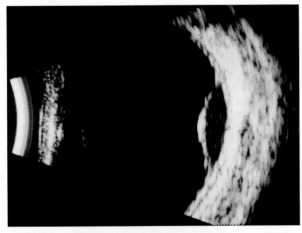

Figure 10-39. B-scan ultrasonogram showing dome-shaped mass with acoustic hollowness, characteristic of melanoma and a thickness of 3.5 mm.

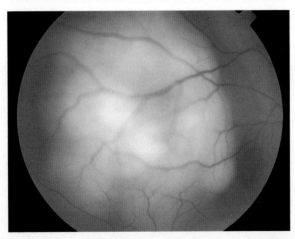

Figure 10-40. Appearance of lesion immediately after the first session of thermotherapy showing whitening of superficial portions of the tumor.

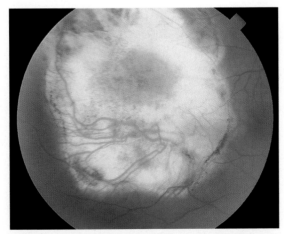

Figure 10-41. Appearance of the lesion after four sessions of thermotherapy showing complete disappearance of the tumor.

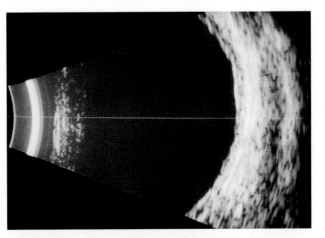

Figure 10-42. Follow-up B-scan ultrasonogram showing no evidence of residual tumor elevation.

Plaque Radiotherapy for Posterior Uveal Melanoma—Plaque Designs and Applications

Plaque radiotherapy can be difficult and requires excellent cooperation among the ophthalmic oncologist, radiation oncologist, and radiation physicist. The ophthalmic oncologist must provide the radiation oncologist with precise tumor measurements, and the radiation oncologist can custom-design the plaque to meet the specific clinical situation and make precise dosimetry calculations. The surgical technique is described in Chapter 22. Approximately 35,000 cGy are delivered to the tumor base and 8,000 cGy to the tumor apex. There are many plaque designs and sizes and only selected ones are shown here.

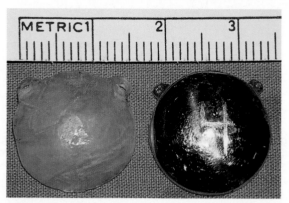

Figure 10-43. Standard, round, 15-mm, iodine-125 plaque. The dummy plaque is to the *left* and the shielded active plaque is to the *right*.

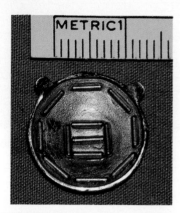

Figure 10-44. Opposite side of the active plaque showing the iodine-125 seeds. This side is directed toward the sclera at the time of plaque application.

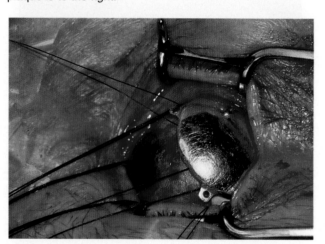

Figure 10-45. Standard round plaque being positioned at the time of surgery.

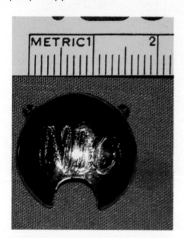

Figure 10-46. Notched plaque for treatment of juxtapapillary tumors.

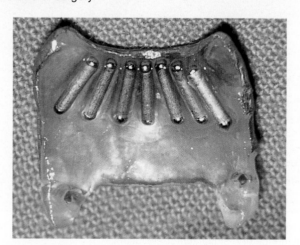

Figure 10-47. Custom-designed ciliary body plaque with lead shield.

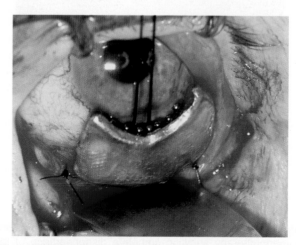

Figure 10-48. Ciliary body plaque being positioned at the time of surgery.

Choroidal Melanomas Amenable to Radiotherapy

Plaque radiotherapy and charged particle irradiation can be used to manage selected posterior uveal melanoma. Each case must be individualized, but radiotherapy often is employed for melanomas that are less than 9 mm in thickness and 18 mm in diameter and that do not invade the optic nerve. When a melanoma is greater than 18 mm in diameter or 9 mm in thickness, enucleation generally is more prudent because of the morbidity of irradiating larger tumors. Illustrated are wide-angle fundus photographs of melanomas that would be amenable to plaque radiotherapy.

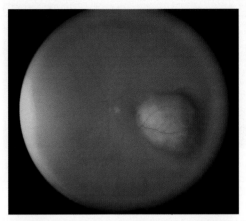

Figure 10-49. Dome-shaped melanoma temporal to the fovea measuring about 12 × 12 × 5 mm in a 66-year-old man.

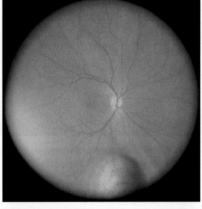

Figure 10-50. Dome-shaped melanoma near the equator inferiorly measuring about 9 × 8 × 5 mm in a 41-year-old woman.

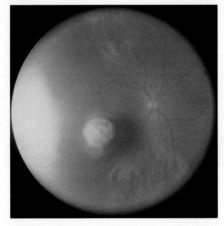

Figure 10-51. Mushroom-shaped melanoma inferotemporal to the fovea measuring about 10 × 10 × 6 mm in a 45-year-old woman.

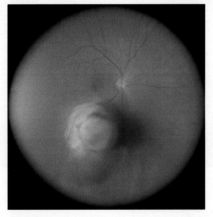

Figure 10-52. Slightly larger, mushroom-shaped melanoma inferior to the fovea measuring about 13 × 12 × 7 mm in a 31-year-old man.

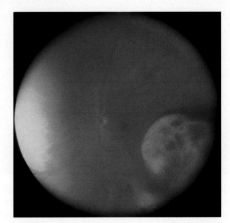

Figure 10-53. Inferotemporal ciliochoroidal melanoma measuring about 14 × 14 × 6 mm in a 53-year-old man.

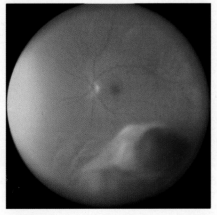

Figure 10-54. Slightly larger inferotemporal ciliochoroidal melanoma measuring about 16 × 14 × 8 mm in a 57-year-old woman.

Choroidal Melanomas Amenable to Plaque Radiotherapy Combined with Thermotherapy or Laser

Choroidal melanomas that are located near the optic nerve or fovea and are too large for thermotherapy can be managed with combined plaque and thermotherapy or laser treatment as an alternative to enucleation. Examples are cited in standard fundus photographs.

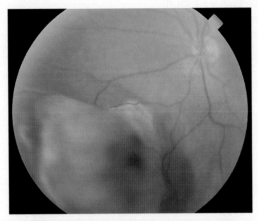

Figure 10-55. Choroidal melanoma measuring about 12 × 11 × 5 mm located inferonasal to the optic disc in a 47-year-old woman.

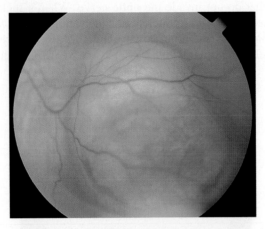

Figure 10-56. Choroidal melanoma measuring about 11 × 7 × 4 mm extending inferior to the fovea in a 68-year-old woman.

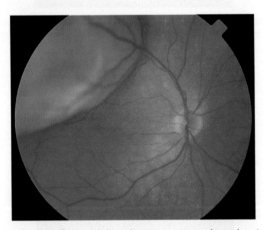

Figure 10-57. Choroidal melanoma measuring about 12 × 12 × 6 mm located superotemporal to the optic disc and fovea in a 30-year-old man.

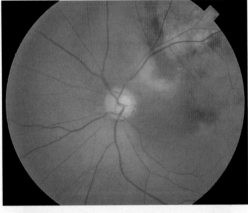

Figure 10-58. Choroidal melanoma measuring about 8 × 7 × 3 mm extending superotemporally from the optic disc in a 66-year-old woman.

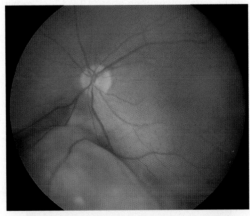

Figure 10-59. Choroidal melanoma measuring about 13 × 12 × 7 mm extending inferior from the optic disc in a 47-year-old woman.

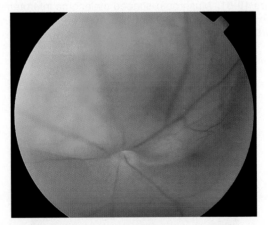

Figure 10-60. Choroidal melanoma measuring about 13 × 13 × 7 mm overhanging superior portion of the optic disc in a 59-year-old woman. This tumor probably could be controlled by plaque radiotherapy and thermotherapy, but a poor visual outcome is anticipated. Enucleation is also an appropriate option.

Plaque Radiotherapy for Choroidal Melanoma—Long-term Follow-up

Although ocular irradiation frequently is associated with radiation complications, some patients withstand the treatment remarkably well. The patient shown here had a cobalt-60 plaque in 1980 and has had excellent tumor control with no significant complications after 18 years.

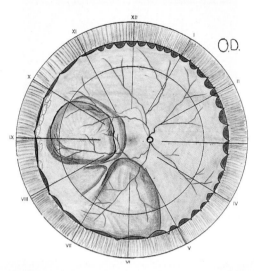

Figure 10-61. Fundus drawing showing melanoma just temporal to the foveal area with a large secondary retinal detachment in a 51-year-old man. The tumor measured 12 × 12 × 6 mm and its margin was less than 3 mm from the foveola.

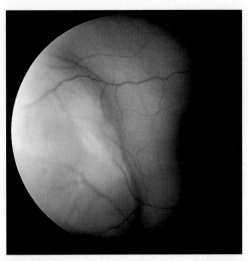

Figure 10-62. Standard photograph showing the posterior margin of the tumor.

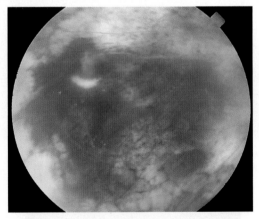

Figure 10-63. Photograph of the center of the tumor after 10 years showing complete tumor control.

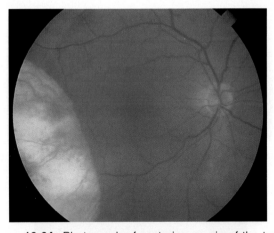

Figure 10-64. Photograph of posterior margin of the tumor after 17 years showing intact foveal region with no appreciable radiation retinopathy.

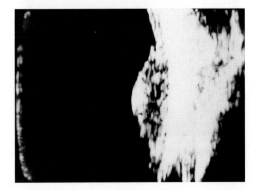

Figure 10-65. B-scan ultrasonography prior to treatment.

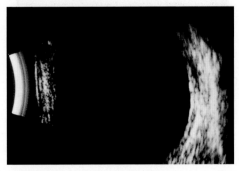

Figure 10-66. B-scan ultrasonography after 17 years showing no elevation.

Early Response of Choroidal Melanoma to Plaque Radiotherapy

Most patients treated with radiotherapy show a good initial response. However, radiation complications eventually develop in such cases.

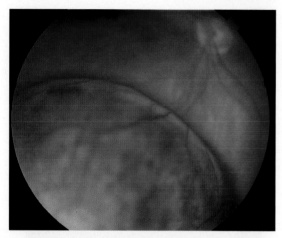

Figure 10-67. Pretreatment appearance of inferotemporal melanoma in a 35-year-old man.

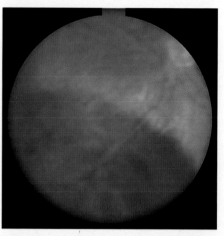

Figure 10-68. Appearance of the lesion shown in Fig. 10-67, 4 months after treatment.

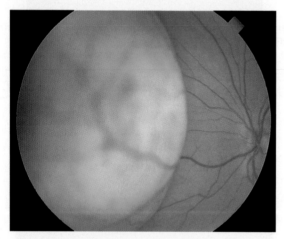

Figure 10-69. Pretreatment appearance of temporal melanoma in a 35-year-old man.

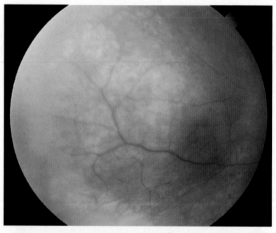

Figure 10-70. Appearance of the lesion shown in Fig. 10-69, 7 months after treatment.

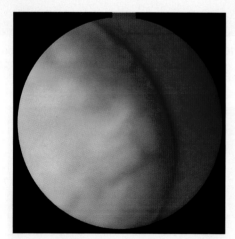

Figure 10-71. Pretreatment appearance of temporal melanoma in a 29-year-old man.

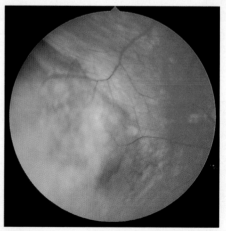

Figure 10-72. Appearance of the lesion shown in Fig. 10-71, 13 months after treatment.

Wide-angle Photography Showing Response of Choroidal Melanoma to Plaque Radiotherapy

With wide-angle photography, one can better appreciate the overall resolution of a melanoma following plaque radiotherapy.

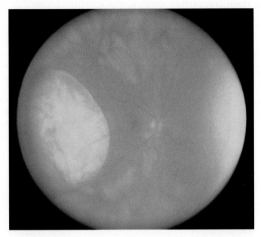

Figure 10-73. Pretreatment appearance of the melanoma shown in Fig. 10-71.

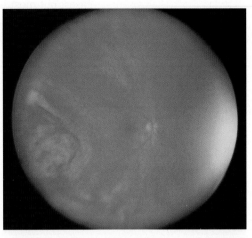

Figure 10-74. Posttreatment appearance of the melanoma shown in Fig. 10-71 after 13 months.

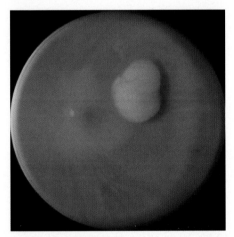

Figure 10-75. Pretreatment appearance of temporal melanoma in a 57-year-old woman.

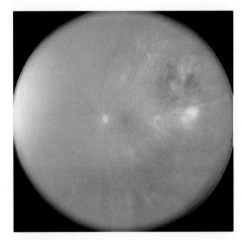

Figure 10-76. Posttreatment appearance of the melanoma shown in Fig. 10-75 after 3 years.

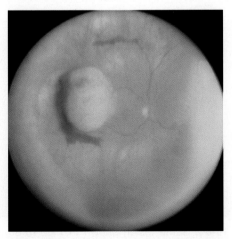

Figure 10-77. Pretreatment appearance of melanoma in a 76-year-old woman.

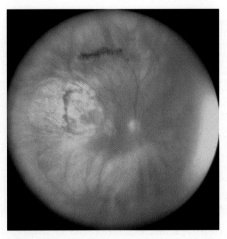

Figure 10-78. Posttreatment appearance of the melanoma shown in Figure 10-77 after 3 years.

Plaque Radiotherapy for Juxtapapillary Melanoma, Ciliary Body Melanoma, and Melanoma with Extraocular Extension

Plaque radiotherapy also can be employed to treat tumors that touch the optic disc, that arise in the ciliary body, and that extend extrasclerally. Complications such as radiation papillopathy, cataract, and scleral melting sometimes can occur in such cases, but most patients can retain their eye, often with some useful vision

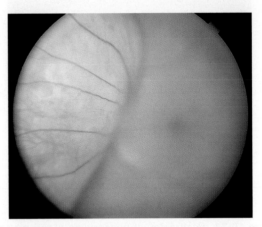

Figure 10-79. Large melanoma overhanging the optic disc on the nasal side in a 49-year-old woman.

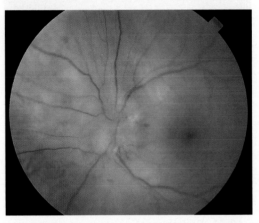

Figure 10-80. Tumor shown in Fig. 10-79 showing marked regression 6 months after notched plaque radiotherapy. Note, however, the radiation papillopathy.

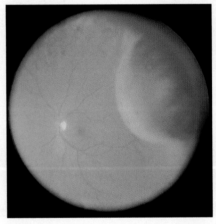

Figure 10-81. Wide-angle photograph of a ciliary body melanoma in a 58-year-old man. The tumor measured 12 mm in thickness.

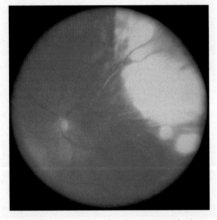

Figure 10-82. Wide-angle photograph of the same eye shown in Fig. 10-81 11 years later, showing complete tumor destruction. The patient had a cataract removed and his pseudophakic visual acuity is 6/18 (20/60).

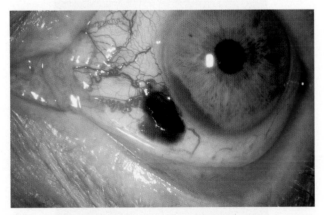

Figure 10-83. Extrascleral extension of large ciliary body melanoma. Note the iris extension. No biopsy was done and the patient was treated with an iodine-125 plaque.

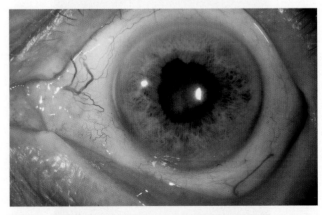

Figure 10-84. Same lesion shown in Fig. 10-83, 2 years after plaque radiotherapy, showing regression of the extraocular and iris components of the neoplasm.

Plaque Radiotherapy Combined with Laser or Thermotherapy for Juxtapapillary Choroidal Melanoma

Juxtapapillary choroidal melanoma is known to carry a small risk for recurrence following techniques of radiotherapy. To decrease the rate of recurrence, juxtapapillary melanomas can be treated with notched plaque radiotherapy combined with either laser photocoagulation or transpupillary thermotherapy (TTT). TTT is most often employed today. The first session of laser or TTT is given at the time of plaque removal, and two or three additional treatments are given at 3- to 4-month intervals.

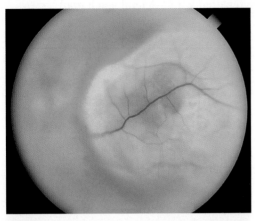

Figure 10-85. Choroidal melanoma nasal to the optic disc in a 52-year-old woman.

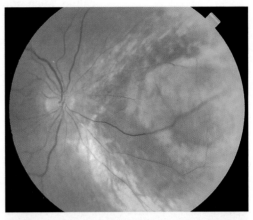

Figure 10-86. Appearance of the lesion almost 2 years after plaque and 1 year after completion of argon laser photocoagulation.

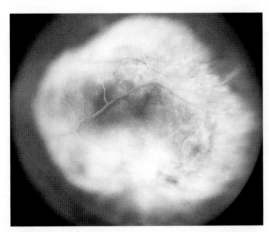

Figure 10-87. Late fluorescein angiogram of the lesion shown in Fig. 10-85 showing hyperfluorescence of the melanoma prior to treatment.

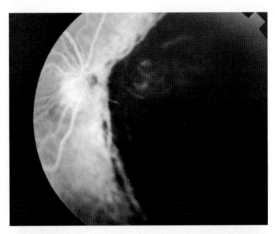

Figure 10-88. Late fluorescein angiogram of the lesion shown in Figure 10-86 demonstrating hypofluorescence of the lesion after completion of treatment.

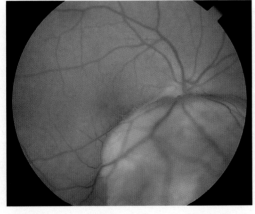

Figure 10-89. Juxtapapillary melanoma inferior to the optic disc in a 32-year-old woman.

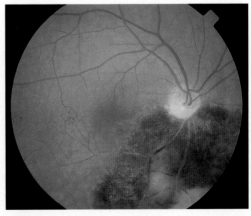

Figure 10-90. Appearance of the lesion shown in Fig. 10-89 after completion of plaque radiotherapy and transpupillary thermotherapy.

Complications of Radiotherapy for Posterior Uveal Melanoma

Most radiation complications occur between 1 and 5 years after radiotherapy. Radiation treatment of melanoma in the posterior aspect of the choroid is likely to induce clinically significant radiation maculopathy and papillopathy. Treatment of anterior choroidal and ciliary body lesions is likely to induce cataract and, rarely, melting of the overlying sclera, particularly if a rectus muscle was removed during plaque application. Such scleral melting can be repaired with a scleral patch graft.

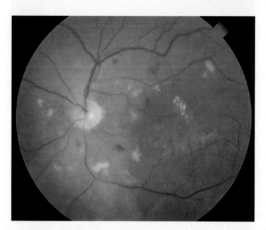

Figure 10-91. Radiation retinopathy showing nerve fiber layer infarctions and hemorrhages in the posterior pole adjacent to treated melanoma.

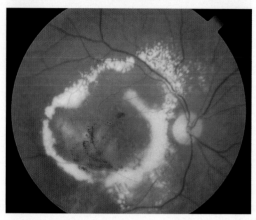

Figure 10-92. Radiation retinopathy with accumulation of yellow subretinal and intraretinal exudation surrounding the residual melanoma in the posterior pole.

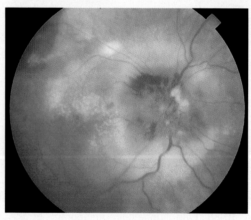

Figure 10-93. Severe radiation papillopathy following treatment of a melanoma superior to the foveal area.

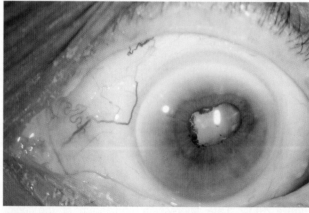

Figure 10-94. Radiation cataract and posterior synechiae secondary to anterior segment ischemic inflammation after radiotherapy.

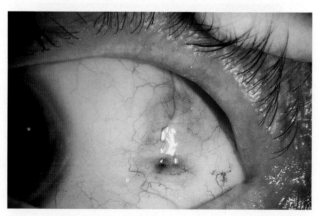

Figure 10-95. Scleral melting secondary to plaque radiotherapy of a ciliochoroidal melanoma. A scleral patch graft was performed at that time.

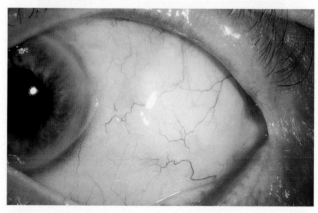

Figure 10-96. Appearance of the area shown in Fig. 10-95, 8 years after a successful scleral patch graft.

Local Resection of Ciliochoroidal Melanoma by Partial Lamellar Sclerouvectomy

Melanoma and other tumors that involve the peripheral choroid and ciliary body can be removed by PLSU. The surgery is difficult and requires experience, but the results can be gratifying. The technique of PLSU is discussed in Chapter 22. The goal of surgery is to remove the tumor intact while preserving the outer sclera, retina, and vitreous. PLSU is particularly applicable for a peripheral choroidal of ciliary body melanoma greater than 6 mm in thickness, in which case radiotherapy would necessitate a higher dose of irradiation to normal ocular structures.

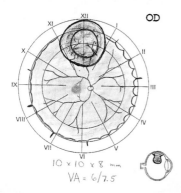

Figure 10-97. Fundus drawing of a mushroom-shaped melanoma at the equator superiorly in a 69-year-old man.

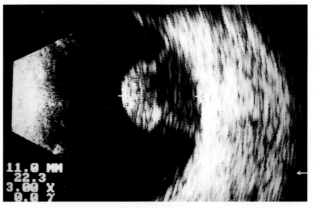

Figure 10-98. B-scan ultrasonogram of the tumor shown in Fig. 10-97 showing mushroom-shaped lesion.

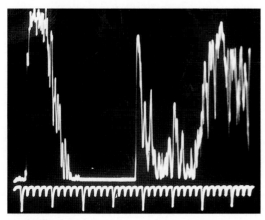

Figure 10-99. A-scan ultrasonogram of the same tumor showing characteristic melanoma pattern.

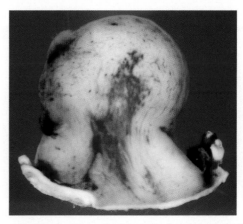

Figure 10-100. Sectioned same mushroom-shaped melanoma after removal by partial lamellar sclerouvectomy.

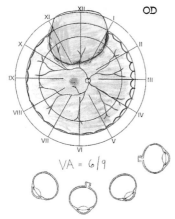

Figure 10-101. Postoperative fundus drawing showing flat retina posteriorly with normal optic disc and macular region.

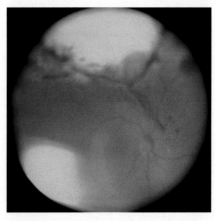

Figure 10-102. Postoperative wide-angle fundus photograph showing resected area above and the normal posterior segment. The inferior bright area is due to the transilluminator used to take the photograph.

Partial Lamellar Sclerouvectomy for a Peripheral Choroidal Melanoma with an Extensive Retinal Detachment

Extensive retinal detachment should not be considered a contraindication to PLSU. In fact, the presence of a retinal detachment may facilitate removing the tumor without damage to the sensory retina.

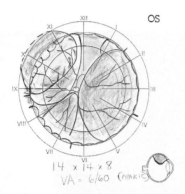

Figure 10-103. Fundus drawing of peripheral choroidal and ciliary body melanoma and retinal detachment (drawn in blue) in a 68-year-old woman.

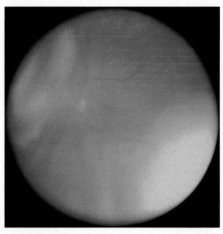

Figure 10-104. Wide-angle photograph of the lesion shown in Fig. 10-103.

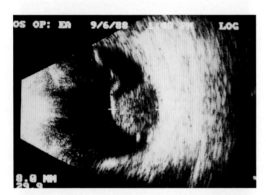

Figure 10-105. B-scan ultrasonogram showing melanoma with extensive retinal detachment.

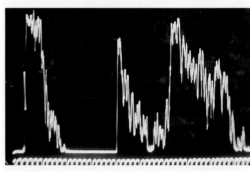

Figure 10-106. A-scan ultrasonogram showing typical melanoma pattern.

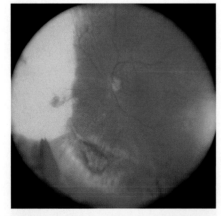

Figure 10-107. Wide-angle photograph after resection of tumor showing resected area (superonasally) and normal disc and macular area. The retinal detachment is gone.

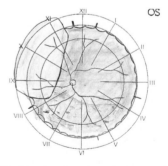

Figure 10-108. Fundus drawing after resection of the tumor.

Results of Partial Lamellar Sclerouvectomy for Posterior Uveal Melanomas

Although PLSU has potential complications such as vitreous hemorrhage, retinal detachment, and cataract, it usually provides gratifying results and avoids enucleation and radiotherapy.

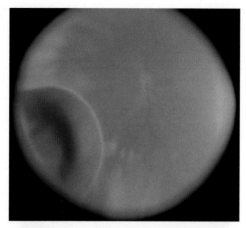

Figure 10-109. Wide-angle photograph of inferotemporal ciliochoroidal melanoma in a 59-year-old woman.

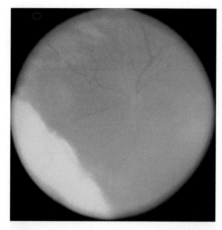

Figure 10-110. Appearance of the same eye shown in Fig. 10-109 after partial lamellar sclerouvectomy showing resection site and flat retina.

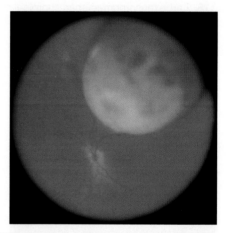

Figure 10-111. Wide-angle photograph of superotemporal choroidal melanoma in a 26-year-old woman who declined enucleation.

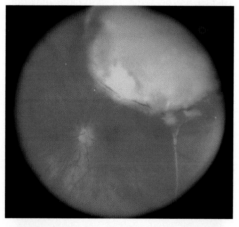

Figure 10-112. Appearance of the eye shown in Fig. 10-111, after partial lamellar sclerouvectomy, showing resection site and flat retina.

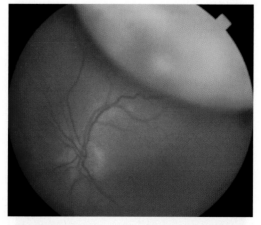

Figure 10-113. Standard 45-degree photograph of the same lesion shown in Fig. 10-111 showing proximity of the tumor to the fovea.

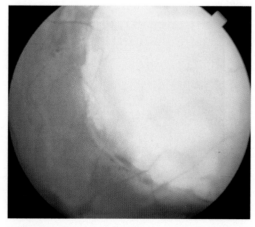

Figure 10-114. Postoperative photograph of the same area shown in Fig. 10-113. Note the clear margins of the resected area.

Large Choroidal Melanomas Managed by Enucleation

There are no firm rules regarding when enucleation should be used for choroidal melanoma. The entire clinical situation must be taken into account. In general, tumors greater than 16 mm in diameter and 10 mm in thickness are best managed by enucleation because of the morbidity of treating such large tumors with radiotherapy or PLSU. However, in older patients whose melanoma is located in their better eye, enucleation may be deferred and irradiation employed. The following wide-angle photographs depict examples in which enucleation probably is justified.

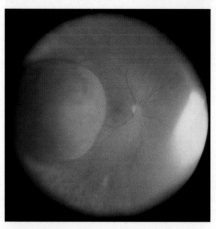

Figure 10-115. Large temporal choroidal melanoma measuring about 18 × 17 × 10 mm in a 40-year-old woman.

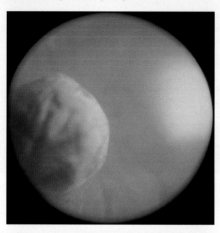

Figure 10-116. Large mushroom-shaped choroidal melanoma measuring about 20 × 19 × 12 mm in a 35-year-old man.

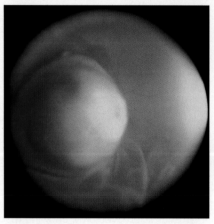

Figure 10-117. Large nasal melanoma measuring about 19 × 19 × 12 mm with a secondary total retinal detachment in a 58-year-old woman.

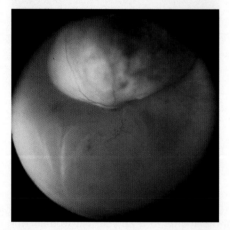

Figure 10-118. Large superior melanoma measuring about 19 × 17 × 11 mm with a secondary total retinal detachment in a 72-year-old man.

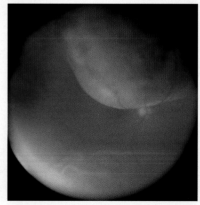

Figure 10-119. Large superior melanoma measuring about 20 × 19 × 13 mm with a secondary total retinal detachment in a 45-year-old man.

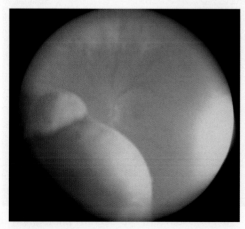

Figure 10-120. Large bilobed ciliochoroidal melanoma measuring about 22 × 18 × 12 mm in a 23-year-old woman.

Medium-sized and Small Choroidal Melanomas Managed by Enucleation

Some small and medium-sized melanomas often are managed best by enucleation. This is true when they occur in young people with a poor visual prognosis, when they invade the optic nerve, or when they assume a diffuse growth pattern.

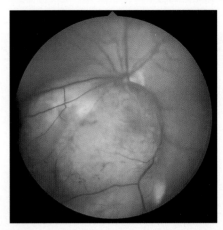

Figure 10-121. Choroidal melanoma in the macular area and overhanging optic disc in a 34-year-old woman. The patient could be treated with plaque radiotherapy, but the tumor location and her young age favor enucleation.

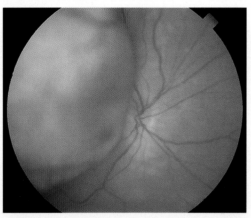

Figure 10-122. Choroidal melanoma in the macular area in a 14-year-old girl. Once again, the tumor location and the young age of the patient are factors that favor enucleation.

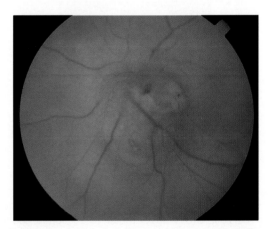

Figure 10-123. Small choroidal melanoma with optic nerve invasion.

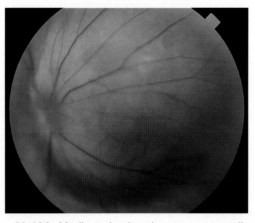

Figure 10-124. Medium-sized melanoma surrounding and invading the optic nerve.

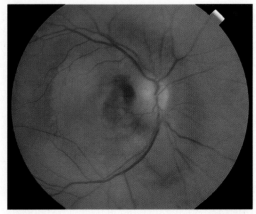

Figure 10-125. Small circumpapillary diffuse choroidal melanoma.

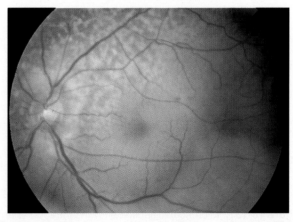

Figure 10-126. Larger circumpapillary, subfoveal diffuse melanoma. Tumor occupied the entire superior fundus.

Management of Choroidal Melanoma by Modified Enucleation Using Lateral Orbitotomy Approach

Occasionally a small choroidal melanoma exhibits circumscribed orbital extension. In such cases, orbital exenteration is controversial and the entire tumor sometimes can be removed intact using a lateral orbitotomy approach. An enucleation orbital implant and prosthesis then can be employed.

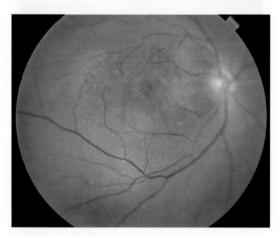

Figure 10-127. Small macular melanoma with orange pigment on the surface.

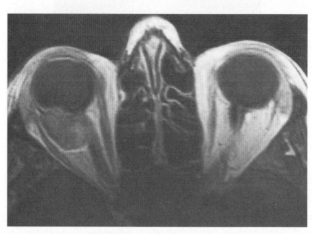

Figure 10-128. Magnetic resonance imaging of orbits showing circumscribed orbital tumor behind the globe.

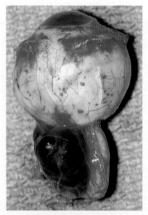

Figure 10-129. Gross appearance of the specimen following removal by a lateral canthotomy approach. Note the intact black tumor in the orbit and the long section of optic nerve.

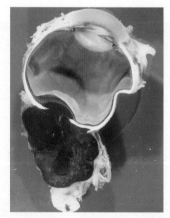

Figure 10-130. Gross appearance of sectioned specimen demonstrating intraocular and orbital components of the tumor.

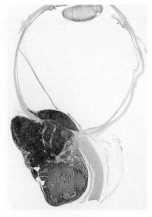

Figure 10-131. Microscopic section showing intraocular and orbital components of the tumor. It proved to be a mixed cell–type melanoma.

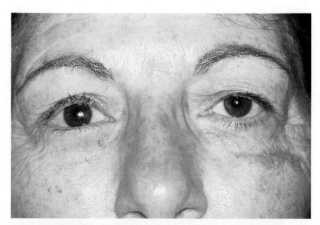

Figure 10-132. Appearance of the patient 6 years after enucleation, hydroxyapatite implant, and peg placement. She is healthy without evidence of metastasis.

Orbital Exenteration for Uveal Melanoma with Massive Orbital Extension

Orbital exenteration generally is considered the treatment of choice for melanoma with massive transcleral extension into the orbital soft tissues. The technique is illustrated in Chapter 22.

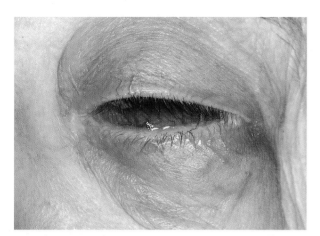

Figure 10-133. Appearance of the left ocular region in a 62-year-old woman showing proptosis and eyelid swelling.

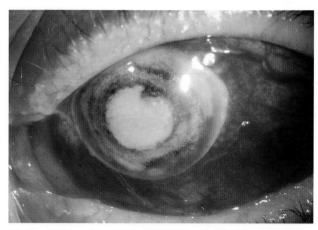

Figure 10-134. Closer view of the left eye showing epibulbar injection, flat anterior chamber, iris atrophy, and cataract.

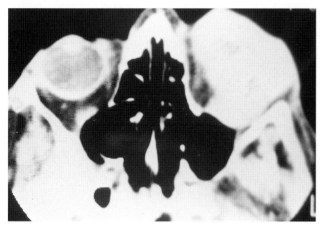

Figure 10-135. Axial computed tomogram of orbit showing globe and orbit filled by a mass.

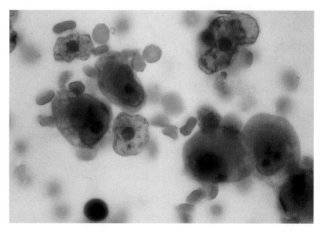

Figure 10-136. Cytology of fine-needle aspiration biopsy performed through the inferior conjunctival fornix showing epithelioid melanoma cells (Papanicolaou, original magnification × 300).

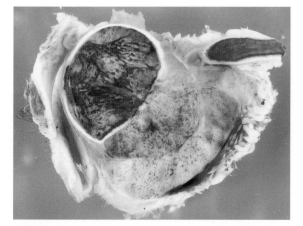

Figure 10-137. Sectioned exenteration specimen showing melanoma filling the globe and orbit, and infiltrating the optic nerve. The optic nerve was subsequently resected to the chiasm and there was no residual tumor.

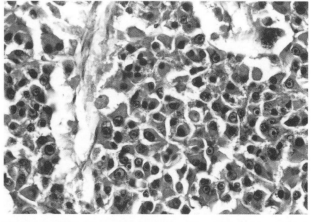

Figure 10-138. Histopathology showing epithelioid cell–type melanoma (hematoxylin–eosin, original magnification × 250). The patient did not develop metastatic disease but died 5 years later of another cause.

CHAPTER 11

Nonneoplastic Conditions That Can Simulate Posterior Uveal Melanoma

NONNEOPLASTIC CONDITIONS THAT CAN SIMULATE POSTERIOR UVEAL MELANOMA

A number of conditions can clinically simulate posterior uveal melanoma (1–6). Other tumors that can resemble melanoma are discussed in detail in their respective chapters. This section covers a few selected nonneoplastic simulating conditions that are not discussed elsewhere in this textbook. These include bilateral diffuse uveal melanocytic proliferation (BDUMP), inflammatory conditions, hemorrhagic lesions, and a variety of other conditions

BDUMP is a peculiar paraneoplastic syndrome that occurs in patients with systemic malignancy, particularly ovarian cancer, small-cell carcinoma of the lung, and several other neoplasms (1,2). Both eyes usually develop a diffuse irregular thickening of the uveal tract with multiple pigmented lesions of variable size, throughout the choroid, and sometimes the ciliary body and iris. There is disruption of the retinal pigment epithelium and a typical mottling seen clinically and with fluorescein angiography, sometimes called a "giraffe-like" fundus. The affected eye usually has signs of low-grade inflammation and rapid onset and progression of cataract. The pathogenesis is unknown, and treatment with corticosteroids and irradiation does not appear to be helpful.

Inflammatory conditions such as nodular posterior scleritis, tuberculosis, sarcoidosis, and idiopathic choroidal granuloma can cause a choroidal or ciliary body granuloma that may simulate an amelanotic melanoma. Hemorrhagic conditions can appear as a dark mass that can resemble a pigmented melanoma. Age-related macular and extramacular degeneration and bleeding retinal macroaneurysm are hemorrhagic conditions that may be very similar to melanoma ophthalmoscopically. Finally, a number of degenerative and miscellaneous conditions can closely resemble posterior uveal melanoma (4–6). Selected examples are cited.

SELECTED REFERENCES

1. Shields JA, Shields CL. *Intraocular tumors. A text and atlas.* Philadelphia: WB Saunders, 1992:137–153.
2. Gass JDM, Gieser RG, Wilkinson CP, Beahm DE, Pautler SE. Bilateral diffuse uveal melanocytic proliferation in patients with occult carcinoma. *Arch Ophthalmol* 1990;108:527–533.
3. Shields JA, Shields CL. *Intraocular tumors. A text and atlas.* Philadelphia: WB Saunders, 1992:50–52.
4. Shields JA, Zimmerman LE. Lesions simulating malignant melanomas of the posterior uvea. *Arch Ophthalmol* 1973;89:466–471.
5. Shields JA, Augsburger JJ, Brown GC, Stephens RF. The differential diagnosis of posterior uveal melanoma. *Ophthalmology* 1980;87:543–548.
6. Benson WE, Shields JA, Tasman WS, Crandall AS. Posterior scleritis. *Arch Ophthalmol* 1979;97:1482–1486.

Bilateral Diffuse Uveal Melanocytic Proliferation

BDUMP can affect the entire uveal tract with typical amelanotic diffuse uveal thickening with more elevated foci that are more deeply pigmented. Depicted is a case of BDUMP in a 66-year-old woman with ovarian cancer.

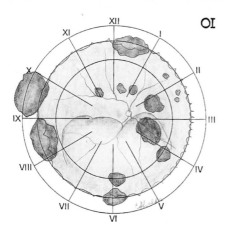

Figure 11-1. Fundus drawing of the right eye showing numerous pigmented nodules and an inferior retinal detachment.

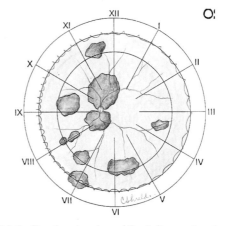

Figure 11-2. Fundus drawing of the left eye showing numerous pigmented nodules and no retinal detachment.

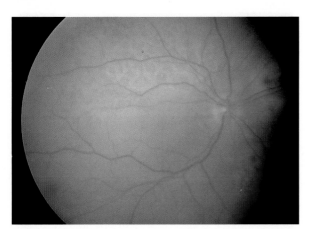

Figure 11-3. Macular area of the right eye showing retinal detachment and minimal retinal pigment epithelial alterations.

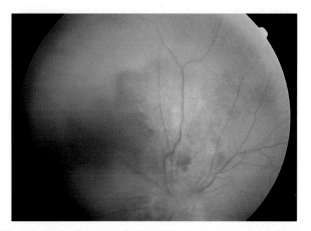

Figure 11-4. Fundus photograph of area superior to the optic disc in the left eye showing typical diffuse uveal pigmentation.

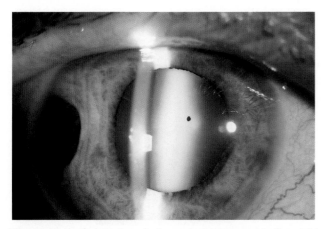

Figure 11-5. Cataract and pigmented iris tumor in the right eye of the same patient.

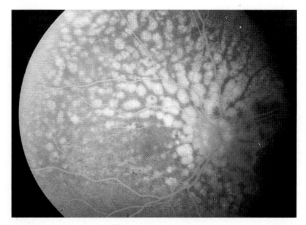

Figure 11-6. Late fluorescein angiogram of the right eye showing typical mottled hyperfluorescence that characterizes bilateral diffuse uveal melanocytic proliferation.

Bilateral Diffuse Uveal Melanocytic Proliferation—Clinical Variations

In addition to the ocular pigmentation, affected patients can develop cutaneous and mucous membrane pigmentation in nonocular areas.

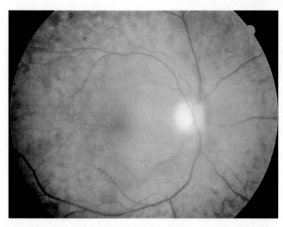

Figure 11-7. Posterior pole of the right eye of a 62-year-old African-American patient with widespread metastasis of "undifferentiated carcinoma." The patient also had recently acquired pigmentation of conjunctiva, buccal mucosa, and hard palate. (Courtesy of Dr. Howard Schatz).

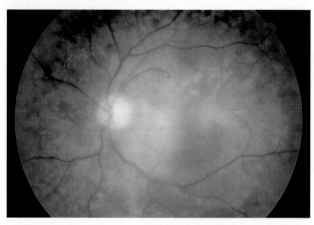

Figure 11-8. Posterior pole of the left eye of the patient shown in Fig. 11-7 showing similar mottled appearance of the macular region and several more deeply pigmented choroidal lesions. (Courtesy of Dr. Howard Schatz.)

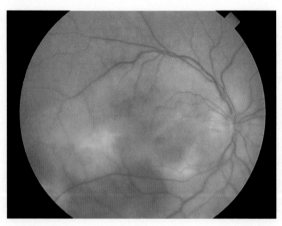

Figure 11-9. Posterior pole of the right eye of a 60-year-old patient with bilateral diffuse uveal melanocytic proliferation associated with metastatic renal-cell carcinoma. Note the irregular area of choroidal pigmentation.

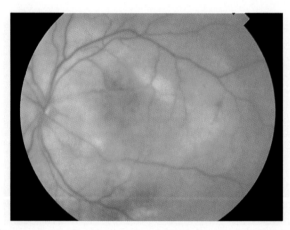

Figure 11-10. Posterior pole of the left eye of the patient shown in Fig. 11-9 showing similar findings.

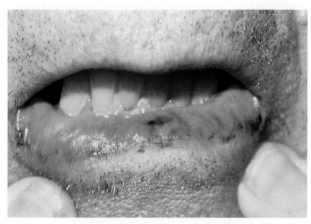

Figure 11-11. Acquired pigmentation of the lip in the patient with bilateral diffuse uveal melanocytic proliferation. (Courtesy of Dr. J. Donald M. Gass.)

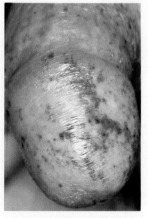

Figure 11-12. Acquired pigmentation of the penis in the patient shown in Fig. 11-10. (Courtesy of Dr. J. Donald M. Gass.)

Nodular Posterior Scleritis Simulating Choroidal Melanoma

Nodular posterior scleritis can manifest as a mass that appears to be within the choroid. Hence, it can closely simulate an intraocular tumor, particularly an amelanotic choroidal melanoma. A case example is shown.

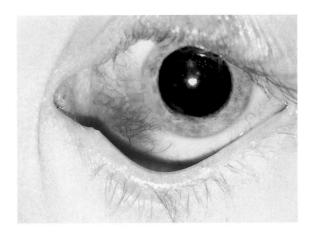

Figure 11-13. Epibulbar injection inferonasally in a 30-year-old woman.

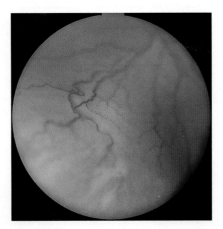

Figure 11-14. Standard fundus photograph of the eye shown in Fig. 11-13 showing inferonasal amelanotic mass.

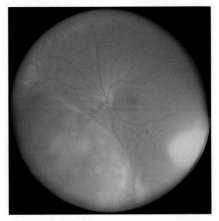

Figure 11-15. Wide-angle photograph showing the full extent of the inferonasal lesion.

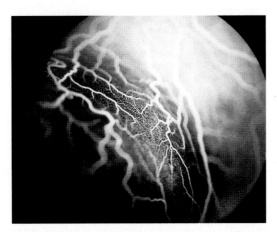

Figure 11-16. Fluorescein angiogram in venous filling phase showing hypofluorescence of the mass. There was mild late hyperfluorescence.

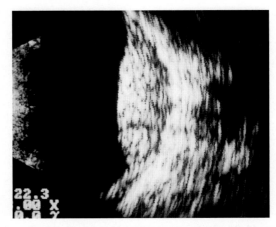

Figure 11-17. B-scan ultrasonogram showing mass with high internal reflectivity secondary to choroidal thickening.

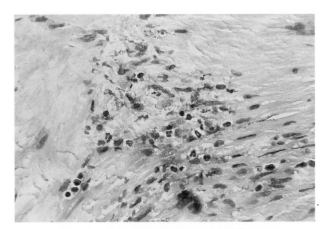

Figure 11-18. Histopathology of scleral biopsy in the same patient showing chronic inflammatory cells within scleral collagen (hematoxylin–eosin, original magnification ×100).

Choroidal Granuloma Simulating Choroidal Melanoma

Granulomatous inflammation of the choroid can manifest as a localized mass that sometimes can be confused clinically with a nonpigmented melanoma. Many cases prove to be "idiopathic" but sometimes a specific etiology such as sarcoidosis or tuberculosis can be proven.

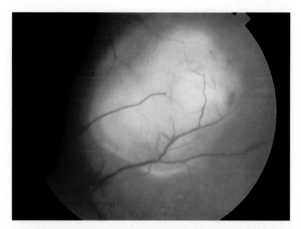

Figure 11-19. Large presumed granuloma in a 30-year-old man. Systemic evaluation failed to reveal a specific etiology.

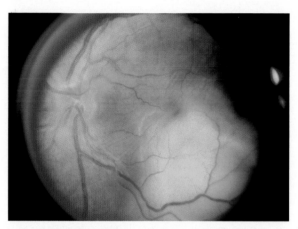

Figure 11-20. Sarcoidosis. Posterior choroidal granuloma secondary to sarcoidosis.

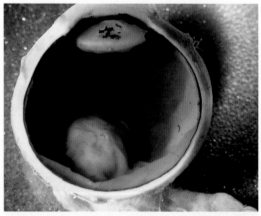

Figure 11-21. Tuberculosis. Posterior choroidal mass in a 34-year-old man. The eye was enucleated elsewhere because of suspected melanoma. (Courtesy of Dr. Robert Peiffer.)

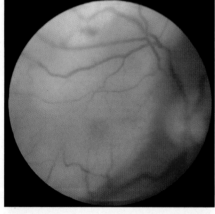

Figure 11-22. Tuberculosis. Gross appearance of enucleated eye showing posterior ocular mass. Histopathologically, it proved to be a localized granuloma containing acid-fast bacilli. (Courtesy of Dr. Robert Peiffer.)

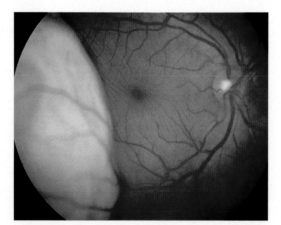

Figure 11-23. Tuberculosis. Amelanotic choroidal mass temporal to the foveal area. Although a neoplasm was considered, systemic evaluation disclosed tuberculosis. (Courtesy of Dr. A. Verbeek.)

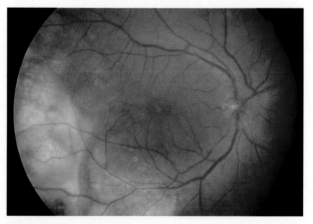

Figure 11-24. Appearance of the lesion shown in Fig. 11-23 after tuberculosis therapy showing excellent resolution of the lesion. (Courtesy of Dr. A. Verbeek.)

Hemorrhagic Lesions Simulating Choroidal Melanoma

Hemorrhagic lesions can closely resemble a pigmented melanoma. However, fresh blood is generally smooth and homogeneous and is hypofluorescent with angiography; resolving blood has a variegated appearance with yellow areas of resolving blood, findings not generally seen with melanoma. Furthermore, blood generally resolves with time. In a practice of ocular oncology, it is common to see a patient with a hemorrhagic macular or extramacular disciform process that was initially diagnosed as a choroidal melanoma. Limited choroidal hemorrhage can occur after cataract surgery, and localized hemorrhage can occur secondary to intraretinal macroaneurysm.

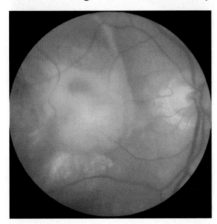

Figure 11-25. Hemorrhagic disciform lesion simulating melanoma as part of age-related macular degeneration in an 80-year-old man.

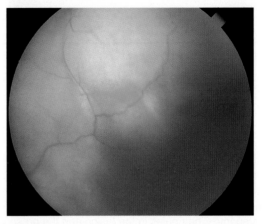

Figure 11-26. Peripheral hemorrhagic disciform lesion as part of age-related extramacular degeneration ("peripheral disciform lesion") in a 76-year-old man.

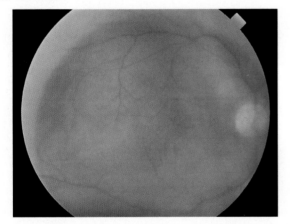

Figure 11-27. Limited choroidal hemorrhage following cataract surgery. This lesion frequently is misdiagnosed as melanoma, but it generally disappears in a few weeks.

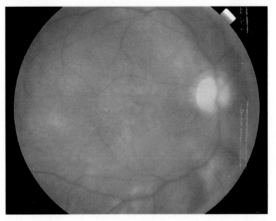

Figure 11-28. Same area depicted in Fig. 11-27 a few months later showing resolution of the choroidal blood.

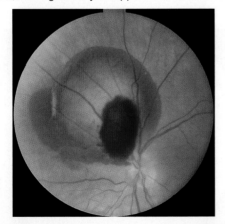

Figure 11-29. Subretinal and preretinal hemorrhage probably secondary to intraretinal arterial macroaneurysm in a 60-year-old woman. The patient was referred with the diagnosis of mushroom-shaped melanoma.

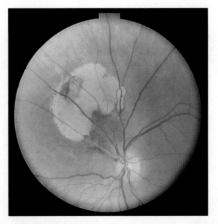

Figure 11-30. Same lesion shown in Fig. 11-29 after 3 months showing resolution of the hemorrhage. The macroaneurysm also had resolved.

Miscellaneous Conditions That Can Simulate Posterior Uveal Melanoma

Other conditions that can simulate melanoma include rhegmatogenous retinal detachment, choroidal detachment, uveal effusion syndrome, and vortex vein varix (1–5). Uveal effusion syndrome occurs unilaterally or bilaterally as combined choroidal and retinal detachment of uncertain origin. Vortex vein varix is a dilation of the ampulla of a vortex vein. Fluorescein and indocyanine green angiography can confirm that the lesion is a dilated blood vessel.

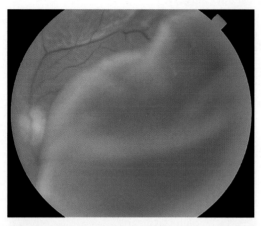

Figure 11-31. Rhegmatogenous retinal detachment simulating melanoma. The ripples in the lesion and the presence of a retinal hole should differentiate this condition from melanoma.

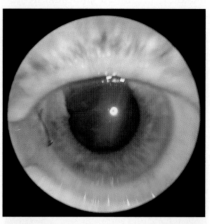

Figure 11-32. Ciliochoroidal detachment after cataract surgery simulating a ciliochoroidal melanoma. In contrast to melanoma, this lesion readily transmits light with transillumination techniques.

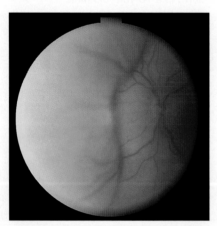

Figure 11-33. Peripheral choroidal detachment as part of the idiopathic uveal effusion syndrome in a 69-year-old man. The patient also had a nonrhegmatogenous retinal detachment extending posteriorly.

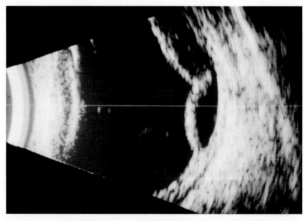

Figure 11-34. B-scan ultrasonogram of idiopathic uveal effusion syndrome showing typical choroidal detachment.

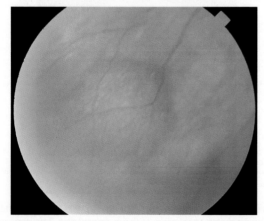

Figure 11-35. Vortex vein varix simulating melanoma located at the equator inferotemporally in a 65-year-old woman.

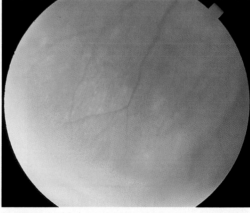

Figure 11-36. Same area shown in Fig. 11-35 with movement of eyes in a different direction. Note that the varix has flattened.

Miscellaneous Conditions That Can Simulate Posterior Uveal Melanoma

The benign conditions shown below all prompted referral because of suspected melanoma.

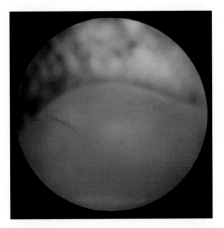

Figure 11-37. Bullous retinoschisis simulating choroidal melanoma. In contrast to melanoma, the normal choroidal vascular pattern can be seen through the lesion. Pigment clumping around the outer layer holes can cause further confusion with melanoma.

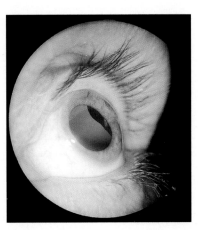

Figure 11-38. Postcataract extraction ciliary body cyst simulating melanoma.

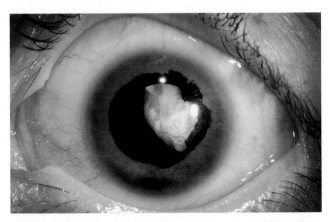

Figure 11-39. Subluxated mature cataract resembling ciliary body melanoma.

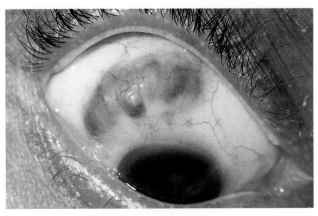

Figure 11-40. Scleral staphyloma simulating ciliary body melanoma with extraocular extension.

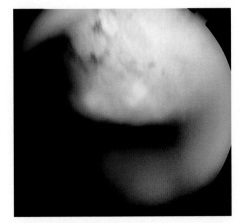

Figure 11-41. Scleral buckle from retinal detachment surgery initially diagnosed as a choroidal melanoma.

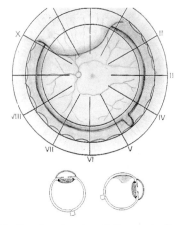

Figure 11-42. Fundus drawing of the case shown in Fig. 11-41 showing elevated scleral buckle superiorly and encircling band.

CHAPTER 12

Metastatic Tumors to the Uvea, Retina, and Optic Disc

METASTATIC TUMORS TO THE INTRAOCULAR STRUCTURES

Metastatic cancer probably represents the most common form of intraocular malignancy. However, in a practice of ocular oncology it is not encountered as frequently as uveal melanoma, possibly because many affected patients have advanced systemic cancer and do not come to the attention of an ophthalmologist. Metastatic cancer reaches the intraocular structures through hematogenous routes and most commonly develops in the uveal tract, with more than 90% involving the posterior aspect of the choroid and less than 10% arising in the iris and/or ciliary body (1–4). Metastasis to the retina, optic disc, and vitreous are relatively uncommon.

Most intraocular metastases are carcinomas, with sarcomas and melanomas being less common primary malignancies. The majority of uveal metastases originate from breast cancer in women and lung cancer in men. Less often, the primary malignancy arises from carcinoma of the alimentary tract, kidney, thyroid gland, pancreas, prostate, and other organs. Cutaneous melanoma and bronchial carcinoid tumors occasionally metastasize to the uveal tract and have distinctive features. Of patients who present to the ophthalmologist with uveal metastasis, about 25% have no known history of systemic cancer. After subsequent systemic evaluation, about 10% have no detectable primary (i.e., occult) cancer. Hence, the clinician should be familiar with the clinical manifestations of intraocular metastatic disease.

The clinical features of an intraocular metastasis vary with the location of the tumor (1–8). Iris metastasis appears as one or more yellow, white, or pink nodules in the iris stroma. It tends to be a friable tumor that can seed cells into the aqueous, producing a clinical picture of intraocular inflammation. A ciliary body metastasis is often more difficult to detect clinically. It can appear as a solitary mass or it can produce inflammatory signs, simulating an iridocyclitis. Choroidal metastasis usually appears as one or more yellow-colored lesions. It has a tendency to affect the posterior choroid, frequently in the macular area. In contrast to iris and ciliary body metastasis, choroidal metastasis tends not to produce inflammatory signs but usually causes a secondary serous retinal detachment. Although choroidal metastasis usually has a yellow color, metastasis from melanoma often has a gray or brown color, and metastasis from carcinoid tumor, thyroid cancer, and renal cell carcinoma often has an orange color. Retinal metastasis can simulate an occlusive vasculitis and can seed into the vitreous. Optic disc metastasis can occur by contiguous spread from juxtapapillary choroidal metastasis or it can involve only the optic nerve where it produces a unilateral elevation of the optic disc. Secondary glaucoma frequently occurs, particularly with iris and ciliary body tumors.

The diagnosis of intraocular metastasis generally is made by taking a history of prior cancers and by careful slit lamp biomicroscopy and ophthalmoscopy. Ancillary studies such as fluorescein angiography and ultrasonography can be of assistance in diagnosis. Fluorescein angiography of a choroidal metastasis generally shows beginning hyperfluorescence of the mass in the late venous phase, usually later than with choroidal hemangioma or melanoma. With ultrasonography it shows high internal reflectivity with A-scan and acoustic solidity with B-scan, a pattern similar to that seen with choroidal hemangioma. In difficult cases that cannot be diagnosed with the aforementioned methods, fine-needle aspiration with cytologic evaluation of the aspirate can be used to establish the diagnosis (9).

Management options for uveal metastasis vary with the clinical situation. Small asymptomatic tumors or those that have responded to prior or concurrent chemotherapy may require no immediate treatment and can be followed periodically. Larger symptomatic tumors may require external beam irradiation or plaque radiotherapy. The systemic prognosis varies with the type of tumor. Patients with choroidal metastasis from breast cancer often have a more favorable prognosis, whereas those from lung cancer or melanoma have a worse prognosis. Patients with metastasis from carcinoid tumor often have a much better prognosis.

SELECTED REFERENCES

1. Ferry AP, Font RL. Carcinoma metastatic to the eye and orbit. I. Clinicopathologic study of 227 cases. *Arch Ophthalmol* 1975;92:276–286.
2. Shields JA, Shields CL. *Intraocular tumors. A text and atlas.* Philadelphia: WB Saunders, 1992:207–238.
3. Shields CL, Shields JA, Gross N, Schwartz G, Lally S. Survey of 520 uveal metastases. *Ophthalmology* 1997; 104:1265–1276.
4. Shields JA, Shields CL, Kiratli H, De Potter P. Metastatic tumors to the iris in 40 patients. *Am J Ophthalmol* 1995;119:422–430.
5. Mewes L, Young SE. Breast carcinoma metastatic to the choroid: analysis of 67 patients. *Ophthalmology* 1982;89:147–151.
6. Gallie BL, Graham JE, Hunter WS. Optic nerve head metastasis. *Arch Ophthalmol* 1975;19;983–987.
7. Robertson DM, Wilkinson CP, Murray JL, et al. Metastatic tumor to the retina and vitreous cavity from primary melanoma of the skin: treatment with systemic and subconjunctival chemotherapy. *Ophthalmology* 1981;88:1296–1301.
8. Gunduz K, Shields JA, Shields CL, Eagle RC Jr. Cutaneous melanoma metastatic to the vitreous cavity. *Ophthalmology* 1998;105:600–605.
9. Shields JA, Shields CL, Ehya H, Eagle RC Jr, De Potter P. Fine needle aspiration biopsy of suspected intraocular tumors. The 1992 Urwick Lecture. *Ophthalmology* 1993;100:1677–1684.

Iris Metastasis

Iris metastasis appears clinically as one or more nodules in the iris stroma. Unlike choroidal metastasis, it is often a friable lesion that tends to seed tumor cells into the surrounding area, leading to a picture of intraocular inflammation. The tumor cells can settle inferiorly, causing a "pseudohypopyon," or the tumor can bleed, leading to a hyphema. Most iris metastases, particularly those from breast, lung, and gastrointestinal primary sites, have a creamy-yellow to white color and commonly show blood vessels and hemorrhage.

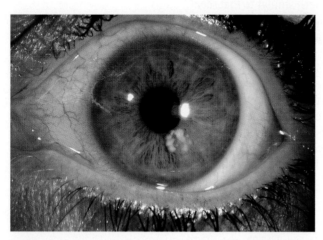

Figure 12-1. Small irregular iris metastasis from breast carcinoma.

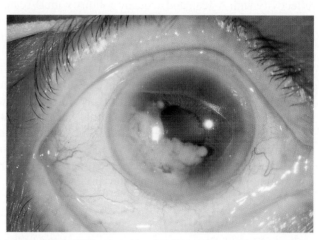

Figure 12-2. Diffuse multinodular iris metastasis from breast carcinoma.

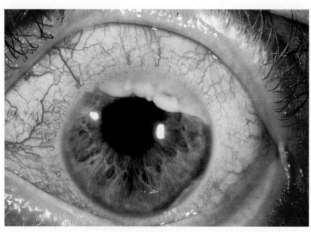

Figure 12-3. Superior diffuse iris metastasis from breast carcinoma.

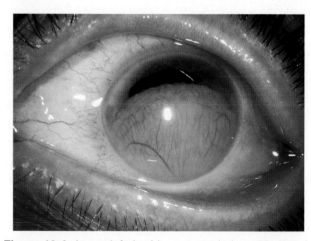

Figure 12-4. Large inferior iris metastasis in a 60-year-old woman with breast carcinoma.

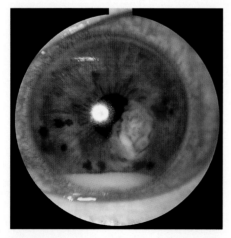

Figure 12-5. Nodular metastasis from stomach cancer with a pseudohypopyon secondary to seeding from the main tumor.

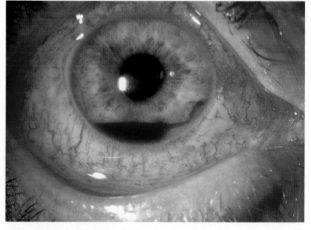

Figure 12-6. Iris metastasis from lung cancer with bleeding and secondary hyphema.

Iris metastasis can take several clinical variations and some forms of iris metastasis have a rather typical color. Metastatic carcinoid tumor may be orange, and metastatic melanoma may be brown to black. Fine-needle aspiration biopsy can be helpful in establishing the diagnosis in difficult cases. Iris metastasis generally is responsive to chemotherapy or radiotherapy.

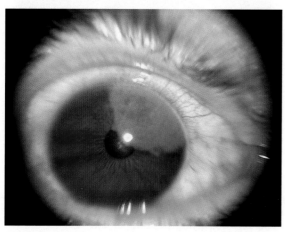

Figure 12-7. Metastatic bronchial carcinoid tumor to the iris showing the characteristic fleshy pink–orange color.

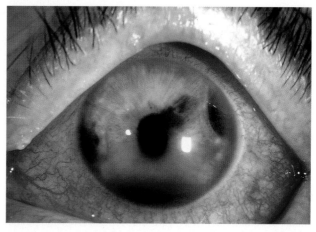

Figure 12-8. Metastatic cutaneous melanoma to the iris. Note that there is a pigmented lesion in the iris both nasally and temporally. Note also the secondary hyphema admixed with loosely cohesive melanoma cells.

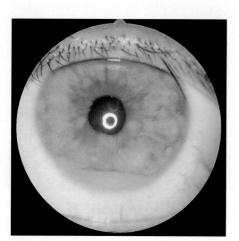

Figure 12-9. Iris metastasis from Ewing's sarcoma of the femur in a 19-year-old woman. Note that the friable tumor has assumed a "pseudohypopyon" appearance.

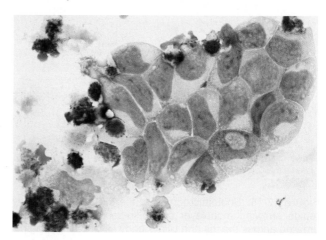

Figure 12-10. Preparation of fine-needle aspiration biopsy specimen from the lesion shown in Fig. 12-9 showing malignant cells (original magnification × 1,000).

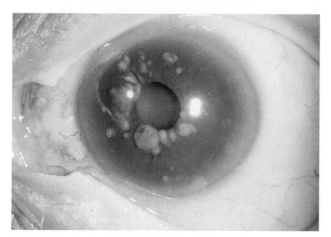

Figure 12-11. Multiple iris metastases from small-cell carcinoma of the lung in a 78-year-old woman.

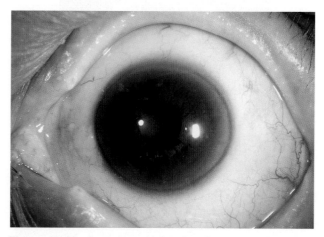

Figure 12-12. Same eye depicted in Fig. 12-11 after external beam radiotherapy showing resolution of the tumors.

Iridociliary and Ciliary Body Metastasis

Metastatic tumors to the ciliary body and peripheral iris are more difficult to visualize and may masquerade as an idiopathic iridocyclitis and secondary glaucoma, often resulting in a delay in diagnosis.

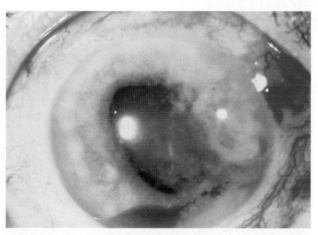

Figure 12-13. Severe intraocular inflammation and hyphema secondary to a diffuse metastasis from mucin-secreting intestinal carcinoma in a 67-year-old woman. The blind painful eye was enucleated.

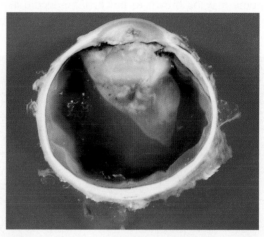

Figure 12-14. Gross appearance of the enucleated eye showing tumor cells in the ciliary body region, surrounding the lens, and occupying the anterior chamber.

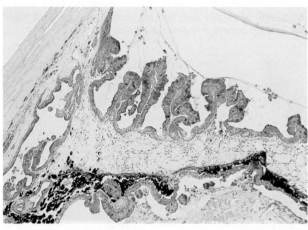

Figure 12-15. Photomicrograph of the iris and ciliary body region showing monolayer of mucin-secreting tumor cells growing across the iris and ciliary body (Alcian blue, original magnification × 20).

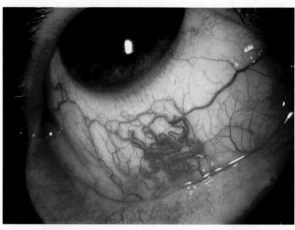

Figure 12-16. Sentinel blood vessels on sclera in the ciliary body region of a 62-year-old woman. A systemic evaluation failed to reveal a primary tumor. The blind painful eye was enucleated.

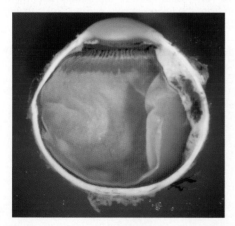

Figure 12-17. Section of enucleated eye shown in Fig. 12-16 showing diffuse tumor of the ciliary body and peripheral choroid.

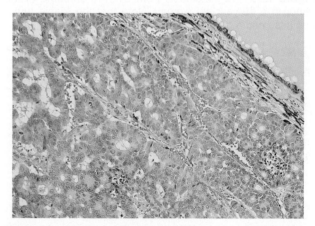

Figure 12-18. Histopathologic section of mucin-secreting adenocarcinoma in the ciliary body (hematoxylin–eosin, original magnification × 200). Several months later, the patient developed evident systemic metastasis, and it was believed that the primary cancer was in the common bile duct.

Choroidal Metastasis

Choroidal metastasis can assume a variety of clinical variations. However, the typical lesion appears as a creamy-yellow sessile or dome-shaped mass in the posterior choroid. Depicted here are examples of typical choroidal metastases.

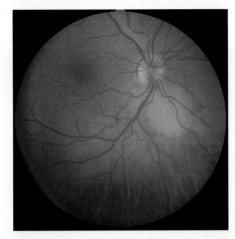

Figure 12-19. Small choroidal metastasis inferior to the optic disc in a 35-year-old woman with metastatic breast cancer.

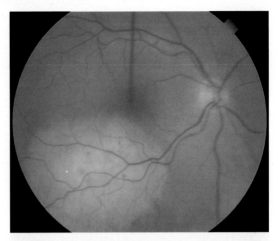

Figure 12-20. Choroidal metastasis in typical location infero-temporal to the fovea in a 67-year-old woman with metastatic breast cancer.

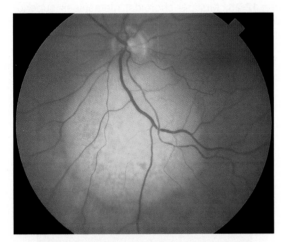

Figure 12-21. Choroidal metastasis inferior to the optic disc in a 55-year-old woman with breast cancer.

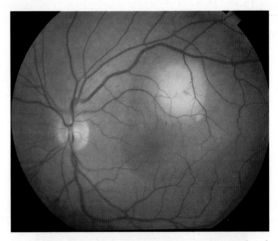

Figure 12-22. Choroidal metastasis superior to the foveal region in a 45-year-old woman with breast cancer. Note the serous detachment of the adjacent fovea. Patients with this finding initially may be misdiagnosed as having central serous chorioretinopathy.

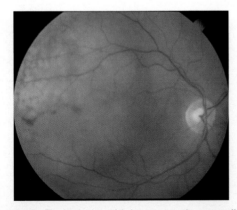

Figure 12-23. Typical choroidal metastasis extending temporally from the foveal area in a 58-year-old woman. She was referred with the diagnosis of central serous chorioretinopathy, had no prior diagnosis of cancer, and denied any knowledge of breast problems. Because the lesion was very suggestive of metastasis, a breast examination was performed.

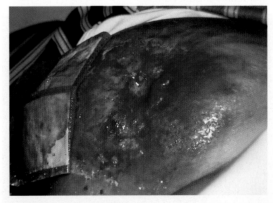

Figure 12-24. Appearance of the breast of the patient shown in Fig. 12-23 showing advanced, ulcerating breast cancer. Although the patient was aware of this lesion, she chose to deny its existence.

Choroidal Metastasis—Clinical Variations

Choroidal metastasis can have several clinical variations. Although it is often a solitary lesion, it can be multifocal and bilateral. Metastatic melanoma to the choroid, from skin or the opposite choroid, is often pigmented.

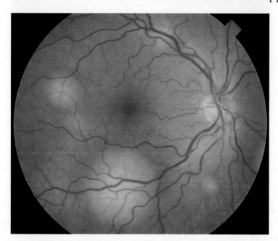

Figure 12-25. Multiple choroidal metastases to the posterior pole of the right eye in a 43-year-old woman with metastatic breast cancer.

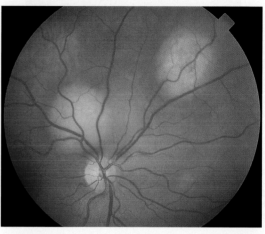

Figure 12-26. Multiple choroidal metastases superior and nasal to the optic disc in a 38-year-old woman with metastatic breast cancer.

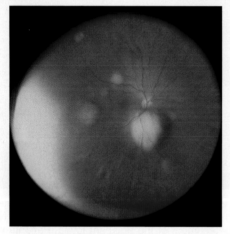

Figure 12-27. Wide-angle photograph showing multiple choroidal metastases in the right eye of a 36-year-old woman with metastatic breast cancer.

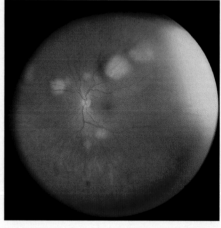

Figure 12-28. Wide-angle photograph of the left eye of the same patient shown in Fig. 12-27 showing similar multiple metastases.

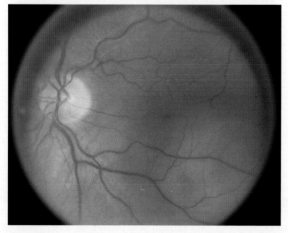

Figure 12-29. Solitary metastasis of cutaneous melanoma to the choroid in a 60-year-old man. The diagnosis was confirmed when the eye was examined postmortem.

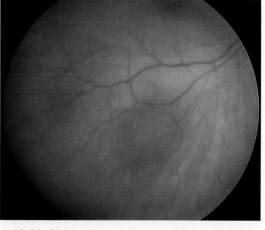

Figure 12-30. Metastatic melanoma to the choroid from a primary choroidal melanoma in the opposite eye. Enucleation was performed about 2 years earlier, and the patient returned with metastasis to the contralateral eyelid, orbit, and choroid.

Choroidal Metastasis—Effects on Adjacent Structures

Choroidal metastasis causes changes in adjacent structures. It can induce pigment epithelial changes, secondary retinal detachment, choroidal detachment, or, rarely, it can assume a nodular configuration, simulating the mushroom shape seen with some primary melanomas.

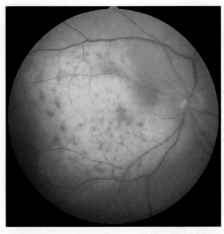

Figure 12-31. Typical pigment clumping over a choroidal metastasis producing the "leopard skin" appearance.

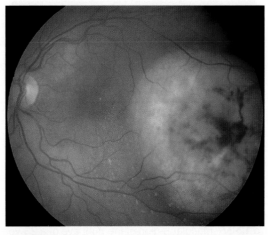

Figure 12-32. Pigment epithelial proliferation over a choroidal metastasis.

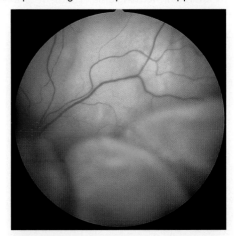

Figure 12-33. Large inferior bullous retinal detachment secondary to a diffuse metastasis in the macular region.

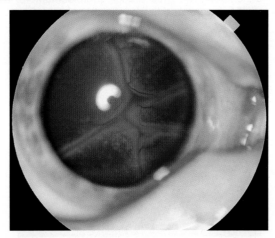

Figure 12-34. Total retinal detachment with retina against the posterior surface of the lens, secondary to a choroidal metastasis. Such a patient may require enucleation because of severe uncontrollable pain.

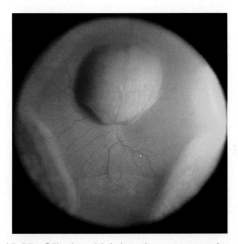

Figure 12-35. Ciliochoroidal detachment secondary to choroidal metastasis. Wide-angle fundus photograph of a metastasis in the superior fundus from lung cancer. Prominent secondary ciliochoroidal detachment for 360 degrees is most pronounced inferotemporally and inferonasally. The mechanism of choroidal detachment in such cases is uncertain.

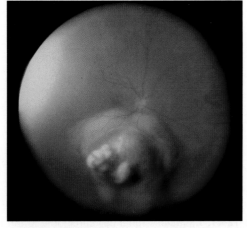

Figure 12-36. Retinal invasion of choroidal metastasis. Wide-angle fundus photograph of a choroidal metastasis inferiorly from lung cancer with nodular surface simulating a mushroom-shaped melanoma.

Orange-colored Choroidal Metastasis

Some forms of choroidal metastasis have an orange color, simulating a choroidal hemangioma. This orange color is seen most often with choroidal metastasis from bronchial carcinoid tumor, thyroid cancer, and renal cell carcinoma. Carcinoid tumor metastasis can be stable or slowly progressive.

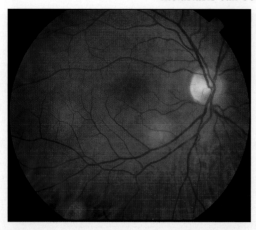

Figure 12-37. Macular region of the right eye of a 23-year-old woman with a history of systemic metastasis from a bronchial carcinoid showing two small orange choroidal tumors. There was a similar lesion nasal to the optic disc of the left eye.

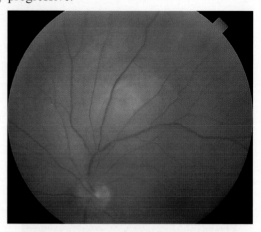

Figure 12-38. Choroidal metastasis from bronchial carcinoid tumor in a 58-year-old woman. Note the similarity of the lesion to a choroidal hemangioma. There were three other choroidal metastases in the same eye.

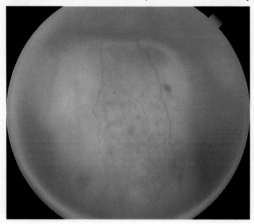

Figure 12-39. Metastatic bronchial carcinoid inferotemporally in the right eye. The diagnosis was confirmed with fine-needle aspiration biopsy.

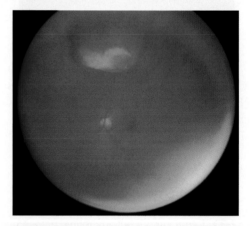

Figure 12-40. Metastatic thyroid cancer to the choroid in the superior fundus showing orange color.

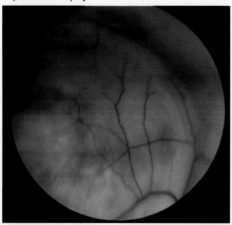

Figure 12-41. Metastatic renal cell carcinoma to the macular area in a man who had nephrectomy 10 years earlier for renal cell carcinoma. The eye was enucleated for suspected choroidal melanoma because the patient failed to reveal the history of renal cell carcinoma. The dark areas in the clinical photograph were due to hemorrhage, a common finding in metastatic renal cell carcinoma.

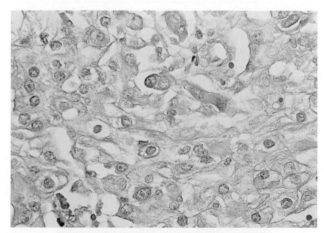

Figure 12-42. Histopathology of the lesion shown in Fig. 12-41 showing clear cells characteristic of renal cell carcinoma (hematoxylin–eosin, original magnification × 200).

Pathology of Choroidal Metastasis

The gross appearance of a choroidal metastasis can vary considerably from case to case. It is usually a nonpigmented yellow or pink lesion with a diffuse or multinodular growth pattern. A detailed discussion of the histopathology of choroidal metastasis is beyond the scope of this text. The microscopic pathology of choroidal metastasis usually reflects the histopathology of the primary tumor.

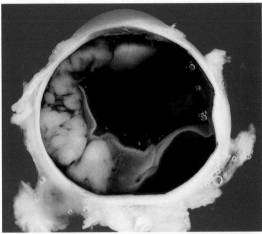

Figure 12-43. Metastatic breast cancer to the choroid with a diffuse, multinodular growth pattern.

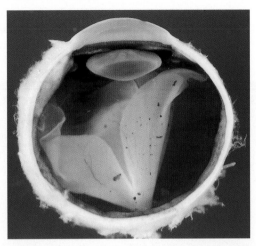

Figure 12-44. Metastatic breast cancer to the choroid with a diffuse, flat growth pattern. Note that the entire posterior uveal tract is only minimally thickened, and there is a total bullous retinal detachment.

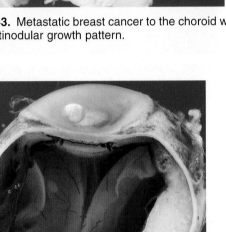

Figure 12-45. Metastatic gastric carcinoma to the choroid.

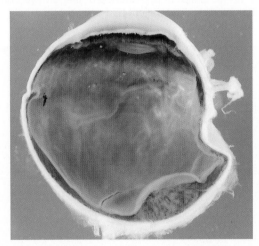

Figure 12-46. Metastatic cutaneous melanoma to the choroid. This is the same case shown in Fig. 12-29.

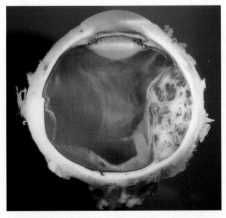

Figure 12-47. Choroidal metastasis presumably from bronchogenic carcinoma. This is a vascular tumor with foci of hemorrhage.

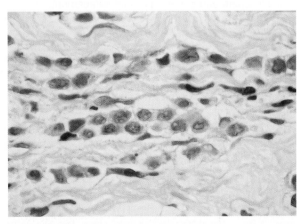

Figure 12-48. Histopathology of metastatic breast cancer showing linear arrangement of malignant cells in a fibrous tissue stroma (hematoxylin–eosin, original magnification × 150).

Clinicopathologic Correlation of Choroidal Metastasis from Uncertain Primary Neoplasm

Choroidal metastasis sometimes can occur in an otherwise healthy person with no history of cancer. In some cases, the primary site of the tumor is never determined. Described here is such a case in a 51-year-old man who developed rapid pain and blindness in his left eye, secondary to a mucous-secreting adenocarcinoma of uncertain origin. The patient died a few weeks later with widespread metastasis; no autopsy was permitted.

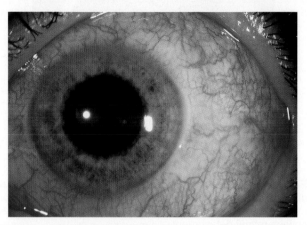

Figure 12-49. External appearance of the left eye showing epibulbar injection. The patient had severe ocular pain.

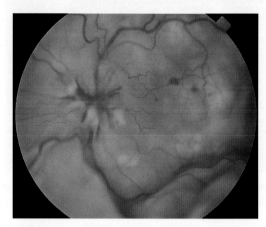

Figure 12-50. Fundus photograph showing diffuse choroidal thickening, edema, and hemorrhage of the optic disc, and inferior retinal detachment.

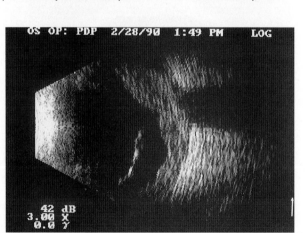

Figure 12-51. B-scan ultrasonogram showing diffuse choroidal thickening and overlying retinal detachment.

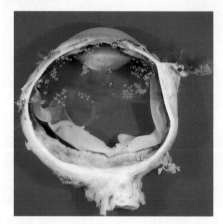

Figure 12-52. Sectioned eye after enucleation showing diffuse choroidal tumor.

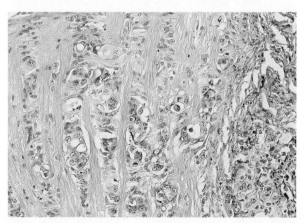

Figure 12-53. Photomicrograph of the optic nerve showing poorly differentiated tumor cells (hematoxylin–eosin, original magnification × 150).

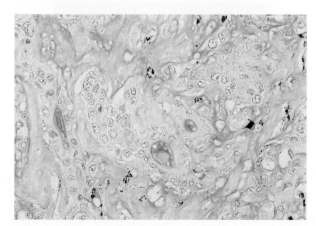

Figure 12-54. Mucin stain showing positive reaction in cytoplasm of tumor cells (Alcian blue, original magnification × 150).

Fluorescein Angiography and Ultrasonography of Choroidal Metastasis

The diagnosis of choroidal metastasis usually is made with ophthalmoscopy. However, ancillary studies may assist in the diagnosis, particularly in difficult cases.

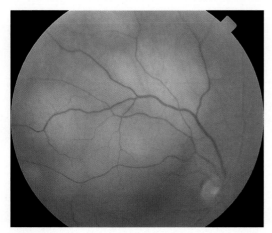

Figure 12-55. Clinical appearance of irregular choroidal metastasis in the macular area of the right eye of a 68-year-old woman.

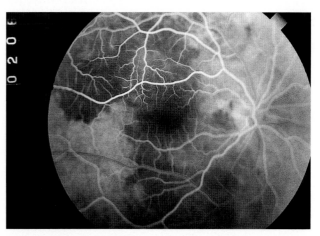

Figure 12-56. Fluorescein angiogram in laminar venous phase showing hypofluorescence of the lesion.

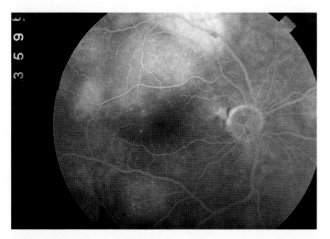

Figure 12-57. Late angiogram showing hyperfluorescence of the lesion.

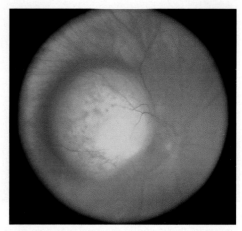

Figure 12-58. Wide-angle photograph of choroidal metastasis in the macular area of a 43-year-old woman.

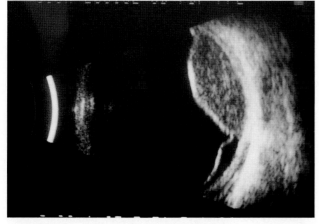

Figure 12-59. B-scan ultrasonogram showing choroidal mass with acoustic solidity and no choroidal excavation. Note the linear echo inferiorly, typical of secondary retinal detachment.

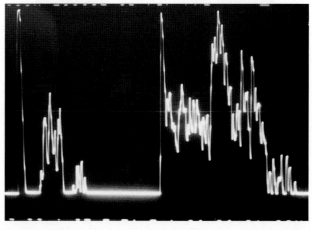

Figure 12-60. A-scan ultrasonogram showing medium internal reflectivity of the tumor.

Computed Tomography, Magnetic Resonance Imaging, and Fine-needle Aspiration Biopsy of Choroidal Metastasis

Computed tomography and magnetic resonance imaging can demonstrate choroidal metastasis but, even with contrast enhancement, they add little information to what is found with clinical examination, fluorescein angiography, and ultrasonography. Fine-needle aspiration biopsy, however, is a very effective method for making the diagnosis in cases where less invasive measures have not established the diagnosis.

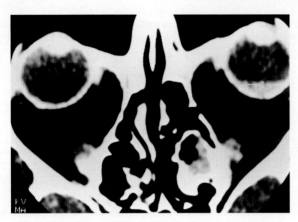

Figure 12-61. Axial computed tomogram showing diffuse posterior choroidal metastasis.

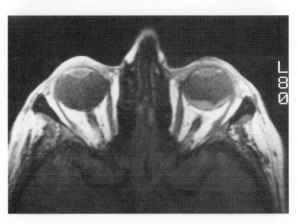

Figure 12-62. Axial magnetic resonance imaging in T1-weighted image showing choroidal mass that is hyperintense to the vitreous.

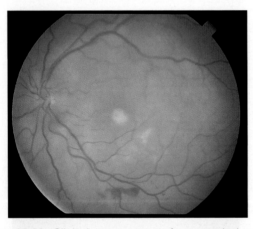

Figure 12-63. Clinical appearance of an atypical yellow-orange choroidal thickening in the posterior pole of an otherwise healthy 61-year-old woman. Systemic evaluation revealed no abnormalities.

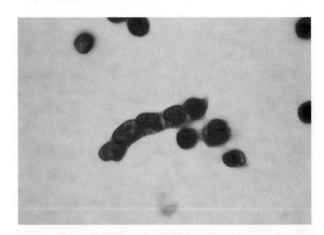

Figure 12-64. Cytology of fine-needle aspiration biopsy showing cells compatible with metastatic breast cancer. Subsequent systemic evaluation of the patient shown in Fig. 12-63 revealed a subtle breast cancer.

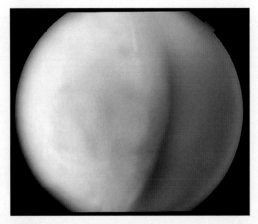

Figure 12-65. Clinical appearance of a large amelanotic ciliochoroidal mass in a 52-year-old woman. The diagnosis was uncertain but primary melanoma was suspected.

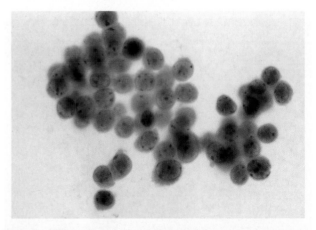

Figure 12-66. Cytology of fine-needle aspiration biopsy showing cells with cytoplasmic granules compatible with metastatic carcinoid tumor. Subsequent systemic evaluation revealed a subtle bronchial carcinoid tumor.

Response of Choroidal Metastasis to Irradiation

Choroidal metastasis may require no treatment if it appears clinically to have regressed spontaneously or from prior treatment. Active choroidal metastasis can be treated with chemotherapy, hormonal therapy, external irradiation, or plaque brachytherapy. The response of the tumor is similar regardless of the treatment employed, with the exception that radiation retinopathy sometimes can occur after radiotherapy.

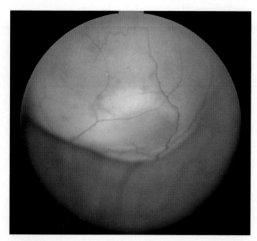

Figure 12-67. External beam irradiation for choroidal metastasis. Choroidal metastasis from thyroid cancer in a 42-year-old man.

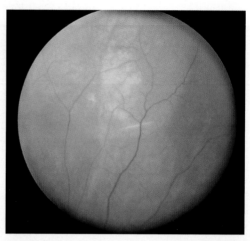

Figure 12-68. Same lesion shown in Fig. 12-67 after external beam irradiation showing excellent tumor regression.

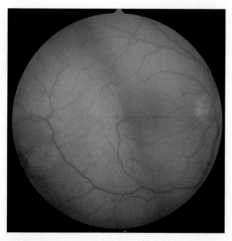

Figure 12-69. Plaque radiotherapy for choroidal metastasis. Choroidal metastasis from breast cancer temporal to the foveal region in a 64-year-old woman.

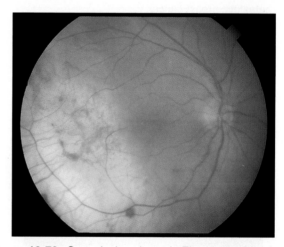

Figure 12-70. Same lesion shown in Fig. 12-69 after plaque radiotherapy showing excellent tumor regression.

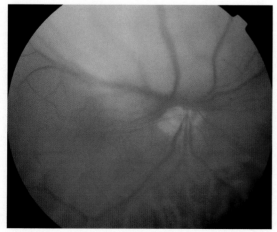

Figure 12-71. Plaque radiotherapy for choroidal metastasis. Choroidal metastasis from lung cancer superior to the optic disc in a 74-year-old man.

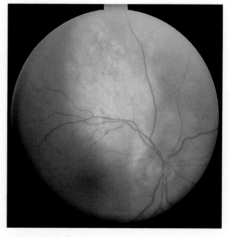

Figure 12-72. Same lesion shown in Fig. 12-71 after plaque radiotherapy showing excellent tumor regression.

Optic-disc Metastasis

Metastatic cancer can affect the optic disc secondary to invasion from juxtapapillary choroidal metastasis, or it can occur on the optic disc as a solitary ocular finding without clinically evident choroidal involvement. It generally is associated with profound visual loss and should be treated promptly with radiotherapy.

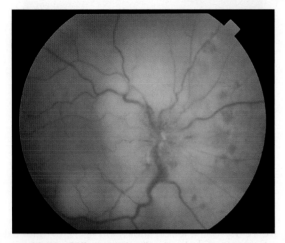

Figure 12-73. Diffuse optic disc involvement secondary to juxtapapillary choroidal metastasis in a 51-year-old woman with metastatic breast cancer.

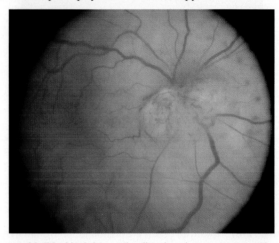

Figure 12-74. Nodular optic disc involvement secondary to juxtapapillary choroidal metastasis in a 60-year-old woman with metastatic breast cancer.

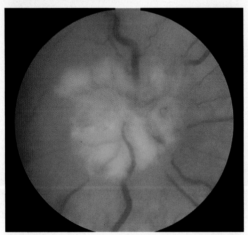

Figure 12-75. Optic disc metastasis from lung cancer in a 50-year-old man. Note the typical solid yellow appearance of the swollen disc.

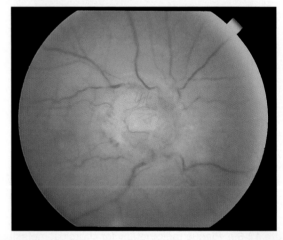

Figure 12-76. Optic disc metastasis from lung cancer in a 78-year-old man.

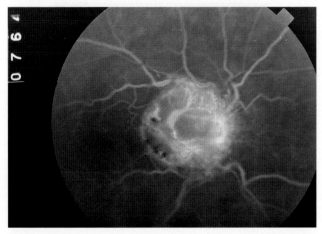

Figure 12-77. Fluorescein angiogram of the lesion shown in Fig. 12-76 in venous phase showing hypofluorescent foci in the lesion.

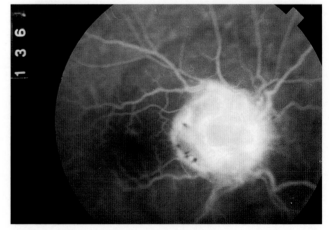

Figure 12-78. Angiogram in recirculation phase showing diffuse hyperfluorescence of the mass.

Retinal and Vitreal Metastasis

Metastasis to the retina and vitreous is rare. It can masquerade as an inflammatory process, and there is often a delay in diagnosis.

Figure 12-82 courtesy of Dr. Frederick Davidorf. From Letson AD, Davidorf FH. Bilateral retinal metastases from cutaneous melanoma. *Arch Ophthalmol* 1982;100: 605–607.

Fig. 83 from Gunduz K, Shields JA, Shields CL, Eagle RC Jr. Cutaneous melanoma metastatic to the vitreous cavity. *Ophthalmology* 1998;105:600–605.

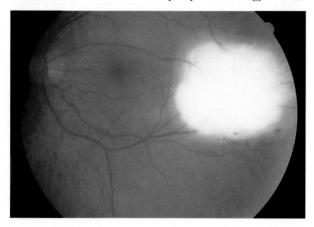

Figure 12-79. Retinal metastasis from small-cell carcinoma. (Courtesy of Dr. Anti Leys.)

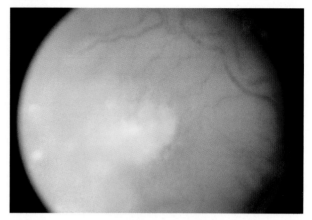

Figure 12-80. Retinal metastasis temporal to the macular area from uncertain primary lesion. (Courtesy of Drs. Robert Kleiner and Ralph C. Eagle Jr.)

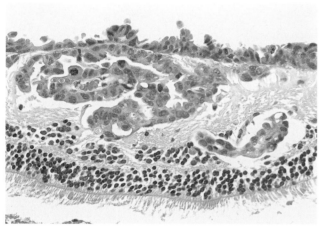

Figure 12-81. Pathology of eyewall biopsy of the lesion shown in Fig. 12-80 showing adenocarcinoma in the inner part of the sensory retina. (Courtesy of Drs. Robert Kleiner and Ralph C. Eagle Jr.)

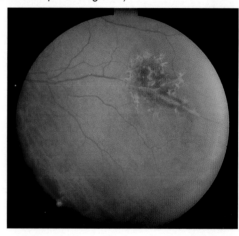

Figure 12-82. Retinal metastasis from cutaneous melanoma.

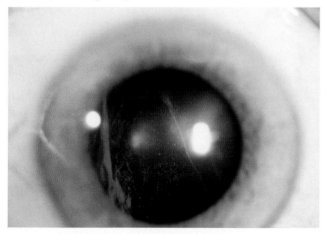

Figure 12-83. Vitreal metastasis from primary cutaneous melanoma. Note the golden-brown cells attached to the vitreous framework.

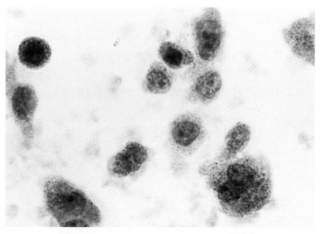

Figure 12-84. Cytology of fine-needle aspiration biopsy of the vitreous showing malignant melanoma cells (Papanicolaou, original magnification × 400).

CHAPTER 13

Vascular Tumors
of the Uvea

CIRCUMSCRIBED CHOROIDAL HEMANGIOMA

Choroidal hemangioma can occur as a circumscribed tumor or as a diffuse lesion in patients with variations of the Sturge–Weber syndrome. Circumscribed choroidal hemangioma almost always is unilateral. It appears as a subtle, red-orange mass in the posterior choroid. It can produce visual loss because of a subfoveal location or a secondary retinal detachment that involves the fovea (1–4). It can induce hyperplasia and fibrous metaplasia of the overlying pigment epithelium that sometimes can lead to diagnostic confusion with melanoma. In addition to retinal detachment, secondary retinoschisis commonly occurs over or adjacent to the tumor. Occasionally, neovascular glaucoma can develop and the subsequent pain may necessitate enucleation (5).

Fluorescein angiography typically shows hyperfluorescence of the tumor blood vessels in the prearterial phase and diffuse late staining of the mass (1,6). Indocyanine green angiography shows early filling of the lesion and a characteristic "wash out" of the hyperfluorescence in the later frames (7). A-scan ultrasonography shows high internal reflectivity within the tumor, and B-scan shows a placoid or rounded choroidal mass pattern with acoustic solidity. Ultrasonography occasionally shows a highly reflective plaque over the tumor surface, which corresponds to fibrous or osseous metaplasia of the overlying retinal pigment epithelium (1). Computed tomography and magnetic resonance imaging also can demonstrate choroidal hemangioma, but the results are not necessarily diagnostic.

Grossly, a circumscribed choroidal hemangioma is a red placoid or ovoid choroidal tumor. Microscopically, it is usually composed of large congested vessels separated by rather thin intervascular septae. If the affected patient is asymptomatic, no treatment is necessary. When there is visual loss because of a serous detachment of the fovea, surface laser treatment can induce resolution of the subretinal fluid (1,2,5,8,9). Plaque or external beam radiotherapy can be employed in cases with more advanced detachment (10–12). In rare instances, neovascular glaucoma may necessitate enucleation.

SELECTED REFERENCES

1. Gass JDM. *Stereoscopic atlas of macular diseases.* St. Louis: CV Mosby, 1997:208–212.
2. Shields JA, Shields CL. *Intraocular tumors. A text and atlas.* Philadelphia: WB Saunders, 1992:252–255.
3. Witschel H, Font RL. Hemangioma of the choroid. A clinicopathologic study of 71 cases and a review of the literature. *Surv Ophthalmol* 1976;20:415–431.
4. Anand R, Augsburger JJ, Shields JA. Circumscribed choroidal hemangiomas. *Arch Ophthalmol* 1989;107: 1338–1342.
5. Shields JA, Stephens RF, Eagle RC Jr, Shields CL, De Potter P. Progressive enlargement of a circumscribed choroidal hemangioma. A clinicopathologic correlation. *Arch Ophthalmol* 1992;110:1276–1278.
6. Norton EWD, Gutman F. Fluorescein angiography of hemangiomas of the choroid. *Arch Ophthalmol* 1967; 78:121–125.
7. Shields CL, Shields JA, De Potter P. Patterns of indocyanine green angiography of choroidal tumors. *Br J Ophthalmol* 1995;79:237–245.
8. Sanborn GE, Augsburger JJ, Shields JA. Treatment of circumscribed choroidal hemangiomas. *Ophthalmology* 1982;89:1374–1380.
9. Shields JA. The expanding role of laser photocoagulation for intraocular tumors. The 1993 H. Christian Zweng Memorial Lecture. *Retina* 1994;14:310–322.
10. Zografos L, Bercher L, Chamot L, Gailloud C, Raimondi S, Egger E. Cobalt-60 treatment of choroidal hemangiomas. *Am J Ophthalmol* 1996;121:190–199.
11. Hannouche D, Frau E, Desjardins L, Cassouix N, Habrand JL, Offret H. Efficacy of proton therapy in circumscribed choroidal hemangiomas associated with serous retinal detachment. *Ophthalmology* 1997;104: 100–103.
12. Shields JA. Radiotherapy of circumscribed choroidal hemangiomas. *Ophthalmology* 1997;104:1784.

Circumscribed Choroidal Hemangioma—Clinical Features

In most instances, the characteristic orange color of a circumscribed choroidal hemangioma strongly suggests the diagnosis.

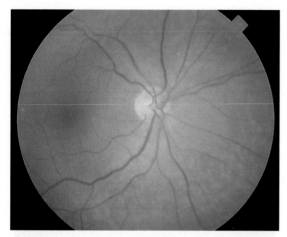

Figure 13-1. Asymptomatic, subtle choroidal hemangioma located nasal to the optic disc in a 69-year-old woman.

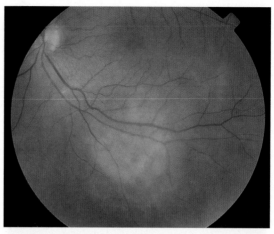

Figure 13-2. Choroidal hemangioma inferior to the fovea in a 47-year-old woman.

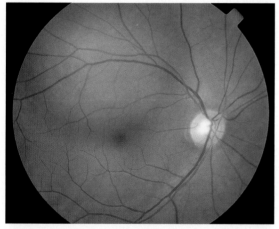

Figure 13-3. Choroidal hemangioma superior to the fovea in a 46-year-old man.

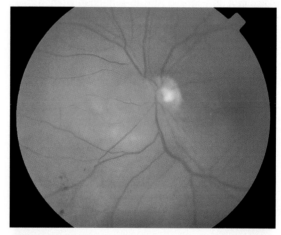

Figure 13-4. Subtle choroidal hemangioma nasal to the optic disc and slightly overhanging the disc in a 39-year-old woman.

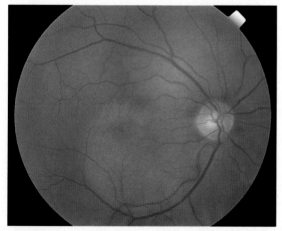

Figure 13-5. Choroidal hemangioma superior to the optic disc causing visual loss due to a secondary serous detachment of the retina, extending into the foveal area.

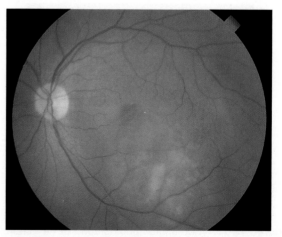

Figure 13-6. Choroidal hemangioma inferior to the fovea causing visual loss due to the foveal elevation by the tumor.

Circumscribed Choroidal Hemangioma—Effects on Adjacent Structures

In some instances, circumscribed choroidal hemangioma can cause secondary hyperplasia or metaplasia of the retinal pigment epithelium, retinal detachment, or retinoschisis.

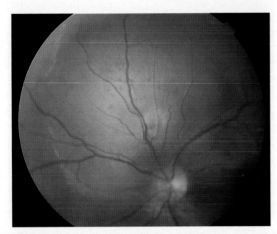

Figure 13-7. Foci of proliferation of the retinal pigment epithelium on the surface of a choroidal hemangioma superior to the optic disc in a 30-year-old African-American woman.

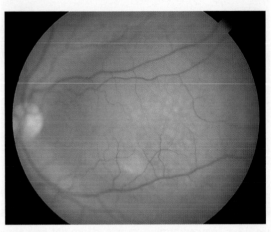

Figure 13-8. Subtle retinal pigment epithelium hyperplasia and fibrous metaplasia over a macular choroidal hemangioma in a 30-year-old woman.

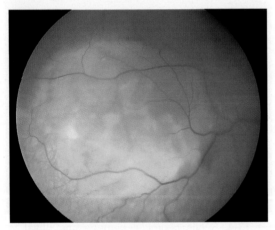

Figure 13-9. Moderate fibrous metaplasia over a choroidal hemangioma in a 30-year-old man.

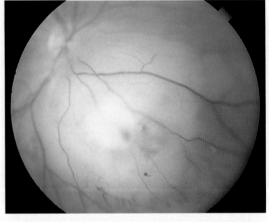

Figure 13-10. Severe fibrous metaplasia over a choroidal hemangioma in a 24-year-old woman.

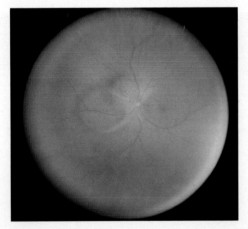

Figure 13-11. Wide-angle photograph of a choroidal hemangioma superonasal to the optic disc and a secondary overlying retinoschisis presenting as an intraretinal cyst. There was also serous detachment of the fovea.

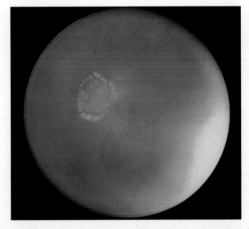

Figure 13-12. Lesion shown in Fig. 13-11 immediately after delimiting and tumor surface photocoagulation to the tumor surface. The retinal cyst collapsed at the time of laser treatment, and the serous retinal detachment resolved.

Fluorescein and Indocyanine Green Angiography of Circumscribed Choroidal Hemangioma

Although the findings are not pathognomonic, fluorescein angiography and indocyanine green angiography often can be helpful in differentiating a choroidal hemangioma from amelanotic melanoma, choroidal metastasis, and other nonpigmented fundus tumors.

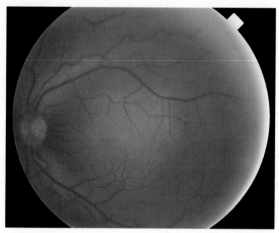

Figure 13-13. Choroidal hemangioma located in the central macular area.

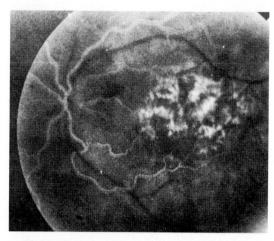

Figure 13-14. Standard fluorescein angiogram in early arterial phase showing reticular hyperfluorescence corresponding to filling of choroidal vessels in the tumor.

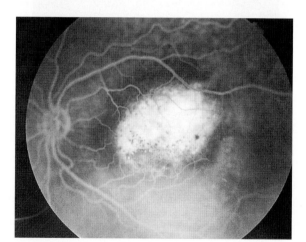

Figure 13-15. Recirculation phase demonstrating marked hyperfluorescence of the lesion.

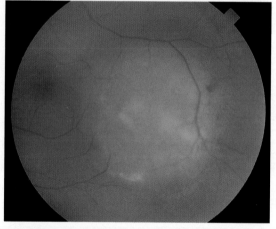

Figure 13-16. Choroidal hemangioma temporal to the foveal region in the left eye of a 39-year-old man.

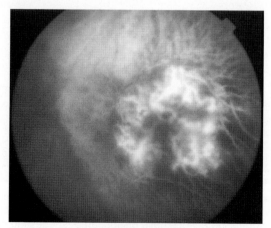

Figure 13-17. Early indocyanine green angiogram showing reticular hyperfluorescence of the lesion.

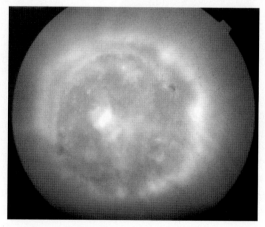

Figure 13-18. Late indocyanine green angiogram showing halo of hyperfluorescence and central "wash out" phenomenon.

Ultrasonography of Circumscribed Choroidal Hemangioma

Ultrasonography of choroidal hemangioma generally shows high internal reflectivity with A-scan and acoustic solidity with B-scan. Fibrous or osseous metaplasia of the overlying pigment epithelium can produce a highly reflective echo.

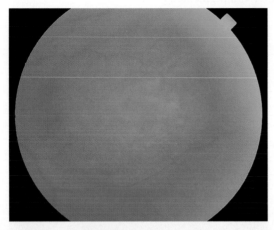

Figure 13-19. Clinical appearance of tumor in the macular area of a 70-year-old woman.

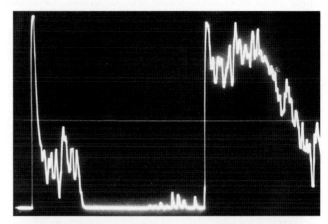

Figure 13-20. A-scan ultrasonogram showing high initial spike and high internal reflectivity in the tumor.

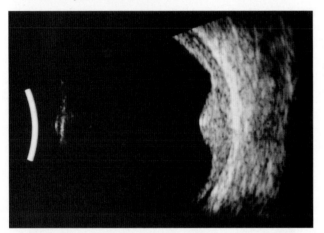

Figure 13-21. B-scan ultrasonogram showing acoustic solidity and lack of choroidal excavation.

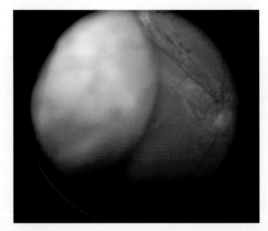

Figure 13-22. Large circumscribed choroidal hemangioma with severe overlying fibrous and/or osseous metaplasia of retinal pigment epithelium in a 9-year-old boy.

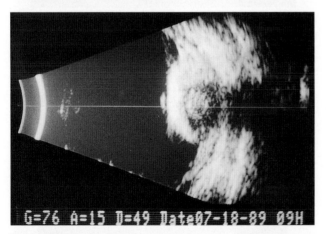

Figure 13-23. B-scan ultrasonogram of the lesion shown in Fig. 13-22 showing highly reflective plaque on the tumor surface.

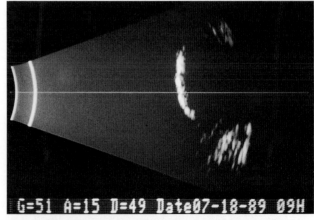

Figure 13-24. B-scan ultrasonogram at lowered sensitivity showing persistence of the echo from the surface plaque after soft-tissue echoes have disappeared, suggesting calcification of the overlying plaque.

Computed Tomography and Magnetic Resonance Imaging of Circumscribed Choroidal Hemangioma

Computed tomography and magnetic resonance imaging can demonstrate characteristic, but not pathognomonic, features of circumscribed choroidal hemangioma. In most instances, the diagnosis can be established without these modalities, but they can be helpful in difficult cases. The case of a 16-year-old girl with a circumscribed choroidal hemangioma that was studied with computed tomography and magnetic resonance imaging is shown.

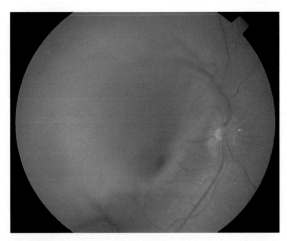

Figure 13-25. Large red choroidal hemangioma temporal to the macular area.

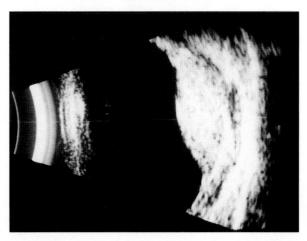

Figure 13-26. B-scan ultrasonogram showing characteristic acoustic solidity.

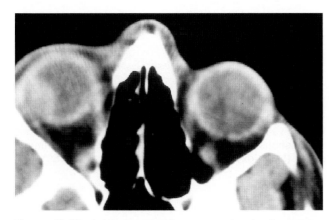

Figure 13-27. Axial computed tomogram showing large intra-ocular mass.

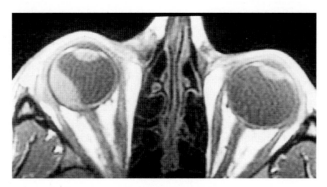

Figure 13-28. Axial magnetic resonance imaging (T1-weighted image) showing mass hyperintense to the vitreous.

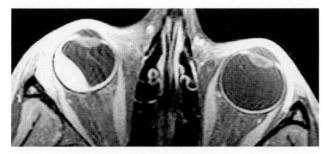

Figure 13-29. Axial magnetic resonance imaging (T1-weighted image with gadolinium enhancement) showing marked enhancement of the mass.

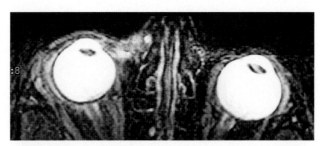

Figure 13-30. Axial magnetic resonance imaging (T2-weighted image) showing poor visibility of the mass because it is isointense to the vitreous.

Pathology of Circumscribed Choroidal Hemangioma

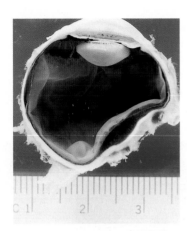

Figure 13-31. Gross photograph of sectioned eye containing a choroidal hemangioma showing the sessile reddish tumor.

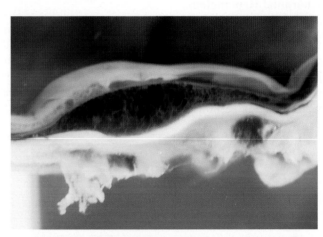

Figure 13-32. Closer view of the lesion shown in Fig. 13-31 showing spongy vascular mass and overlying cystic changes in the sensory retina.

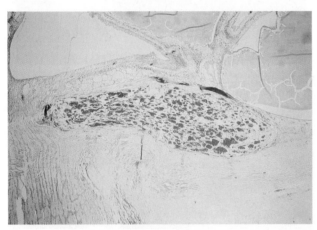

Figure 13-33. Low-magnification photomicrograph of choroidal hemangioma showing vascular choroidal lesion and overlying retinal detachment (hematoxylin–eosin, original magnification × 10).

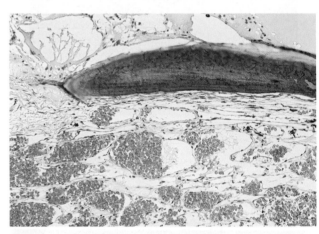

Figure 13-34. Photomicrograph showing plaque of fibrous and osseous metaplasia over a cavernous choroidal hemangioma (hematoxylin–eosin, original magnification × 50).

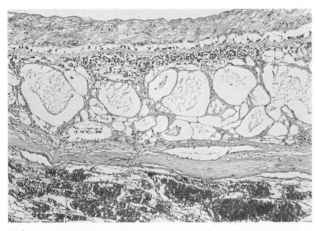

Figure 13-35. Photomicrograph showing cystic changes in the sensory retina over a cavernous choroidal hemangioma (hematoxylin–eosin, original magnification × 50).

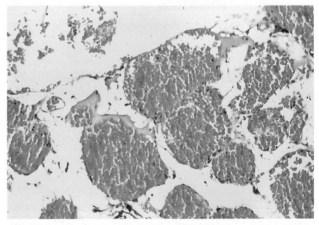

Figure 13-36. Photomicrograph showing large dilated, thin-walled vascular channels (hematoxylin–eosin, original magnification × 100).

Clinicopathologic Correlation of Progressively Enlarging Choroidal Hemangioma

The majority of circumscribed choroidal hemagiomas are stable lesions that show no significant growth. Occasionally, this tumor can show progressive enlargement, possibly due to vascular engorgement. This is particularly likely to occur during pregnancy. A case of progressive growth of circumscribed choroidal hemangioma that ultimately necessitated enucleation is illustrated.

From Shields JA, Stephens RF, Eagle RC Jr, Shields CL, De Potter P. Progressive enlargement of a circumscribed choroidal hemangioma. A clinicopathologic correlation. *Arch Ophthalmol* 1992;110:1276–1278.

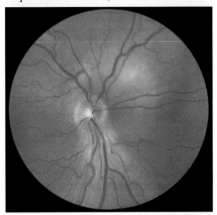

Figure 13-37. Choroidal hemangioma superonasal to the optic disc in a 30-year-old man as seen in 1981. It was treated with laser because of a shallow serous detachment of the fovea.

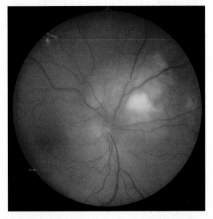

Figure 13-38. Lesion 3 years later in 1984 showing apparent increase in size and fibrous metaplasia of the retinal pigment epithelium.

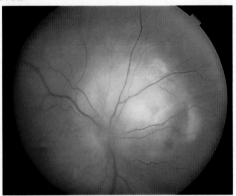

Figure 13-39. Appearance of the lesion in 1989 showing further enlargement. A retinal detachment progressed in spite of further laser treatment.

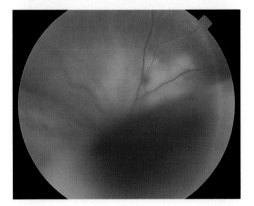

Figure 13-40. Appearance of the lesion in 1990 showing futher enlargement and large bullous retinal detachment. Pain secondary to glaucoma and low suspicion of atypical choroidal melanoma prompted enucleation of the blind eye.

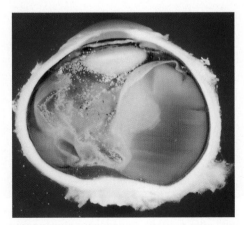

Figure 13-41. Gross photograph of the sectioned eye showing red tumor in the posterior pole and overlying total retinal detachment.

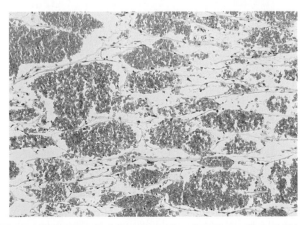

Figure 13-42. Photomicrograph showing large dilated, thin-walled vascular channels (hematoxylin–eosin, original magnification × 100).

Laser Photocoagulation of a Choroidal Hemangioma

Laser photocoagulation is indicated when a circumscribed choroidal hemangioma causes visual loss due to a serous detachment of the sensory retina. The goal of treatment is to create a chorioretinal adhesion over the tumor to allow resorption of the subretinal fluid. Heavy treatment to destroy the tumor could lead to excessive retinal damage.

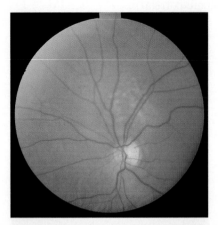

Figure 13-43. Circumscribed choroidal hemangioma superior to the optic disc in a 59-year-old man. There was decreased vision due to a serous detachment of the fovea.

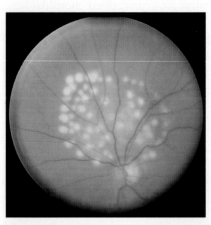

Figure 13-44. Appearance of the lesion immediately after argon laser photocoagulation showing laser-induced lesions near the tumor surface.

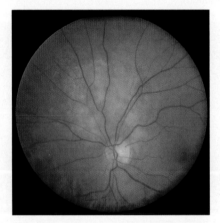

Figure 13-45. Appearance 1 month after laser treatment. The vision had returned from 6/12 to 6/6.

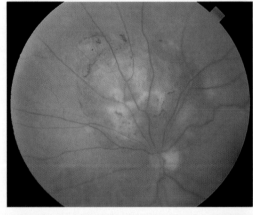

Figure 13-46. Appearance 12 years after treatment. The retinal detachment is controlled and good vision is retained.

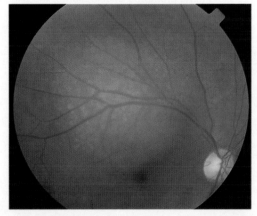

Figure 13-47. Circumscribed choroidal hemangioma superior to the foveal area in a 48-year-old man. There was visual loss due to a serous detachment of the fovea.

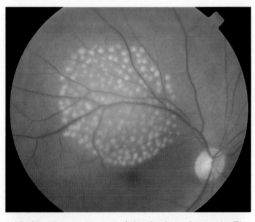

Figure 13-48. Appearance of the lesion shown in Fig. 13-47 immediately after properly placed laser photocoagulation.

Plaque Radiotherapy for Circumscribed Choroidal Hemangioma

Plaque brachytherapy or proton beam irradiation can be employed for circumscribed choroidal hemangiomas that produce a serous retinal detachment that cannot be controlled with standard laser treatment.

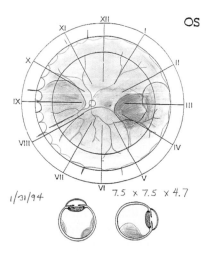

Figure 13-49. Fundus drawing of cavernous hemangioma temporal to the foveal region in a 39-year-old man. Note the hemiretinal detachment inferiorly. The detachment could not be controlled with laser treatment.

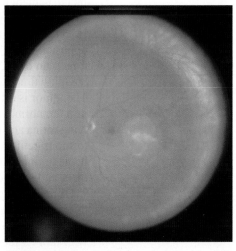

Figure 13-50. Wide-angle fundus photograph of the tumor shown in Fig. 13-49.

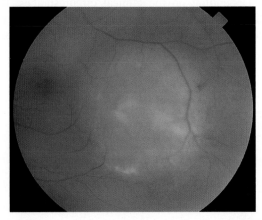

Figure 13-51. Fundus photograph showing typical clinical appearance of a circumscribed choroidal hemangioma.

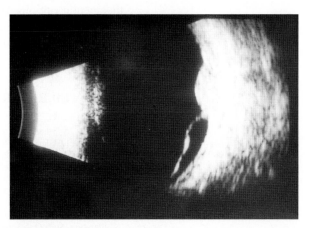

Figure 13-52. B-scan ultrasonogram of the lesion showing acoustically solid mass typical of choroidal hemangioma. Note the linear echo representing a retinal detachment inferior to the lesion.

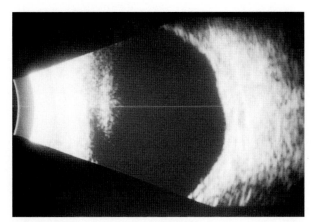

Figure 13-53. B-scan ultrasonogram about 1 year after plaque radiotherapy showing complete resolution of the elevated mass.

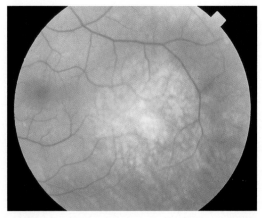

Figure 13-54. Clinical appearance of the lesion 1 year after plaque radiotherapy showing complete resolution of the mass.

DIFFUSE CHOROIDAL HEMANGIOMA

Diffuse choroidal hemangioma frequently is located ipsilateral to a facial hemangioma, usually as a component of the Sturge–Weber syndrome (1–3). It generally is diagnosed when the affected patient is young (median age 8 years), either because the facial hemangioma prompts a fundus examination or because of visual loss from hyperopic amblyopia or secondary retinal detachment. The ipsilateral pupil characteristically shows a bright red reflex (tomato catsup fundus) in contrast to the normal opposite pupil (4). The facial nevus flammeus and the choroidal hemangioma sometimes can occur bilaterally (5).

Ophthalmoscopy reveals a diffuse red-orange thickening of the posterior choroid. The tumor is often thickest in the macular area and it sometimes blends imperceptibly into the normal choroid anteriorly near the equator. Cystoid degeneration of the overlying retina and disruption of the retinal pigment epithelium commonly occur. Dilated, tortuous retinal blood vessels frequently are present in eyes with diffuse choroidal hemangioma. Diffuse choroidal hemangioma also can produce total retinal detachment and secondary neovascular glaucoma.

Ultrasonography of a diffuse choroidal hemangioma demonstrates a markedly thickened choroid, often with an overlying retinal detachment. Fluorescein angiography shows diffuse leakage similar to the circumscribed choroidal hemangioma but with more widespread involvement. Pathologically, diffuse choroidal hemangioma is identical to the circumscribed type, except that it is more diffuse and less well defined (6).

The management of diffuse choroidal hemangioma can be extremely difficult and therapeutic options are reported. Depending on the clinical circumstances, it can involve observation, amblyopic therapy, laser photocoagulation, irradiation, retinal detachment surgery, or even enucleation when there is severe secondary neovascular glaucoma (1,2).

SELECTED REFERENCES

1. Shields JA, Shields CL. *Intraocular tumors. A text and atlas.* Philadelphia: WB Saunders, 1992:252–255.
2. Shields JA, Shields CL. *Intraocular tumors. A text and atlas.* Philadelphia: WB Saunders, 1992:528–533.
3. Sullivan TJ, Clarke MP, Morin JD. The ocular manifestations of the Sturge–Weber syndrome. *J Pediatr Ophthalmol Strabismus* 1992;29:349–356.
4. Susac JO, Smith JL, Scelfo RJ. The "tomato-catsup" fundus in Sturge–Weber syndrome. *Arch Ophthalmol* 1974;92:69–70.
5. Lindsey PS, Shields JA, Goldberg RE, Augsburger JJ, Frank PE. Bilateral choroidal hemangiomas and facial nevus flammeus. *Retina* 1981;1:88–95.
6. Witschel H, Font RL. Hemangioma of the choroid. A clinicopathologic study of 71 cases and a review of the literature. *Surv Ophthalmol* 1976;20:415–431.

Diffuse Choroidal Hemangioma and Sturge–Weber Syndrome

Diffuse choroidal hemangioma usually occurs ipsilateral to a facial nevus flammeus, often as a part of the Sturge–Weber syndrome. Other ocular components of the syndrome include ipsilateral tortuous dilated epibulbar and retinal vessels, retinal detachment, retinoschisis, and congenital or juvenile glaucoma.

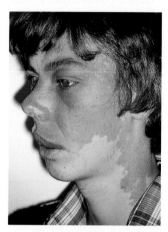

Figure 13-55. Left facial hemangioma (nevus flammeus). This lesion generally is distributed along the course of the ramifications of the trigeminal nerve.

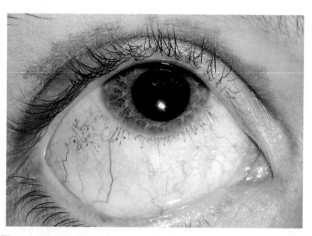

Figure 13-56. Epibulbar vascular lesion in the patient shown in Fig. 13-55. This excess vascular tissue usually is located in the episclera but can involve the conjunctiva as well.

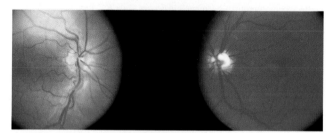

Figure 13-57. Fundus appearance of the "tomato catsup" fundus secondary to a diffuse choroidal hemangioma. The right eye is normal and the left eye shows a more red background color. With time, a secondary retinal detachment frequently develops in such cases.

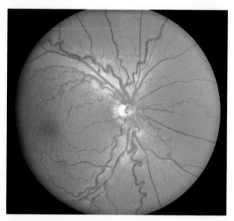

Figure 13-58. Tortuous retinal vessels in a patient with ipsilateral nevus flammeus and choroidal hemangioma.

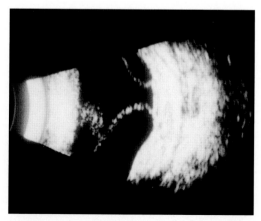

Figure 13-59. B-scan ultrasonogram showing diffuse choroidal thickening due to choroidal hemangioma in a patient with Sturge–Weber syndrome. Note the secondary retinal detachment.

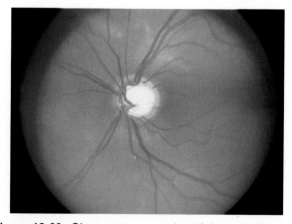

Figure 13-60. Glaucomatous cupping of the optic disc in a 28-year-old man with Sturge–Weber syndrome and diffuse choroidal hemangioma.

CAPILLARY HEMANGIOMA (HEMANGIOBLASTOMA) OF THE POSTERIOR UVEA

The majority of uveal hemangiomas are circumscribed or diffuse tumors that are composed of large dilated choroidal blood vessels, and they are classified as cavernous hemangiomas (1,2). Histopathologic studies have disclosed that many circumscribed and most diffuse hemangiomas also have a component of small-caliber capillary-type vessels and are classified as mixed types (2). Pure capillary hemangioma (hemangioblastoma) is well known to occur in the retina in association with the von Hippel–Lindau syndrome (3). However, capillary hemangioma of the choroid and ciliary body are rare, and they have not been associated with the von Hippel–Lindau syndrome.

Capillary hemangioma of the choroid has been seen in association with a nearby cutaneous capillary hemangioma (4). It can be large and lead to secondary retinal detachment. Hemangioblastoma also has been recognized in the ciliary body as an isolated lesion unassociated with the von Hippel–Lindau syndrome (5).

SELECTED REFERENCES

1. Witschel H, Font RL. Hemangioma of the choroid. A clinicopathologic study of 71 cases and a review of the literature. *Surv Ophthalmol* 1976;20:415–431.
2. Shields JA, Shields CL. *Intraocular tumors. A text and atlas.* Philadelphia: WB Saunders, 1992:252–255.
3. Shields JA, Shields CL. *Intraocular tumors. A text and atlas.* Philadelphia: WB Saunders, 1992:393–419.
4. Gass JDM. Ipsilateral facial and uveal arteriovenous and capillary angioma, microphthalmos, heterochromia of the iris and hypotony: an oculocutaneous syndrome simulating Sturge–Weber syndrome. *Trans Am Ophthalmol Soc* 1997;94:227–239.
5. Jefferies P, Clemett R. An unusual ciliary body tumour: a haemangioblastoma. *Aust N Z J Ophthalmol* 1991; 19:183–186.

Capillary Hemangioma (Hemangioblastoma) of the Posterior Uvea

Capillary vascular tumors of the uvea are rare and poorly understood. Cases of infantile capillary hemangioma of the choroid and a presumed hemangioblastoma of the ciliary body, which occurred as an acquired tumor in an adult, are depicted.

Figs. 13-61 through 13-64 courtesy of Dr. J. Donald M. Gass. From Gass JDM. Ipsilateral facial and uveal arteriovenous and capillary angioma, microphthalmos, heterochromia of the iris and hypotony: an oculocutaneous syndrome simulating Sturge–Weber syndrome. *Trans Am Ophthalmol Soc* 1997;94:227–239.

Figs. 13-65 and 13-66 courtesy of Dr. Richard Clemett. From Jefferies P, Clemett R. An unusual ciliary body tumour: a haemangioblastoma. *Aust N Z J Ophthalmol* 1991;19:183–186.

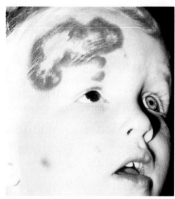

Figure 13-61. Congenital capillary hemangioma on forehead above the right eye.

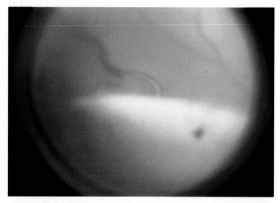

Figure 13-62. Red color of background fundus in the right eye of the patient shown in Fig. 13-61. Note also the secondary retinal detachment inferiorly. The eye eventually was enucleated after unsuccessful attempts at retinal detachment repair.

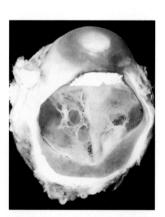

Figure 13-63. Section of enucleated eye from the patient shown in Fig. 13-61. Note the red choroidal tumor that occupies most of the choroid.

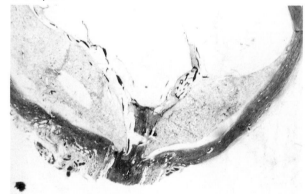

Figure 13-64. Microscopic section of eye showing spongy vascular choroidal mass (Masson trichrome, original magnification × 2).

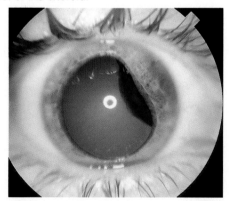

Figure 13-65. Hemangioblastoma of the ciliary body. Clinically, the lesion cannot be differentiated from an amelanotic melanoma or leiomyoma.

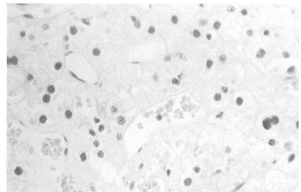

Figure 13-66. Histopathology of the lesion shown in Fig. 13-65 following removal of the tumor by iridocyclectomy. Note the round cells with uniform nuclei and abundant cytoplasm. Special studies supported the diagnosis of hemangioblastoma (hematoxylin–eosin, original magnification × 200).

UVEAL HEMANGIOPERICYTOMA

Hemangiopericytoma, a tumor composed of a proliferation of vascular pericytes, is extremely rare in the uveal tract, with only a few reported cases (1–3). It can develop in the ciliary body or choroid as an amelanotic mass that may be clinically similar to an amelanotic melanoma, choroidal hemangioma, or metastatic carcinoma. With fluorescein angiography, it seems to show early hyperfluorescence and marked late hyperfluorescence. A-scan ultrasonography generally demonstrates low to medium internal reflectivity, and B-scan shows acoustic hollowness and choroidal excavation. Histopathologically, it is composed of sinusoidal vascular channels separated by spindle-shaped cells that have immunohistochemical and electron microscopic features compatible with pericytes (1–3).

SELECTED REFERENCES

1. Shields JA, Shields CL. *Intraocular tumors. A text and atlas.* Philadelphia: WB Saunders, 1992:252–255.
2. Gieser SC, Hufnagel TJ, Jaros PA, MacRae D, Khodadoust AA. Hemangiopericytoma of the ciliary body. *Arch Ophthalmol* 1988;106:1269–1272.
3. Papale JJ, Frederick AR, Albert DM. Intraocular hemangiopericytoma. *Arch Ophthalmol* 1983;101:1409–1415.

Uveal Hemangiopericytoma

Uveal hemangiopericytoma is rare, with only a few well-documented cases in the literature. A clinicopathologic correlation of such a case is depicted.

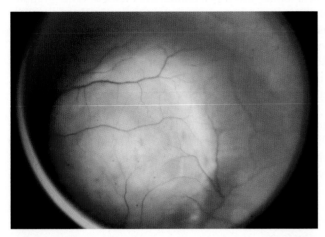

Figure 13-67. Fundus photograph of amelanotic fundus tumor. (Courtesy of Dr. Oscar Croxatto.)

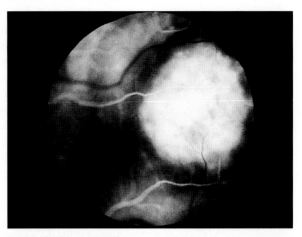

Figure 13-68. Late fluorescein angiogram showing intense hyperfluorescence of the lesion. (Courtesy of Dr. Oscar Croxatto.)

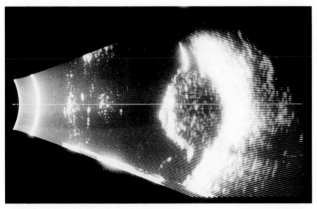

Figure 13-69. B-scan ultrasonogram showing choroidal mass with moderate acoustic hollowness and choroidal excavation. The lesion was removed by local resection. (Courtesy of Dr. Oscar Croxatto.)

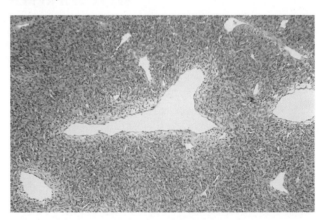

Figure 13-70. Photomicrograph showing closely compact cells with branching "staghorn" vessels (hematoxylin–eosin, original magnification × 100). (Courtesy of Dr. Oscar Croxatto.)

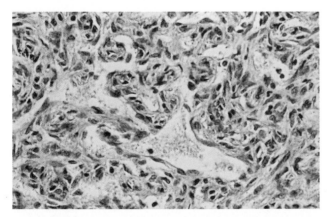

Figure 13-71. Higher-magnification photomicrograph showing spindle-shaped cells with small- and medium-caliber vascular channels (hematoxylin–eosin, original magnification × 250). (Courtesy of Dr. Oscar Croxatto.)

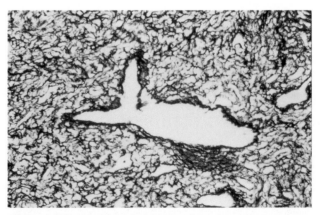

Figure 13-72. Photomicrograph of reticulin-stained section showing that the tumor cells are outside the basement membrane of blood vessels, characteristic of hemangiopericytoma (Reticulin, original magnification × 250). (Courtesy of Dr. Oscar Croxatto.)

IRIS HEMANGIOMA

In 1972, Ferry (1) reported his review of reported cases of iris hemangioma and concluded that almost all of them had been misdiagnosed histopathologically and that they actually were vascular melanomas, juvenile xanthogranulomas, or other granulomas. He raised some doubts about the existence of iris hemangioma. However, there have been a number of cases of iris hemangioma that are acceptable (2–6). Like hemangioma of the retina, iris hemangioma can be classified into capillary, cavernous, and racemose types. Capillary hemangioma rarely is seen in children with a congenital periocular cutaneous capillary hemangioma (4,5). It tends to regress spontaneously, similar to its cutaneous counterpart. Cavernous hemangioma of the iris is typically very small and located near the pupillary. It is subtle, must be detected with slit-lamp biomicroscopy, and is difficult to photograph. It occasionally can be the cause of hyphema (3). Although we have observed such lesions, they are small and difficult to demonstrate with photography. Racemose hemangioma is actually an anomalous arteriovenous communication with a tangle of vascular channels at the site of the communication (6).

Iris hemangioma rarely comes to histopathologic confirmation. Most are benign and nonprogressive and require no treatment. They usually are sporadic and not associated with the vascular phakomatoses.

SELECTED REFERENCES

1. Ferry AP. Hemangiomas of the iris and ciliary body. Do they exist? A search for a histologically proved case. *Int Ophthalmol Clin* 1972;12:177–194.
2. Shields JA, Shields CL. *Intraocular tumors. A text and atlas.* Philadelphia: WB Saunders, 1992:255–257.
3. Prost M. Cavernous hemangioma of the iris. *Ophthalmologica* 1987;195:183–187.
4. Ruttum MS, Mittelman D, Singh P. Iris hemangiomas in infants with periorbital capillary hemangiomas. *J Pediatr Strabismus* 1993;30:331–333.
5. Naidoff MA, Kenyon DR, Green WR. Iris hemangioma and abnormal retinal vasculature in a case of diffuse congenital hemangiomatosis. *Am J Ophthalmol* 1971;72:633–644.
6. Shields JA, Shields CL, O'Rourk T. Racemose hemangioma of the iris. *Br J Ophthalmol* 1996;80:770–771.

Iris Hemangioma

Figs. 13-73 through 13-75 courtesy of Dr. Mark Ruttum. From Ruttum MS, Mittelman D, Singh P. Iris hemangiomas in infants with periorbital capillary hemangiomas. *J Pediatr Strabismus* 1993;30:331–333.

Figs. 13-76 through 13-78 from Shields JA, Shields CL, O'Rourk T. Racemose hemangioma of the iris. *Br J Ophthalmol* 1996;80:770–771.

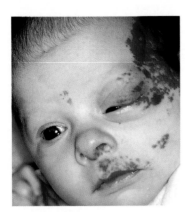

Figure 13-73. Facial capillary hemangioma involving the left eyelid in an infant.

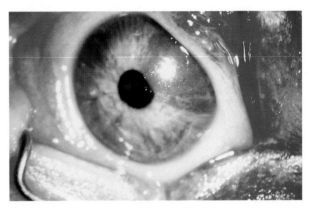

Figure 13-74. Capillary hemangioma involving the superotemporal quadrant of the ipsilateral iris in the child shown in Fig. 13-73.

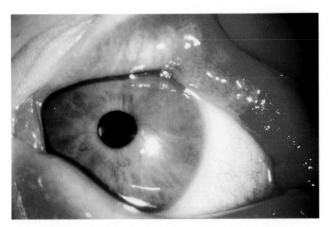

Figure 13-75. Appearance of the iris after spontaneous regression of the cutaneous and iris lesion.

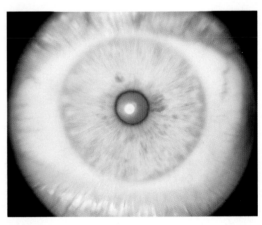

Figure 13-76. Racemose hemangioma of the iris in a 40-year-old man.

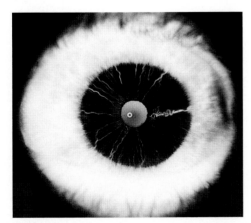

Figure 13-77. Early fluorescein angiogram of the iris lesion shown in Fig. 13-76 depicting a tortuous artery feeding the vascular anomaly.

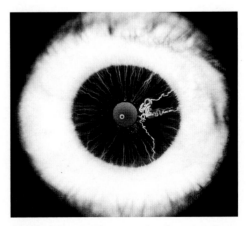

Figure 13-78. Later angiogram showing complex vascular lesion and draining vein inferiorly.

CHAPTER 14

Osseous, Myogenic, Neurogenic, Fibrous, and Histiocytic Tumors of the Uvea

CHOROIDAL OSTEOMA

Choroidal osteoma is a benign tumor that is composed of bone (1–6). It can be unilateral or bilateral and most often is diagnosed in young adult females (7). Familial cases have been seen (8,9). It appears as a yellow-orange placoid, juxtapapillary, or macular lesion with well-defined margins that may show pseudopodia-like projections. It can show slow enlargement (10), become decalcified (11), and develop choroidal neovascularization.

Fluorescein angiography shows patchy early hyperfluorescence and intense late staining of the lesion (1–5). Vascular tufts sometimes are seen emerging through the bone. A-scan and B-scan ultrasonography show a highly reflective echo that persists at lower sensitivity. Computed tomography reveals a choroidal plaque with bone density. Magnetic resonance imaging shows the tumor to be hyperintense to vitreous on the T1-weighted image and hypointense to vitreous on the T2-weighted image (12). The pathogenesis of choroidal osteoma is unknown. Serum calcium, phosphorus, and alkaline phosphatase levels generally are normal.

Histopathologically, choroidal osteoma is composed of pure bone at the level of the choroid. The overlying retinal pigment epithelium usually is intact (1–3). It usually is managed by observation. If subretinal neovascularization threatens vision, laser photocoagulation can be employed (13,14). The visual prognosis is unpredictable. Most patients retain fair vision in spite of a subfoveal tumor location. Bilateral total blindness has been recognized (15).

SELECTED REFERENCES

1. Gass JDM, Guerry RK, Jack RL, et al. Choroidal osteoma. *Arch Ophthalmol* 1978;96:428–435.
2. Shields JA, Shields CL. *Intraocular tumors. A text and atlas.* Philadelphia: WB Saunders, 1992:261–271.
3. Williams AT, Font RL, Van Dyk HJ, et al. Osseous choristoma of the choroid simulating a choroidal melanoma. *Arch Ophthalmol* 1978;96:1874–1877.
4. Joffe L, Shields JA, Fitzgerald JR. Osseous choristoma of the choroid. *Arch Ophthalmol* 1978;96:1809–1812.
5. Shields CL, Shields JA, Augsburger JJ. Choroidal osteoma. *Surv Ophthalmol* 1988;33:17–27.
6. Augsburger JJ, Shields JA, Rife CJ. Bilateral choroidal osteoma after nine years. *Can J Ophthalmol* 1979;14: 281–284.
7. Fava GE, Brown GC, Shields JA, Brooker G. Choroidal osteoma in a 6-year-old child. *J Pediatr Ophthalmol Strabismus* 1980;17:203–205.
8. Cunha SL. Osseous choristoma of the choroid. A familial disease. *Arch Ophthalmol* 1984;102:1052–1054.
9. Noble KG. Bilateral choroidal osteoma in three siblings. *Am J Ophthalmol* 1990;109:656–660.
10. Shields JA, Shields CL, De Potter P, Belmont JB. Progressive enlargement of a choroidal osteoma. *Arch Ophthalmol* 1995;113:819–820.
11. Trimble SB, Schatz H, Schneider GB. Spontaneous decalcification of a choroidal osteoma. *Ophthalmology* 1988;95:631–634.
12. De Potter P, Shields JA, Shields CL, Rao V. Magnetic resonance imaging of choroidal osteoma. *Retina* 1991; 11:221–223.
13. Grand MG, Burgess DB, Singerman LJ, Ramsey J. Choroidal osteoma. Treatment of associated subretinal neovascular membranes. *Retina* 1984;4:84–90.
14. Morrison DL, Magargal LE, Ehrlich DR, Goldberg RE, Robb-Doyle E. Review of choroidal osteoma: successful krypton red laser photocoagulation of an associated subretinal neovascular membrane involving the fovea. *Ophthal Surg* 1987;18:299–303.
15. Shields JA, Shields CL, Ellis J, De Potter P. Bilateral choroidal osteoma associated with bilateral total blindness. *Retina* 1996;16:445–447.

Choroidal Osteoma—Clinical Features

Figs. 14-5 and 14-6 from Shields JA, Shields CL, De Potter P, Belmont JB. Progressive enlargement of a choroidal osteoma. *Arch Ophthalmol* 1995;113:819–820.

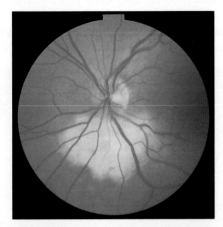

Figure 14-1. Small choroidal osteoma inferior to the optic disc in a 30-year-old woman. The patient was suspected to have a choroidal metastasis elsewhere, and a breast biopsy was done in hopes of locating the primary tumor.

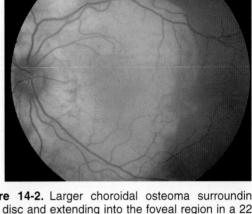

Figure 14-2. Larger choroidal osteoma surrounding the optic disc and extending into the foveal region in a 22-year-old woman.

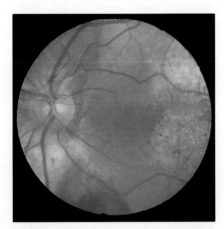

Figure 14-3. Irregular choroidal osteoma inferior to the optic disc and extending into the foveal region in a 16-year-old girl.

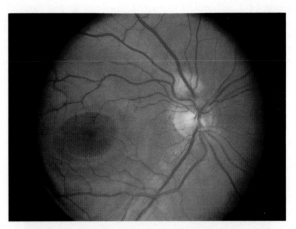

Figure 14-4. Opposite eye of the patient shown in Fig. 14-3 showing small early choroidal osteoma superior to the optic disc. The same area was photographed 2 years earlier and no lesion was seen.

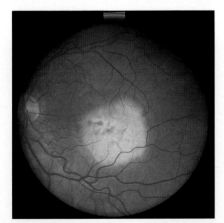

Figure 14-5. Small choroidal osteoma in the foveal region in a 20-year-old woman. The lesion originally was diagnosed as an amelanotic choroidal nevus. The lesion subsequently showed progressive growth.

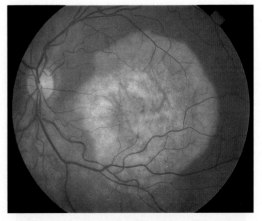

Figure 14-6. Same tumor shown in Fig. 14-5 as it looked 6 years later. Note the significant enlargement.

Choroidal Osteoma—Clinical Variations and Fluorescein Angiography

Figs. 14-7 and 14-8 courtesy of Dr. Larry Magargal. From Morrison DL, Magargal LE, Ehrlich DR, Goldberg RE, Robb-Doyle E. Review of choroidal osteoma: successful krypton red laser photocoagulation of an associated subretinal neovascular membrane involving the fovea. *Ophthal Surg* 1987;18:299–303.

Figs. 14-9 through 14-12 from Shields JA, Shields CL, Ellis J, De Potter P. Bilateral choroidal osteoma associated with bilateral total blindness. *Retina* 1996;16:445–447.

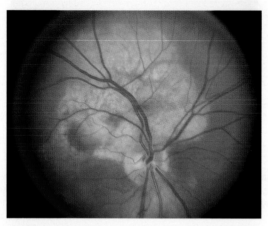

Figure 14-7. Choroidal osteoma superior to the optic disc with choroidal neovascular membrane extending into the foveal region.

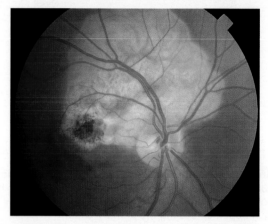

Figure 14-8. Same lesion shown in Fig. 14-7 after laser photocoagulation to the juxtafoveal neovascular membrane. Note the proliferation of the retinal pigment epithelium at the site of the photocoagulation adjacent to the foveola.

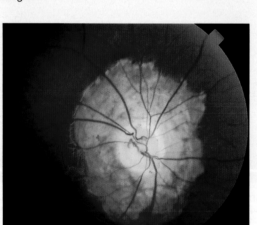

Figure 14-9. Choroidal osteomas associated with bilateral total blindness. Fundus photograph of the right eye showing circumpapillary lesion and optic atrophy.

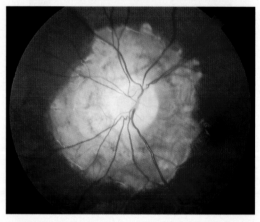

Figure 14-10. Appearance of the left eye showing similar findings.

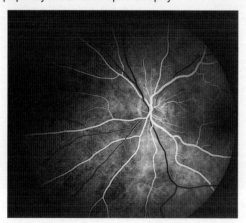

Figure 14-11. Early fluorescein angiogram of the lesion shown in Fig. 14-1 showing minimal fluorescence of the lesion.

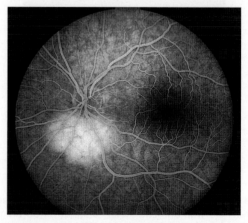

Figure 14-12. Late fluorescein angiogram showing more intense hyperfluorescence of the lesion.

Choroidal Osteoma—Ultrasonography, Computed Tomography, Magnetic Resonance Imaging, and Pathology

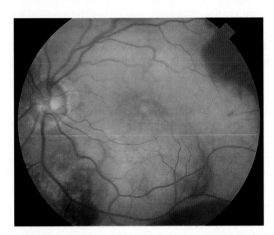

Figure 14-13. Large irregular choroidal osteoma in the macular region of a 43-year-old woman. She had bilateral lesions and previously was diagnosed as having atypical Best's disease at one institution and atypical macular degeneration at another institution.

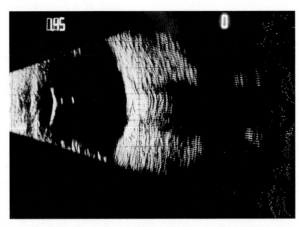

Figure 14-14. B-scan ultrasonogram of the same patient shown in Fig. 14-13 showing placoid lesion in the posterior pole with acoustic shadow in orbital fat posterior to the lesion.

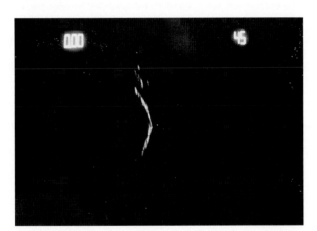

Figure 14-15. B-scan ultrasonogram at lower sensitivity showing persistence of the placoid calcific lesion after soft-tissue echoes have resolved.

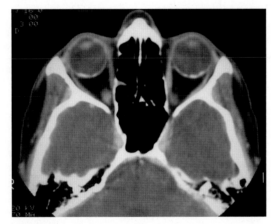

Figure 14-16. Axial computed tomogram of the same patient showing bilateral placoid lesions of bone density in the posterior choroid.

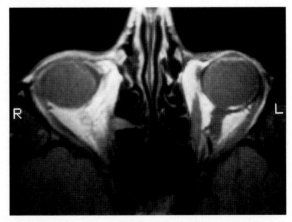

Figure 14-17. Axial magnetic resonance imaging of the same patient showing lesion in the left eye that is hyperintense to vitreous. The osteoma in the right eye is not clearly shown in this cut.

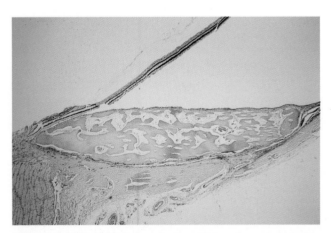

Figure 14-18. Pathology of choroidal osteoma showing plaque of bone causing choroidal thickening (hematoxylin–eosin, original magnification × 20).

MYOGENIC TUMORS

Myogenic tumors of the uvea include leiomyoma and rhabdomyosarcoma. Leiomyoma is a benign, smooth-muscle tumor that generally occurs in the uterus, but can arise in the uveal tract, most often in the iris and ciliary body (1–4). It is clinically similar to an amelanotic melanoma by producing sentinel blood vessels and extending through the sclera (5). Recent observations have suggested that, in contrast to melanoma, it more often occurs in young adult females and may arise in the suprauveal space, rather than in the uveal stroma (3). If the diagnosis can be made clinically, iris tumors usually can be observed without treatment. Larger growing ciliary body tumors may be managed best by local resection of the tumor by a partial lamellar sclerouvectomy (3–5).

Rhabdomyosarcoma, a malignant mesenchymal tumor of childhood, rarely occurs in the uveal tract, but rather usually in the iris or ciliary body (6–8). It has not been described in the choroid. The pathogenesis of skeletal muscle tumors in the eye is uncertain. Although the diagnosis is rarely made clinically, the recommended treatment is local resection of the tumor. Rarely, the tumor may be so large that enucleation is necessary.

SELECTED REFERENCES

1. Green WR. The uveal tract. In: Spencer WH, Font RL, Green WR, Howes EL Jr, Jakobiec FA, Zimmerman LE, eds. *Ophthalmic pathology. An atlas and textbook,* vol. 3, 4th ed. Philadelphia: WB Saunders Co, 1996: 1653.
2. Shields JA, Shields CL. *Intraocular tumors. A text and atlas.* Philadelphia: WB Saunders, 1992:274–281.
3. Shields JA, Shields CL, Eagle RC Jr, De Potter P. Observations on seven cases of intraocular leiomyoma. The 1993 Byron Demorest Lecture. *Arch Ophthalmol* 1994;112:521–528.
4. Shields JA, Shields CL, Eagle RC Jr. Mesectodermal leiomyoma of the ciliary body managed by partial lamellar iridocyclochoroidectomy. *Ophthalmology* 1989;96:1369–1376.
5. Shields CL, Shields JA, Varenhorst M. Transcleral leiomyoma. *Ophthalmology* 1991;98:84–87.
6. Woyke S, Chevinot R. Rhabdomyosarcoma of the iris. Report of the first recorded case. *Br J Ophthalmol* 1972;56:60–64.
7. Elsas FJ, Mroczek EC, Kelly DR, Specht CS. Primary rhabdomyosarcoma of the iris. *Arch Ophthalmol* 1991; 109:982–984.
8. Wilson ME, McClatchey SK, Zimmerman LE. Rhabdomyosarcoma of the ciliary body. *Ophthalmology* 1990;97:1484–1488.

Uveal Leiomyoma—Clinical Variations

Uveal leiomyoma can assume different clinical appearances, but it is usually a nonpigmented tumor of the ciliary body region. Even though it is amelanotic, it can appear pigmented on clinical examination. However, it transmits light readily with transillumination. It occasionally can erode through the sclera and appear in the epibulbar tissues. The clinical features that serve to differentiate leiomyoma from ciliary body melanoma have been described (3). The cases depicted here were all confirmed histopathologically to be leiomyoma.

Figs. 14-23 and 14-24 from Shields CL, Shields JA, Varenhorst M. Transcleral leiomyoma. *Ophthalmology* 1991;98:84–87.

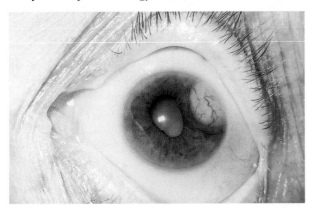

Figure 14-19. Leiomyoma involving the iris in an elderly woman. The lesion also extended to involve the ciliary body, and it is uncertain whether it originated in the iris or the ciliary body.

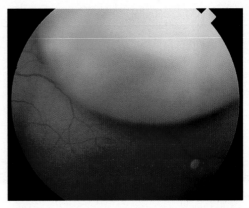

Figure 14-20. Leiomyoma arising from the ciliary body and peripheral choroid in a 24-year-old man. Note the red-orange color to the lesion as it transmits light.

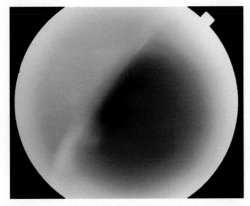

Figure 14-21. Inferotemporal ciliochoroidal leiomyoma in a 68-year-old man. The large mass aroused clinical suspicion of melanoma, and enucleation was performed.

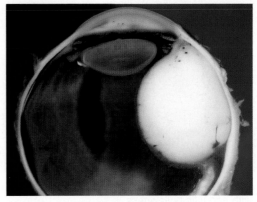

Figure 14-22. Grossly sectioned eye shown in Fig. 14-21. Note that the tumor appears entirely nonpigmented on cross-sectional view.

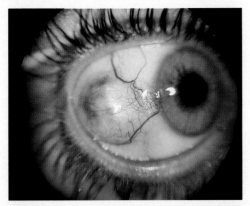

Figure 14-23. Transcleral extension of ciliary body leiomyoma in a 31-year-old woman. The red-orange tumor was removed by local excision. The uveal tract over the lesion was intact and not disrupted at surgery, suggesting that the tumor arose in the suprauveal space.

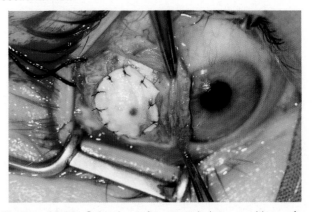

Figure 14-24. Scleral graft sutured into position after removal of the lesion shown in Fig. 14-23. The patient had an excellent recovery. Histopathologically, the lesion proved to be a vascular leiomyoma.

Uveal Leiomyoma—Clinicopathologic Correlation

Figs. 14-25 through 14-30 from Shields JA, Shields CL, Eagle RC. Mesectodermal leiomyoma of the ciliary body managed by partial lamellar iridocyclochoroidectomy. *Ophthalmology* 1989;96:1369–1376.

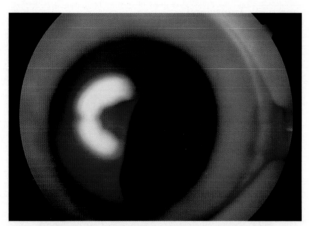

Figure 14-25. Ciliochoroidal mass nasally in the right eye of an 11-year-old girl.

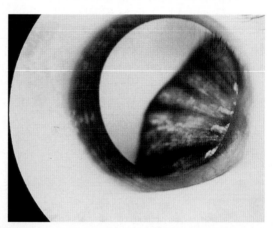

Figure 14-26. Fluorescein angiogram in recirculation phase showing mild hyperfluorescence of the mass.

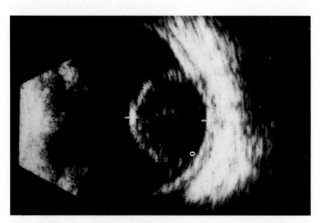

Figure 14-27. B-scan ultrasonogram showing dome-shaped mass with acoustic hollowness.

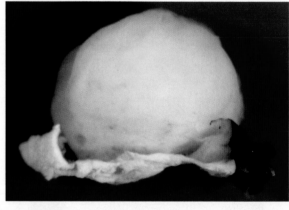

Figure 14-28. Appearance of the tumor after removal by partial lamellar sclerouvectomy showing that the lesion is nonpigmented.

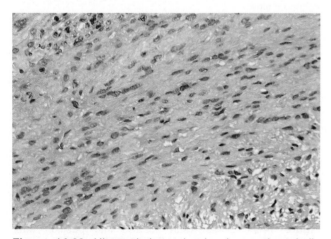

Figure 14-29. Histopathology showing low-grade spindle cells with abundant intercellular collagen.

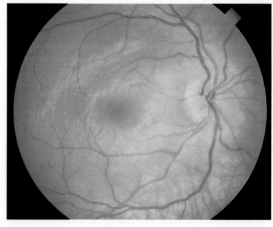

Figure 14-30. Appearance of the posterior pole after 9 years. The patient still maintained excellent vision, and there was no tumor recurrence.

Iris and Ciliary Body Rhabdomyosarcoma

Iris and ciliary body rhabdomyosarcomas are rare, but well-documented cases have been reported (6–8).

Figs. 14-31 through 14-35 courtesy of Dr. Frederick Elsas. From Elsas FJ, Mroczek EC, Kelly DR, Specht CS. Primary rhabdomyosarcoma of the iris. *Arch Ophthalmol* 1991;109:982–984.

Figure 14-36 from Wilson ME, McClatchey SK, Zimmerman LE. Rhabdomyosarcoma of the ciliary body. *Ophthalmology* 1990;97:1484–1488.

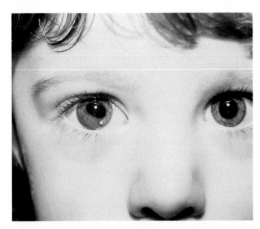

Figure 14-31. Facial photograph of a 2-year-old girl who developed fleshy iris mass inferotemporally in the right eye.

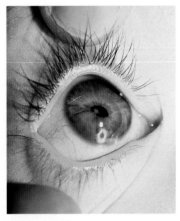

Figure 14-32. Closer view of the same iris lesion.

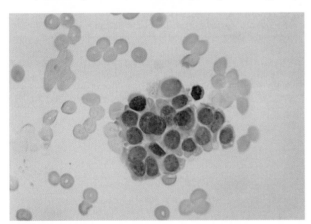

Figure 14-33. Fine-needle aspiration biopsy of the iris lesion showing a clump of malignant cells. The cytopathologist could not make a specific diagnosis (Papanicolaou, original magnification × 250).

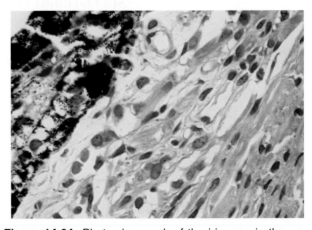

Figure 14-34. Photomicrograph of the iris area in the enucleated eye showing malignant strap cells with abundant eosinophilic cytoplasm (hematoxylin–eosin, original magnification × 200).

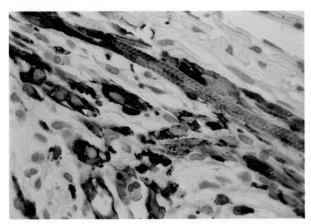

Figure 14-35. Photomicrograph of tumor showing cross-striations in some of the tumor cells (muscle-specific actin, original magnification × 200).

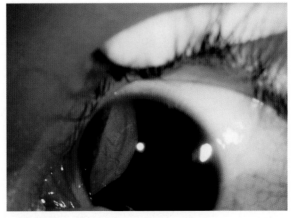

Figure 14-36. Rhabdomyosarcoma of the ciliary body in a 12-year-old boy. The diagnosis was made histopathologically after enucleation.

NEUROGENIC TUMORS

Neural tumors that can arise in the uveal tract include neurilemoma (schwannoma), neurofibroma, and primitive neuroectodermal tumor (1,2).

Uveal neurilemoma is a benign peripheral nerve-sheath tumor that arises from the ciliary nerves in the uveal tract. It can occur in the iris, ciliary body, or choroid, where it appears as a nonpigmented mass that may be impossible to differentiate from amelanotic melanoma. In rare instances, a neurilemoma can be pigmented and appear identical to a pigmented melanoma (3). Although most peripheral nerve-sheath tumors occur in patients with neurofibromatosis, most cases of uveal neurilemoma have been solitary lesions in patients who do not have neurofibromatosis. Most cases have been managed with enucleation or radiotherapy with the presumptive diagnosis of melanoma. Histopathologically, uveal neurilemoma is composed of a pure proliferation of Schwann cells. Fluorescein angiography and ultrasonography show findings similar to melanoma.

Neurofibroma can occur in the uveal tract, usually in association with von Recklinghausen's neurofibromatosis (4). Patients with neurofibromatosis can have glial–melanocytic hamartoma of the iris (Lisch nodules) and a diffuse choroidal thickening due to excess neural and melanocytic tissue in the choroid.

Primitive neuroectodermal tumor and granular cell tumor, a neoplasm of possible Schwann cell origin, also has been recognized in the uvea.

SELECTED REFERENCES

1. Shields JA, Shields CL. *Intraocular tumors. A text and atlas.* Philadelphia: WB Saunders, 1992:285–294.
2. Shields JA, Sanborn GE, Kurz GH, Augsburger JJ. Benign peripheral nerve tumor of the choroid. *Ophthalmology* 1981;88:1322–1329.
3. Shields JA, Font RL, Eagle RC Jr, Shields CL, Gass JDM. Melanotic schwannoma of the choroid: immunohistochemistry and electron microscopic observations. *Ophthalmology* 1994;101:843–849.
4. Klein RM, Glassman L. Neurofibromatosis of the choroid. *Am J Ophthalmol* 1985;99:367–368.

Uveal Neurilemoma

Uveal neurilemoma (schwannoma) may be impossible to differentiate clinically from a nonpigmented choroidal melanoma. A clinicopathologic correlation is shown of a choroidal neurilemoma that was believed clinically to be a melanoma.

Figs. 14-37 through 14-42 from Shields JA, Sanborn GE, Kurz GH, Augsburger JJ. Benign peripheral nerve tumor of the choroid. *Ophthalmology* 1981;88:1322–1329.

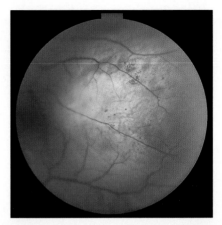

Figure 14-37. Fundus appearance of nonpigmented choroidal mass temporal to the foveal area in a 30-year-old man.

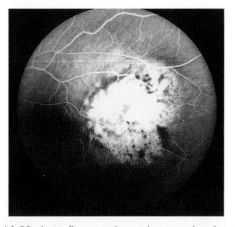

Figure 14-38. Late fluorescein angiogram showing moderately intense hyperfluorescence of the tumor.

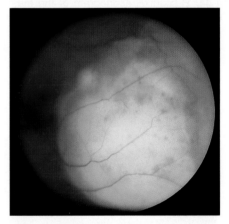

Figure 14-39. Appearance of the lesion 1 year later after it had demonstrated growth in spite of treatment with a radioactive plaque.

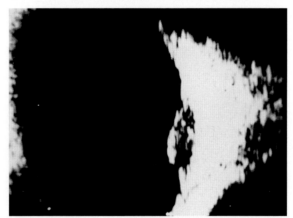

Figure 14-40. B-scan ultrasonogram showing the mass with acoustic hollowness and choroidal excavation.

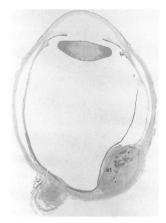

Figure 14-41. Low-power photomicrograph of sectioned eye showing elevated choroidal mass.

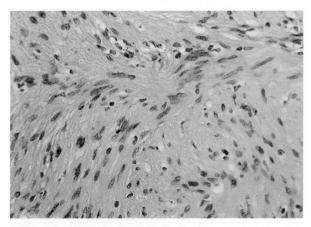

Figure 14-42. Photomicrograph showing abundant uniform spindle cells with abundant extracellular collagen. Electron microscopy confirmed that the tumor was composed of Schwann cells (hematoxylin–eosin, original magnification × 150).

Uveal Melanotic Schwannoma

In some instances, a neurilemoma can be pigmented. In such cases, its differentiation from melanoma may be impossible.

Figs. 14-43 through 14-48 from Shields JA, Font RL, Eagle RC Jr, Shields CL, Gass JDM. Melanotic schwannoma of the choroid: immunohistochemistry and electron microscopic observations. *Ophthalmology* 1994;101:843–849.

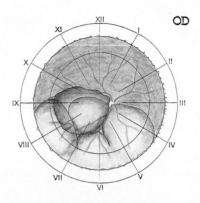

Figure 14-43. Fundus drawing of diffuse pigmented choroidal mass in a 21-year-old woman.

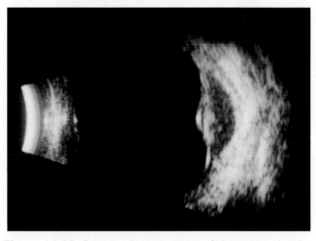

Figure 14-44. B-scan ultrasonogram of the mass showing acoustic hollowness and slight choroidal excavation.

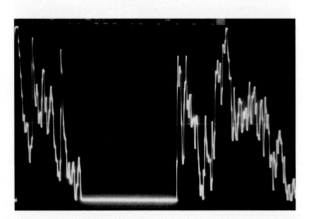

Figure 14-45. A-scan ultrasonogram showing decreasing amplitude reflectivity in the mass.

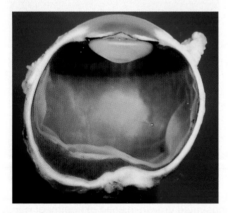

Figure 14-46. Sectioned eye after enucleation showing diffuse pigmented choroidal mass.

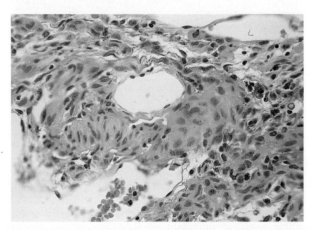

Figure 14-47. Histopathology showing whorls of benign spindle cells (hematoxylin-eosin, original magnification × 150).

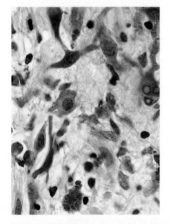

Figure 14-48. Histopathology showing whorls of benign spindle cells, some of which contain dense cytoplasmic pigment (hematoxylin–eosin, original magnification × 250).

Neurofibroma and Primitive Neuroectodermal Tumor

Figs. 14-49 and 14-50 courtesy of Dr. Richard Klein. From Klein RM, Glassman L. Neurofibromatosis of the choroid. *Am J Ophthalmol* 1985;99:367–368.

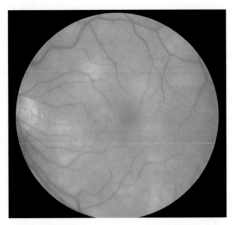

Figure 14-49. Choroidal neurofibromatosis. Diffuse choroidal thickening in a patient with neurofibromatosis.

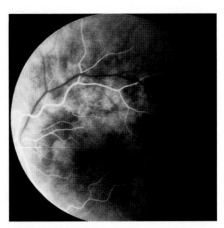

Figure 14-50. Fluorescein angiogram in vascular filling phase of the area shown in Fig. 14-49. Note the diffuse hyperfluorescence due to defects in the retinal pigment epithelium and the thickened choroid from excess neural and melanocytic proliferation.

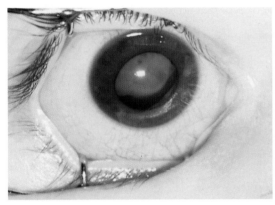

Figure 14-51. Unusual ciliary body tumor, possibly a primitive neuroectodermal tumor of the ciliary body and peripheral choroid. Photomicrograph showing fleshy-pink peripheral fundus mass in a 16-month-old girl. A similar tumor occurred on the child's neck at birth.

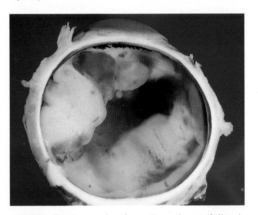

Figure 14-52. Photograph of sectioned eye following enucleation of the eye shown in Fig. 14-51. Note the dome-shaped mass of the ciliary body and peripheral choroid and secondary retinal detachment.

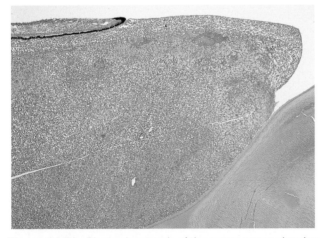

Figure 14-53. Photomicrograph of the same tumor showing mass arising from the ciliary body region.

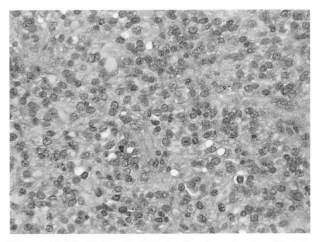

Figure 14-54. Photomicrograph showing sheets of poorly differentiated cells. Although there was no uniform agreement among the ophthalmic pathologists who reviewed the case, most favored the diagnosis of primitive neuroectodermal tumor.

FIBROUS AND HISTIOCYTIC TUMORS

Fibrous and histiocytic tumors of the uveal tract are very uncommon. We are aware of a case of fibrous histiocytoma of the choroid, a tumor that occurs more often in the orbit (1). It has been known to produce a large nonpigmented choroidal mass that simulates an amelanotic melanoma, neurilemoma, or leiomyoma.

Histiocytic disorders sometimes can involve the uveal tract. Juvenile xanthogranuloma usually is considered to be an inflammatory condition, but it is included here because it generally assumes tumorous proportions. It is best known to affect the iris in young children, but it can occur in the posterior uvea as well (2,3). Of the histiocytic X disorders, Letterer–Siwe disease is known to cause a diffuse choroidal infiltration (4,5).

SELECTED REFERENCES

1. Shields JA. *Diagnosis and management of orbital tumors.* Philadelphia: WB Saunders, 1989:199–201.
2. Shields JA, Eagle RC, Shields CL, Collins MLZ, De Potter P. Iris juvenile xanthogranuloma studied by immunohistochemistry and flow cytometry. *Ophthalmic Surg Lasers* 1997;98:40–44.
3. DeBarge LR, Chan CC, Greenberg SC, McLean IW, Yannuzzi LA, Nussenblatt RB. Chorioretinal, iris, and ciliary body infiltration by juvenile xanthogranuloma masquerading as uveitis. *Surv Ophthalmol* 1994;39:65–71.
4. Angell LK, Burton TC. Posterior choroidal involvement in Letterer–Siwe disease. *J Pediatr Ophthalmol Strabismus* 1978;15:79–81.
5. Mittelman D, Apple DJ, Goldberg MF. Ocular involvement in Letterer–Siwe disease. *Am J Ophthalmol* 1973;75:261–265.

Fibrous Histiocytoma, Juvenile Xanthogranuloma, and Histiocytosis X

Figs. 14-57 and 14-58 from Shields JA, Eagle RC Jr, Shields CL, Collins MLZ, De Potter P. Iris juvenile xanthogranuloma studied by immunohistochemistry and flow cytometry. *Ophthalmic Surg Lasers* 1997;98:40–44.

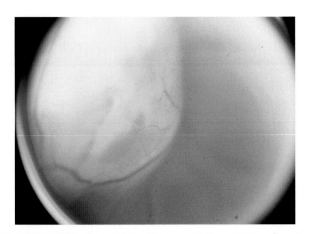

Figure 14-55. Choroidal fibrous histiocytoma. Fundus appearance of nonpigmented choroidal mass. The eye was enucleated because of suspicion of amelanotic choroidal melanoma. (Courtesy of Dr. Oscar Croxatto.)

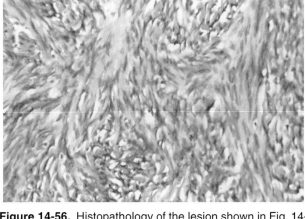

Figure 14-56. Histopathology of the lesion shown in Fig. 14-55 demonstrating the storiform pattern of the benign spindle cells. Special studies supported the diagnosis of fibrous histiocytoma. (Courtesy of Dr. Oscar Croxatto.)

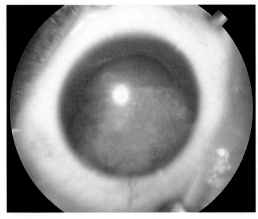

Figure 14-57. Juvenile xanthogranuloma of the iris in a 19-month-old child.

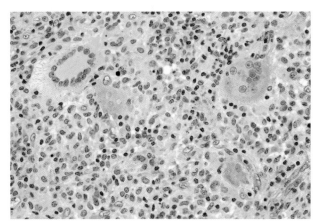

Figure 14-58. Histopathology of the lesion shown in Fig. 14-57 demonstrating granulomatous inflammation with atypical Touton giant cells (hematoxylin–eosin, original magnification × 200).

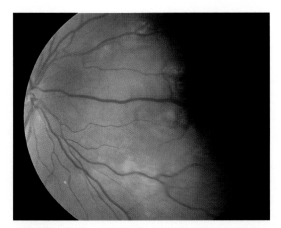

Figure 14-59. Diffuse choroidal thickening due to juvenile xanthogranuloma. There was also histopathologically confirmed iris involvement. The lesion responded to corticosteroids. (Courtesy of Dr. Lawrence Yannuzzi.)

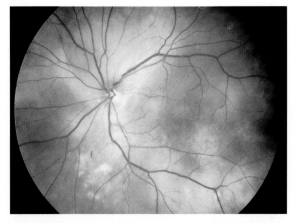

Figure 14-60. Choroidal involvement with histiocytosis X. Diffuse, irregular, posterior choroidal thickening. The patient was diagnosed as having histiocytosis X based on systemic findings and a gingival biopsy. It responded to ocular radiotherapy. (Courtesy of Dr. Thomas Aaberg Sr.)

PART II

Tumors of the Retina
and Optic Disc

CHAPTER 15

Retinoblastoma

RETINOBLASTOMA

Details regarding general principles, clinical features, genetics, differential diagnosis, diagnostic techniques, management, pathology, and prognosis are discussed in detail elsewhere (1). Retinoblastoma is the most common intraocular malignancy of childhood, occurring in about 1 in 15,000 live births. It can be unilateral or bilateral, with the bilateral cases invariably representing germinal mutations. The familial form has been associated with a deletion of the long arm of chromosome 13. Patients with this genetic abnormality are recognized to have a predisposition to develop a number of second tumors, particularly soft-tissue sarcomas (1–3). The familial form of retinoblastoma also is associated with a higher incidence of pinealoblastoma, a tumor that is very similar to retinoblastoma from embryologic, anatomic, and immunologic standpoints (4). Affected patients sometimes can have overt clinical signs of the 13q syndrome and occasionally holoprosencephaly (1).

Clinically, retinoblastoma begins as a small transparent lesion in the sensory retina that easily may be overlooked ophthalmoscopically (1). As the tumor enlarges, it becomes opaque white and develops a dilated retinal feeding artery and draining vein. A secondary retinal detachment can occur. A larger tumor can assume an exophytic growth pattern, endophytic growth pattern, or a combination of the two. The exophytic pattern is characterized by growth of the tumor toward the subretinal space, producing an overlying retinal detachment. The endophytic pattern is characterized by seeding of tumor cells into the overlying vitreous, obscuring a clear view of the retina. The less common diffuse growth pattern is characterized by flat growth of the tumor (5). It can simulate an inflammatory process, which can lead to a long delay in diagnosis.

Retinoblastoma usually is diagnosed in the first 3 years of life, but it can be congenital (6) or it can have its clinical onset in older children (7). More advanced tumors can cause secondary glaucoma (8) or signs of orbital cellulitis (9). It can extend extrasclerally and present as an advanced fungating mass. In some cases, retinoblastoma is known to undergo spontaneous regression or arrest, more commonly called a retinoma or retinocytoma (1,10–12).

Pathologically, retinoblastoma has characteristic gross and microscopic features (1,12). Grossly, it is a white tumor often with foci of chalky calcification. Microscopically, it is a neuroblastic tumor with small round cells. The better-differentiated tumors contain Flexner–Wintersteiner rosettes and fleurettes, signs of photoreceptor differentiation in the tumor.

The diagnosis of retinoblastoma is best made by recognition of its typical clinical features using indirect ophthalmoscopy and slit-lamp biomicroscopy (1). Fluorescein angiography shows a vascular tumor that fills rapidly with fluorescein and shows later hyperfluorescence (13). Ultrasonography and computed tomography can assist in making the diagnosis by demonstrating an intraocular mass that contains calcium. Computed tomography or magnetic resonance imaging can be used to detect gross optic nerve extension or associated pinealoblastoma (1).

Management of retinoblastoma has become a complex issue (1,14). Enucleation and external beam irradiation have been the standard treatments for large tumors (15,16). Cryotherapy (17), laser photocoagulation (18,19), and plaque brachytherapy (20) have been used for smaller tumors. More recently, techniques of chemoreduction or chemothermotherapy have gained popularity (21–23). In many instances, combinations of these treatments are necessary to achieve good tumor control. The management of retinoblastoma generally should be performed by ocular oncologists who have had experience making the complex decisions that are necessary in these cases.

SELECTED REFERENCES

1. Shields JA, Shields CL. *Intraocular tumors. A text and atlas.* Philadelphia: WB Saunders 1992:305–391.
2. Abramson DH, Ellsworth RM, Zimmerman LE. Nonocular cancer in retinoblastoma survivors. *Trans Am Acad Ophthalmol* 1976;81:454–456.
3. Roarty JD, McLean IW, Zimmerman LE. Incidence of second neoplasms in patients with bilateral retinoblastoma. *Ophthalmology* 1988;95:1583–1587.
4. De Potter P, Shields CL, Shields JA. Clinical variations of trilateral retinoblastoma. A report of 13 cases. *J Pediatr Ophthalmol Strabismus* 1994;31:26–31.
5. Shields JA, Shields CL, Eagle RC, Blair CJ. Spontaneous pseudohypopyon secondary to diffuse infiltrating retinoblastoma. *Arch Ophthalmol* 1988;106:1301-1302.
6. Plotsky D, Quinn G, Eagle RC, Shields JA, Granowetter L. Congenital retinoblastoma. *J Pediatr Ophthalmol Strabismus* 1987;24:120–123.
7. Shields CL, Shields JA, Shah P. Retinoblastoma in older children. *Ophthalmology* 1991;98:395–399.
8. Shields CL, Shields JA, Shields MB, Augsburger JJ. Prevalence and mechanisms of secondary intraocular pressure elevation in eyes with intraocular tumors. *Ophthalmology* 1987;94:839–846.
9. Shields JA, Shields CL, Suvarnamani C, Schroeder RP, De Potter P. Retinoblastoma manifesting as orbital cellulitis. *Am J Ophthalmol* 1991;112:442–449.
10. Gallie BL, Phillips RA, Ellsworth RM, Abramson DH. Significance of retinoma and phthisis bulbi for retinoblastoma. *Ophthalmology* 1982;89:1393–1399.
11. Margo C, Hidayat A, Kopelman J, et al. Retinocytoma. A benign variant of retinoblastoma. *Arch Ophthalmol* 1983;101;1519–1531.
12. McLean IW. Retinoblastomas, retinocytomas, and pseudoretinoblastomas. In: Spencer WH, ed. *Ophthalmic pathology. An atlas and textbook,* 4th ed. Philadelphia: WB Saunders, 1996:1340–1375.
13. Shields JA, Sanborn GE, Augsburger JJ, Orlock D, Donoso LA. Fluorescein angiography of retinoblastoma. *Retina* 1982;2:206–214.
14. Shields CL, Shields JA, De Potter P. New treatment modalities for retinoblastoma. *Curr Opin Ophthalmol* 1996;7:20–26.
15. Shields JA, Shields CL, De Potter P. Enucleation technique for children with retinoblastoma. *J Pediatr Ophthalmol Strabismus* 1992;29:213–215.
16. Hungerford JL, Toma NMG, Plowman PN, Kingston JE. External beam radiotherapy for retinoblastoma: I. Whole eye technique. *Br J Ophthalmol* 1995;79:109–111.
17. Shields JA, Parsons H, Shields CL, Giblin ME. The role of cryotherapy in the management of retinoblastoma. *Am J Ophthalmol* 1989;108:260–264.
18. Shields JA, Shields CL, Parsons H, Giblin ME. The role of photocoagulation in the management of retinoblastoma. *Arch Ophthalmol* 1990;108:205–208.
19. Shields CL, Shields JA, Kiratli H, De Potter P. Treatment of retinoblastoma with indirect ophthalmoscope laser photocoagulation. *J Pediatr Ophthalmol Strabismus* 1995;32:317–322.
20. Shields JA, Shields CL, De Potter P, Hernandez C, Brady LW. Plaque radiotherapy of retinoblastoma. *Int Ophthalmol Clin* 1993;33:107–117.
21. Shields CL, De Potter P, Himmelstein B, Shields JA, Meadows AT, Maris J. Chemoreduction in the initial management of intraocular retinoblastoma. *Arch Ophthalmol* 1996;114:1330–1338.
22. Gallie BL, Budning A, DeBoer G, et al. Chemotherapy with focal therapy can cure intraocular retinoblastoma without radiotherapy. *Arch Ophthalmol* 1996;114:1321–1328.
23. Murphree AL, Villablanca JG, Deegan WF, Sato JK, Malogolowkin M, Fisher A, Parker RK, Reed KE, Gomer CJ. Chemotherapy plus focal treatment in the management of intraocular retinoblastoma. *Arch Ophthalmol* 1996;114:1348–1356.

Retinoblastoma—Typical Clinical Features

In the early stages, retinoblastoma is a small transparent lesion in the retina. When it becomes slightly larger, it becomes opaque and more visible and eventually displays a dilated feeding retinal artery and draining vein. Chalky-white foci of calcification sometimes can be seen ophthalmoscopically in the tumor. Tumors in the foveal region can cause loss of visual fixation and strabismus, either esotropia or exotropia. With time, the tumor produces a characteristic white pupillary reflex (leukocoria). Most tumors are diagnosed following the development of leukocoria.

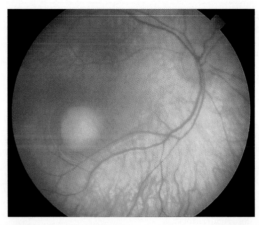

Figure 15-1. Small retinoblastoma inferior to the fovea in the right eye.

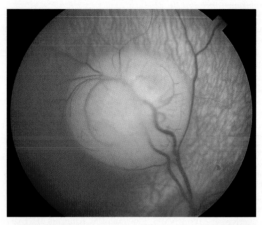

Figure 15-2. Slightly larger retinoblastoma superior to the optic disc. Note the dilated feeding artery and draining vein.

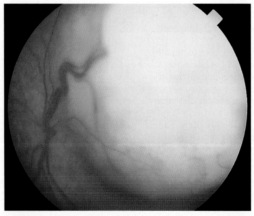

Figure 15-3. Larger retinoblastoma in the superior macular area. Note that the superior vessels coming from the disc are dilated and the inferior vessels are not dilated.

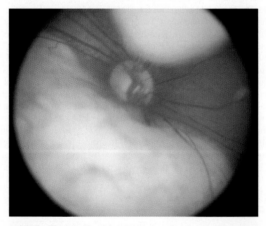

Figure 15-4. Two retinoblastomas adjacent to the optic disc. The superior tumor is seeding the overlying vitreous (endophytic) and the inferior tumor is still within the retina.

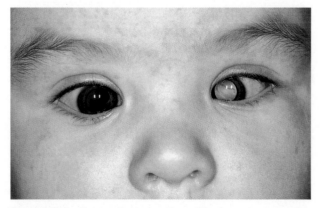

Figure 15-5. Esotropia and unilateral leukocoria secondary to retinoblastoma.

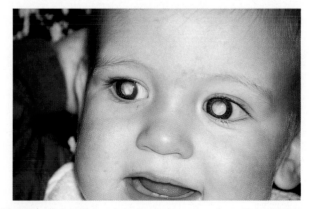

Figure 15-6. Bilateral leukocoria secondary to retinoblastoma.

Retinoblastoma—Exophytic and Endophytic Growth Patterns

Retinoblastoma begins in the sensory retina. With time, it can grow either into the subretinal area (exophytic growth pattern) or into the vitreous cavity (endophytic growth pattern). Advanced tumors may show both endophytic and exophytic components. Endophytic tumors sometimes can seed into the anterior chamber, simulating intraocular inflammation or infection. They often occur in somewhat older children.

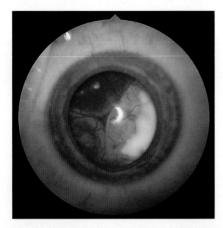

Figure 15-7. Exophytic growth pattern. Note that the solid tumor is to the *right* and a secondary retinal detachment (with subretinal tumor seeds) is to the *left*. Note that the retinal blood vessels are seen posterior to the clear lens.

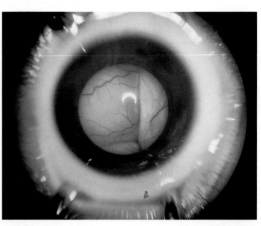

Figure 15-8. Exophytic growth pattern. In this instance, the tumor involves all lobes of the retinal detachment.

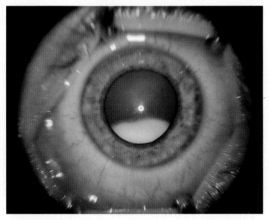

Figure 15-9. Endophytic growth pattern. Note the white tumor inferiorly with no overlying retinal vessels.

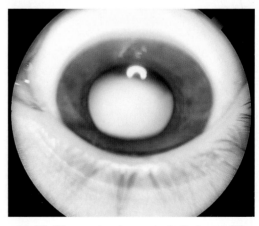

Figure 15-10. More extensive endophytic tumor filling most of the retrolental area.

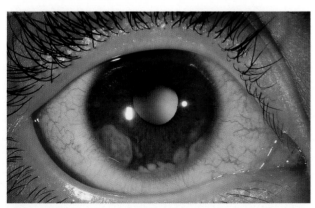

Figure 15-11. Anterior chamber seeding of endophytic retinoblastoma forming semisolid tumor nodules on the iris surface in a 6-year-old child.

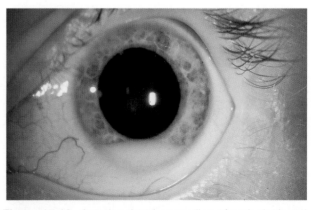

Figure 15-12. Anterior chamber seeding of endophytic retinoblastoma forming a "pseudohypopyon" in the inferior aspect of the anterior chamber.

Retinoblastoma—Diffuse Growth Pattern

Diffuse infiltrating retinoblastoma is an unusual variant in which the tumor grows in a flat, infiltrating pattern and does not appear as an elevated mass. It is usually unilateral and nonfamilial and is diagnosed in older children. Intraocular calcium usually is not demonstrable with ultrasonography or computed tomography. There is often a delay in diagnosis and misdirected therapy in such cases. Optic nerve invasion is frequently present and enucleation is generally the treatment of choice. A clinicopathologic correlation of a diffuse infiltrating retinoblastoma is illustrated.

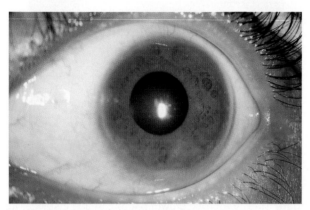

Figure 15-13. Small inferior "pseudohypopyon" in a 7-year-old child.

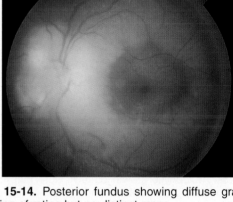

Figure 15-14. Posterior fundus showing diffuse gray-white thickening of retina but no distinct mass.

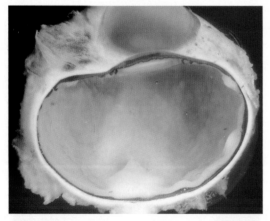

Figure 15-15. Section of enucleated eyes showing diffuse white thickening of retina.

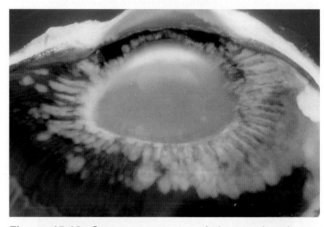

Figure 15-16. Gross appearance of the retrolental area showing characteristic seeding of white tumor cells in the ciliary body and zonule.

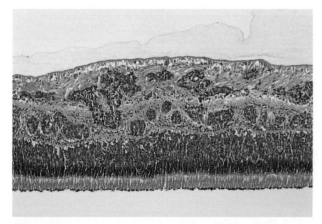

Figure 15-17. Cross-section of retina showing islands of retinoblastoma cells in the inner layers (hematoxylin–eosin, original magnification × 20).

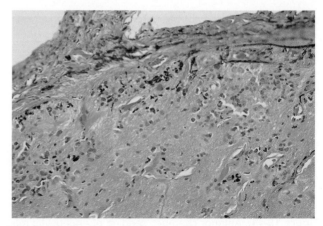

Figure 15-18. Cross-section of optic nerve showing scattered retinoblastoma cells (hematoxylin–eosin, original magnification × 20).

Retinoblastoma—Secondary Glaucoma and Orbital Cellulitis

In some instances, retinoblastoma can induce secondary glaucoma by any of several mechanisms. About 17% of eyes with newly diagnosed retinoblastoma have glaucoma and about 50% that come to enucleation have elevated intraocular pressure, usually secondary to iris neovascularization (neovascular glaucoma). Occasionally, a large retinoblastoma can become necrotic and produce inflammatory signs resembling orbital cellulitis.

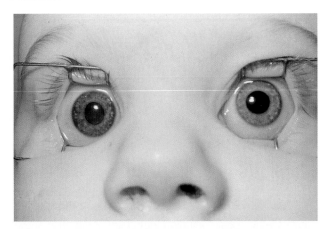

Figure 15-19. Acquired heterochromia iridis secondary to iris neovascularization. Note that the affected right iris is darker.

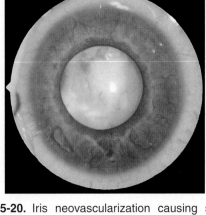

Figure 15-20. Iris neovascularization causing secondary glaucoma in an eye with a large retinoblastoma.

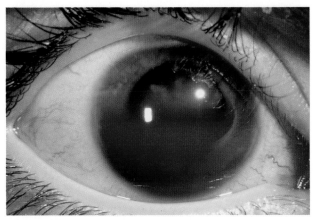

Figure 15-21. Spontaneous hyphema secondary to iris neovascularization in a child with retinoblastoma.

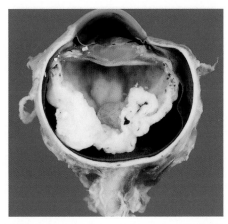

Figure 15-22. Section of enucleated eye shown in Fig. 15-21. Note the hyphema and the diffuse irregular white mass involving the entire sensory retina.

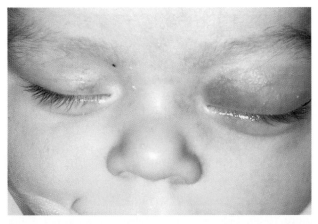

Figure 15-23. Signs of acute orbital cellulitis in the left eye of a child with necrotic retinoblastoma.

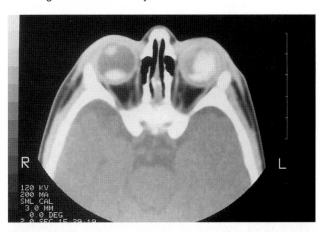

Figure 15-24. Axial computed tomogram of patient shown in Fig. 15-23 revealing retinoblastoma in both eyes. Even though there is periocular soft tissue swelling on the left side, there was no pathologic evidence of extraocular extension of the tumor.

Retinoblastoma—Massive Extraocular Extension

In some advanced instances, retinoblastoma can extend from the eye into the orbital soft tissues and cause massive extraocular involvement by the neoplasm. This is seen most often in underdeveloped countries where medical care is not readily available.

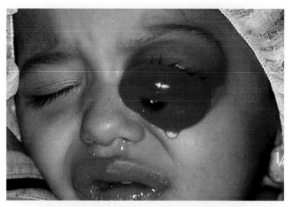

Figure 15-25. Massive proptosis and periocular edema secondary to retinoblastoma. (Courtesy of Dr. Amelda Pifano.)

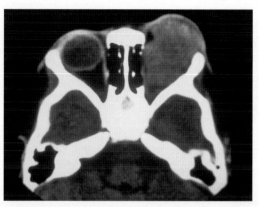

Figure 15-26. Axial computed tomogram of the child shown in Fig. 15-25 showing the globe and orbit filled by the neoplasm. (Courtesy of Dr. Amelda Pifano.)

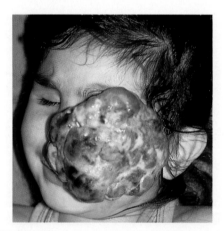

Figure 15-27. Massive extraocular extension of retinoblastoma. The opposite eye had developed phthisis secondary to spontaneous necrosis and regression of retinoblastoma.

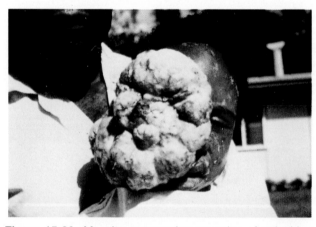

Figure 15-28. Massive extraocular extension of retinoblastoma due to unavailable medical care. (Courtesy of Dr. Jimmy Rodgers.)

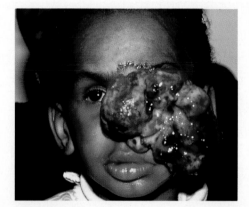

Figure 15-29. Massive extraocular extension of retinoblastoma. Treatment was refused by the parents when the tumor was recognized about 1 year earlier. (Photograph courtesy of Dr. Albert Biglan.)

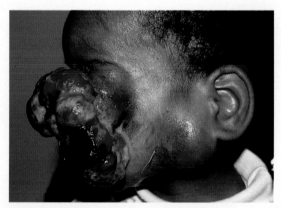

Figure 15-30. Side view of the patient shown in Fig. 15-29 showing metastasis to preauricular lymph nodes. (Courtesy of Dr. Albert Biglan.)

Retinoblastoma—Congenital Aggressive Type

Retinoblastoma generally is diagnosed between age 3 months and 3 years. However, it can be clinically evident at birth. Some congenital retinoblastomas are highly aggressive. An example of sporadic congenital retinoblastoma that eventually led to brain metastasis and death is cited.

Figs. 15-31 through 15-36 from Plotsky D, Quinn G, Eagle RC, Shields JA, Granowetter L. Congenital retinoblastoma. *J Pediatr Ophthalmol Strabismus* 1987;24: 120–123.

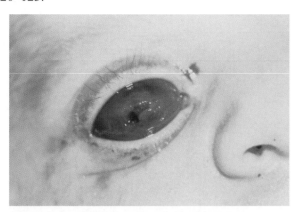

Figure 15-31. Extensive conjunctival and precorneal hemorrhage noted at birth.

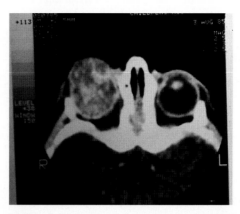

Figure 15-32. Axial computed tomogram showing marked enlargement of the right eye (buphthalmos). In spite of the buphthalmos, the calcified mass appeared to be confined to the eye. Enucleation was performed elsewhere and the globe was ruptured at the time of surgery.

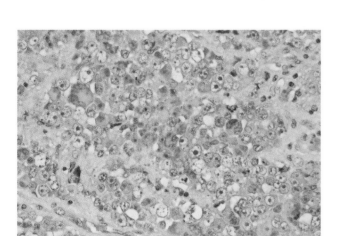

Figure 15-33. Histopathology showing anaplastic retinoblastoma cells (hematoxylin–eosin, original magnification × 200).

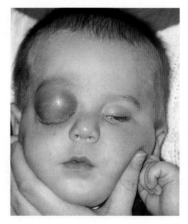

Figure 15-34. Clinical appearance a few months later when the child presented with orbital recurrence in spite of maximal chemotherapy and irradiation.

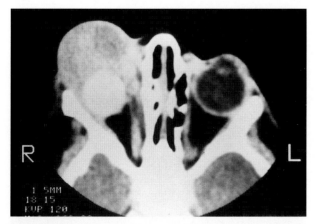

Figure 15-35. Axial computed tomogram showing massive tumor recurrence anterior the spherical orbital implant. Systemic evaluation revealed no metastasis and orbital exenteration was performed.

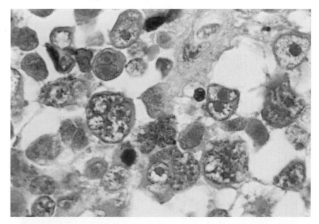

Figure 15-36. Histopathology of orbital recurrence showing highly atypical anaplastic cells. Brain metastasis became apparent a few months later (hematoxylin–eosin, original magnification × 300).

Retinoblastoma in Older Children

Although retinoblastoma generally is diagnosed between age 3 months and 3 years, it is not so widely recognized that retinoblastoma be first diagnosed in older children. The majority of such tumors have an endophytic (often diffuse) growth pattern and are unilateral and sporadic. Examples of retinoblastoma occurring at an older age are depicted.

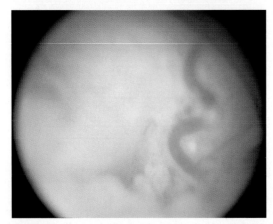

Figure 15-37. Endophytic retinoblastoma in a 6-year-old girl.

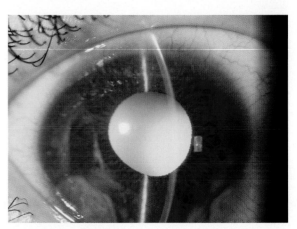

Figure 15-38. Endophytic retinoblastoma in an 8-year-old girl.

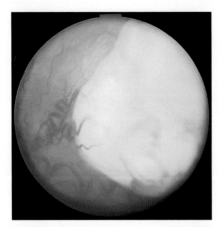

Figure 15-39. Retinoblastoma in a 13-year-old girl.

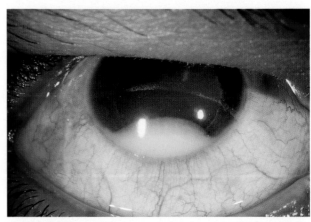

Figure 15-40. Retinoblastoma presenting as a pseudohypopyon in a 16-year-old girl.

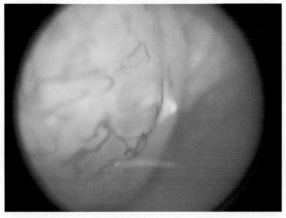

Figure 15-41. Retinoblastoma in a 17-year-old boy.

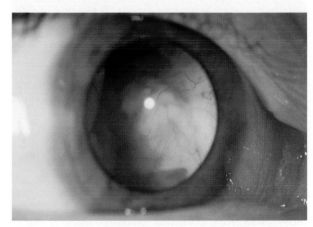

Figure 15-42. Retinoblastoma in an 18-year-old girl.

Retinoblastoma—Spontaneously Arrested and Spontaneously Regressed Tumors ("Retinocytoma")

Some retinoblastomas appear to be stationary and nonprogressive and may represent a "benign" variant of this disease. Terms like retinoma and retinocytoma have been applied to such lesions. We have employed the clinically descriptive terms spontaneously arrested retinoblastoma for tumors that appear clinically to have reached their final size and stopped growing. We prefer the term spontaneously regressed retinoblastoma for those that appear to have reached a certain size and then regressed. The latter appears to have surrounding alterations in the retinal pigment epithelium, similar to a tumor that has been treated successfully. Large spontaneously regressed retinoblastomas can cause phthisis bulbi.

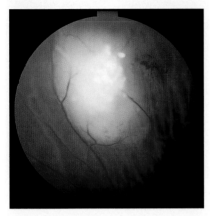

Figure 15-43. Spontaneously arrested retinoblastoma in a 30-year-old man showing calcified central area and surrounding semiopaque "fish-flesh" appearance.

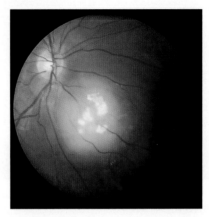

Figure 15-44. Spontaneously arrested retinoblastoma in a 12-year-old girl showing similar features to the one shown in Fig. 15-43.

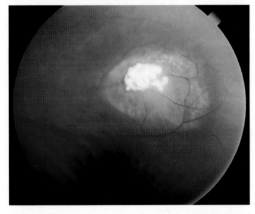

Figure 15-45. Spontaneously arrested retinoblastoma in a 25-year-old woman.

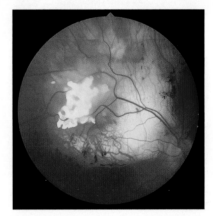

Figure 15-46. Spontaneously regressed retinoblastoma as originally seen in a 6-year-old girl. The lesion has subsequently remained stable for 15 years.

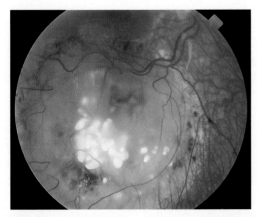

Figure 15-47. Spontaneously regressed retinoblastoma as originally seen in a 6-year-old boy. It has remained stable for 8 years.

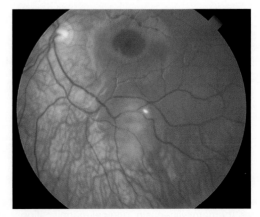

Figure 15-48. Spontaneously arrested retinoblastoma in the opposite eye of the child shown in Fig. 15-47. There was no family history of retinoblastoma.

Malignant Transformation of Retinocytoma

On rare occasions, a retinoblastoma that appears to have been arrested or regressed may show growth and malignant transformation. Such a case is depicted.

Figs. 15-49 through 15-54 from Eagle RC, Shields JA, Donoso LA, Milner RS. Malignant transformation of spontaneously regressed retinoblastoma, retinoma/retinocytoma variant. *Ophthalmology* 1989;96:1389–1395.

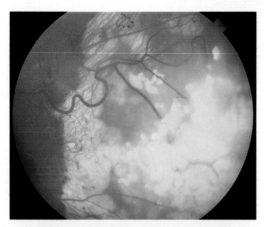

Figure 15-49. Spontaneously regressed retinoblastoma as seen initially in 3-year-old child.

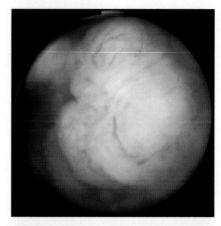

Figure 15-50. Same lesion shown at age 7 when there was florid regrowth of the tumor.

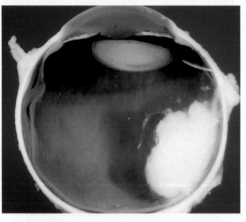

Figure 15-51. Enucleated eye showing fluffy white mass arising from the retina.

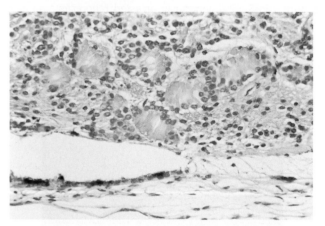

Figure 15-52. Photomicrograph showing well-differentiated tumor cells with fleurette formation (hematoxylin–eosin, original magnification × 100).

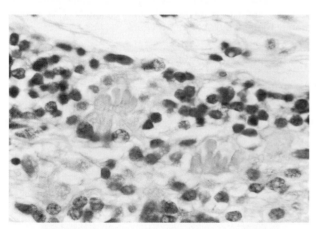

Figure 15-53. Photomicrograph showing a characteristic fleurettes (hematoxylin–eosin, original magnification × 200).

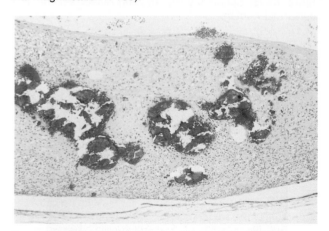

Figure 15-54. Photomicrograph in another area of the tumor showing foci of calcification in an area of viable, well-differentiated tumor cells, a typical feature of retinocytoma (hematoxylin–eosin, original magnification × 100).

Retinoblastoma Associated with Pinealoblastoma ("Trilateral Retinoblastoma")

A number of second tumors are known to occur in patients with the familial form of retinoblastoma. This subject is mentioned in *Atlas of Orbital Tumors*. One form of second tumor, termed trilateral retinoblastoma, is mentioned here. Trilateral retinoblastoma is a term applied to the occurrence, in the same patient, of bilateral retinoblastoma and pinealoblastoma or other parasellar intracranial tumors. A case of familial retinoblastoma in which multiple small tumors in each eye were controlled with radiotherapy but later a pinealoblastoma developed and proved to be fatal is depicted.

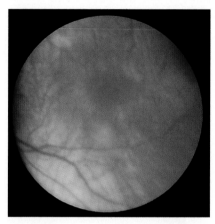

Figure 15-55. Fundus photograph of a small, subtle familial retinoblastoma near the fovea in the left eye of a 4-month-old girl.

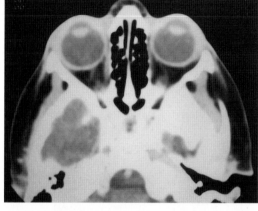

Figure 15-56. Axial computed tomogram after treatment showing normal eyes with no sign of intraocular tumor. The treated tumors were too small to be detected radiographically.

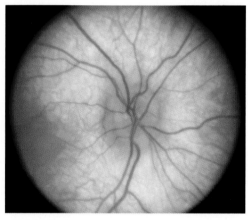

Figure 15-57. Papilledema of the right optic disc at age 36 months when the child developed headaches.

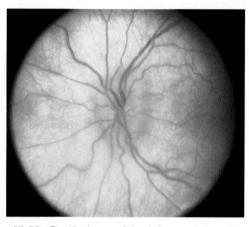

Figure 15-58. Papilledema of the left eye at the same time.

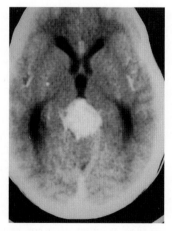

Figure 15-59. Cranial computed tomogram showing large pineal tumor.

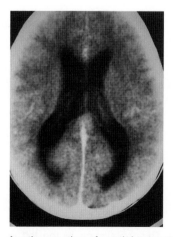

Figure 15-60. Another section of cranial computed tomogram showing dilated ventricles characteristic of hydrocephalus.

Retinoblastoma—Association with 13q Deletion Syndrome and Holoprosencephaly

A gene deletion on the long arm of chromosome 13 is responsible for the development of retinoblastoma. In some instances, detection of physical findings of 13q deletion syndrome, such as low-set ears and typical facies, has led to the early diagnosis of retinoblastoma. Other abnormalities, such as holoprosencephaly, also have been associated with retinoblastoma.

Figs. 15-61 and 15-62 from Seidman DJ, Shields JA, Augsburger JJ, Nelson LB, Ming-Liang L, Sciorra LJ. Early diagnosis of retinoblastoma based on dysmorphic features and karyotype analysis. *Ophthalmology* 1987;94:663–666.

Figs. 15-63 through 15-66 from Desai VN, Shields CL, Shields JA, Donoso LA, Wagner RS. Retinoblastoma associated with holoprosencephaly. *Am J Ophthalmol* 1990;109:355–356.

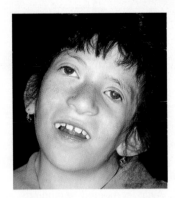

Figure 15-61. Facial appearance of a child with 13q deletion syndrome. This appearance prompted ocular examination and detection of unilateral multifocal retinoblastoma.

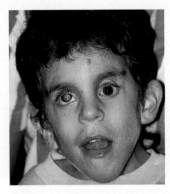

Figure 15-62. Facial appearance of another child with 13q deletion syndrome. This child had bilateral retinoblastoma.

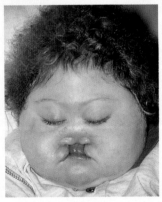

Figure 15-63. Facial appearance of a child with atypical cleft lip and holoprosencephaly.

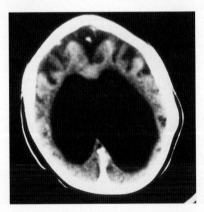

Figure 15-64. Axial cranial computed tomogram of the child shown in Fig. 15-63 showing holoprosencephaly.

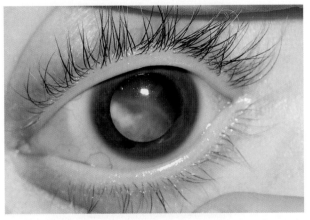

Figure 15-65. Retinoblastoma in the left eye of the child shown in Fig. 15-63.

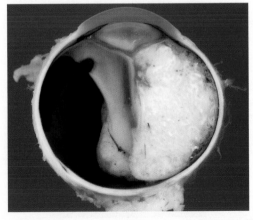

Figure 15-66. Section of enucleated eye shown in Fig. 15-65 showing large exophytic retinoblastoma.

Retinoblastoma—Fluorescein Angiography

Fluorescein angiography has characteristic features with retinoblastoma, which can vary with the growth pattern of the tumor. Intraretinal tumors show marked vascularity, which is less evident in endophytic tumors.

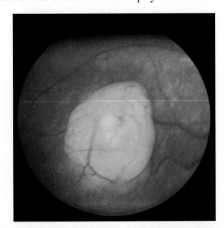

Figure 15-67. Small intraretinal retinoblastoma.

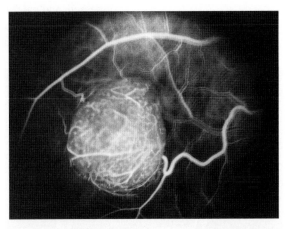

Figure 15-68. Venous phase of the tumor shown in Fig. 15-67 showing large feeding and draining vessels and fine intrinsic vascular channels in the tumor.

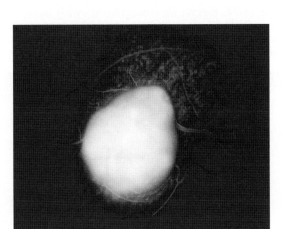

Figure 15-69. Late angiogram of the tumor shown in Fig. 15-67 showing homogeneous intense staining of the well-delineated tumor.

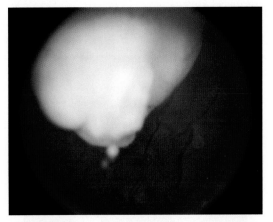

Figure 15-70. Endophytic retinoblastoma in the superior fundus.

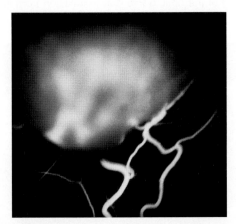

Figure 15-71. Venous phase of the tumor shown in Fig. 15-70 showing hazy hyperfluorescence of the lesion with poor definition of the intrinsic blood vessels.

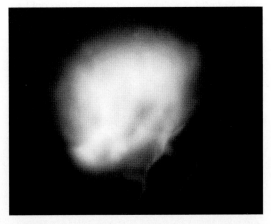

Figure 15-72. Late angiogram of the tumor shown in Fig. 15-70 showing hazy view of the tumor due to fluorescein leakage into the vitreous.

Retinoblastoma—Ultrasonography, Computed Tomography, and Magnetic Resonance Imaging

Ultrasonography and computed tomography show rather characteristic features with retinoblastoma. With these techniques, the size and extent of the tumor(s) can be assessed, and calcium within the lesion can be detected. Magnetic resonance imaging, particularly with contrast enhancement, provides better definition of the soft tissues and may provide early detection of orbital extension and associated pinealoblastoma.

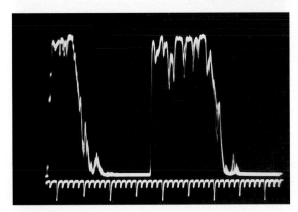

Figure 15-73. A-scan ultrasonogram of retinoblastoma showing markedly high internal reflectivity in the tumor.

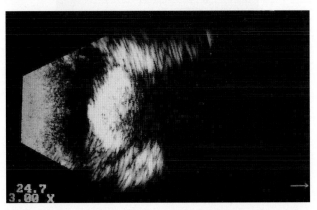

Figure 15-74. B-scan ultrasonogram showing highly reflective mass with a typical shadow in the orbital soft tissues posterior to the tumor. Dense echoes persist in the lesion on lower sensitivities, supporting the presence of calcium in the mass.

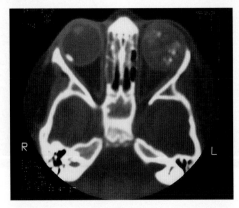

Figure 15-75. Axial computed tomogram of bilateral retinoblastoma. Note the small calcified tumor in the right eye and the extensive calcified tumor in the left eye.

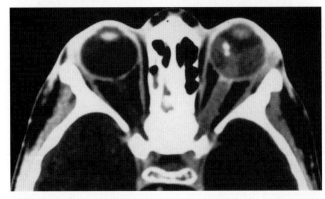

Figure 15-76. Axial computed tomogram showing diffuse thickening of the optic nerve due to invasion from ipsilateral retinoblastoma. (Courtesy of Dr. David Abramson.)

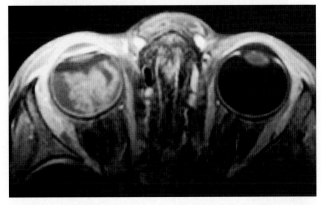

Figure 15-77. Magnetic resonance imaging of retinoblastoma in T1-weighted image with gadolinium enhancement showing the extent of the mass and associated retinal detachment.

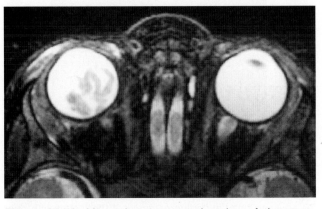

Figure 15-78. Magnetic resonance imaging of the same tumor in T2-weighted image showing that the tumor is hypointense to vitreous.

Retinoblastoma—Pathology

Retinoblastoma has characteristic gross and microscopic features. Grossly, it appears as a chalky-white tumor, frequently with areas of calcification. Microscopically, it is a neuroblastic tumor that can show viable tumor cells with areas of necrosis and calcification. The better-differentiated tumors often show typical Flexner–Wintersteiner rosettes and fleurettes, structures that represent attempts of the tumor toward photoreceptor differentiation.

Photographs courtesy of Dr. Ralph C. Eagle, Jr.

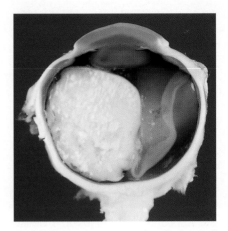

Figure 15-79. Gross appearance of typical exophytic retinoblastoma showing white foci of calcification.

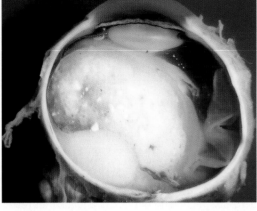

Figure 15-80. Gross appearance of exophytic retinoblastoma with choroidal invasion. Calcification is seen within the retinal portion of the tumor but not in the choroidal portion in the lower part of the photograph.

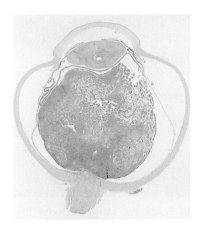

Figure 15-81. Low-magnification photomicrograph showing large exophytic retinoblastoma.

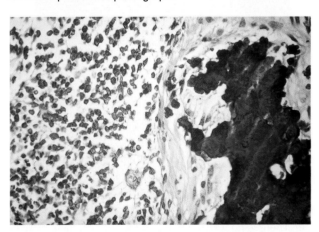

Figure 15-82. Photomicrograph of retinoblastoma showing poorly differentiated viable tumor cells (to the *left*) and dystrophic calcification in an area of necrosis (to the *right*).

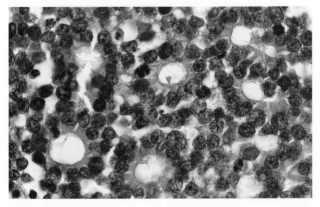

Figure 15-83. Photomicrograph of retinoblastoma showing Flexner–Wintersteiner rosettes (hematoxylin–eosin, original magnification × 200).

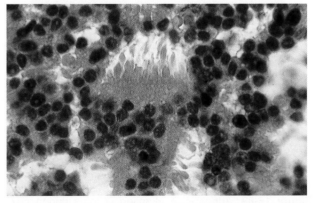

Figure 15-84. Photomicrograph of retinoblastoma showing fleurettes (hematoxylin–eosin, original magnification × 200).

Retinoblastoma—Laser Photocoagulation and Cryotherapy

Laser photocoagulation and cryotherapy can be employed to treat selected small retinoblastomas. The former is used for more posteriorly located tumors and the latter for more peripheral tumors.

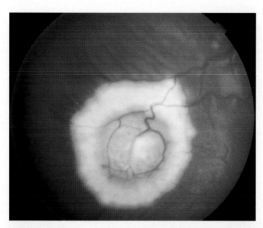

Figure 15-85. Technique of photocoagulation of retinoblastoma showing laser marks around the margin of the tumor.

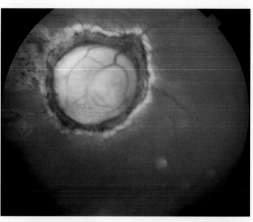

Figure 15-86. Appearance of the lesion 3 weeks later. The tumor is still viable. A second surrounding treatment was performed and tumor control was achieved.

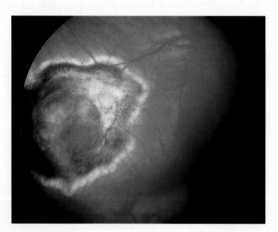

Figure 15-87. Appearance of the same lesion 6 months later. There is no viable tumor and the scar contains proliferated pigment epithelium.

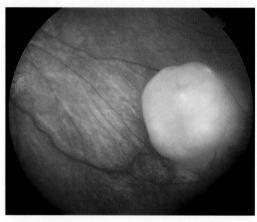

Figure 15-88. Peripheral retinoblastoma that is ideal for treatment with cryotherapy.

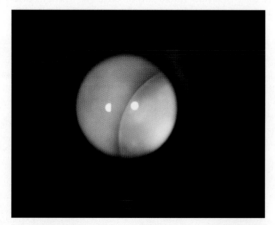

Figure 15-89. Appearance of retinoblastoma during cryotherapy. An ice ball has incorporated the tumor and extends slightly into the overlying vitreous.

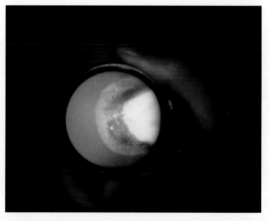

Figure 15-90. Appearance of scar following successful cryotherapy for retinoblastoma.

Retinoblastoma—External Beam Radiotherapy

External beam radiotherapy is an effective method of treating selected retinoblastomas. It sometimes can contribute to the development of second cancers, particularly in children with familial retinoblastoma. It can cause dry-eye symptoms, cataract, radiation retinopathy, and cosmetic problems in the field of radiation. It is used mostly for large tumors or tumors with extensive vitreous or subretinal tumor seeds.

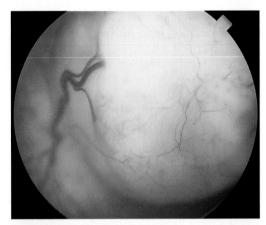

Figure 15-91. Retinoblastoma superotemporal to the optic disc prior to external beam radiotherapy.

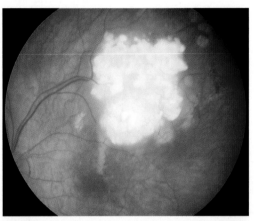

Figure 15-92. Appearance of the same lesion 1 year later showing regression and almost total calcification of the tumor. This is called a type 1 regression pattern. If the lesion shows a fish-flesh appearance without calcification, it is called type 2. A tumor that is partly calcified and partly fish-flesh pattern is called type 3.

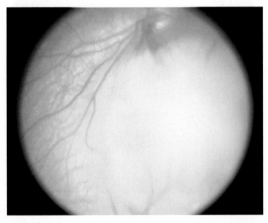

Figure 15-93. Endophytic retinoblastoma inferior to the optic disc.

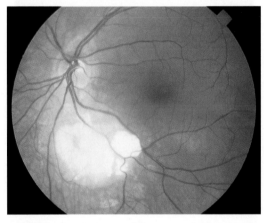

Figure 15-94. Appearance of the same lesion 1 year after external beam radiotherapy showing excellent tumor regression. This is a type 3 regression pattern with partial calcification of the tumor.

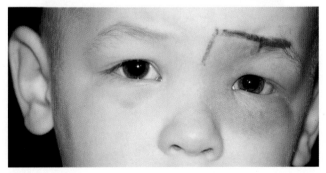

Figure 15-95. Radiation blepharopathy during external beam radiotherapy for retinoblastoma.

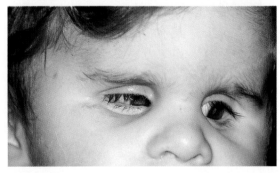

Figure 15-96. Radiation-induced enophthalmos following bilateral external beam radiotherapy for retinoblastoma.

Retinoblastoma—Plaque Radiotherapy

Brachytherapy, using a radioactive plaque, is an effective way of treating selected retinoblastomas, particularly circumscribed tumors without extensive vitreous seeding. It has the advantage over external beam radiotherapy in that it takes only 3 to 4 days to complete the irradiation, appears to have fewer ocular complications, and appears to be less likely to cause radiation-induced second cancers. Plaque radiotherapy is particularly useful for residual or recurrent tumor after failure of other treatment methods. There does not appear to be a higher rate of second cancers using techniques of plaque radiotherapy due to extensive shielding of radiation from surrounding tissues.

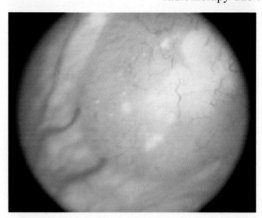

Figure 15-97. Superonasal circumscribed retinoblastoma in a 12-month-old child. The opposite eye had been enucleated for advanced disease.

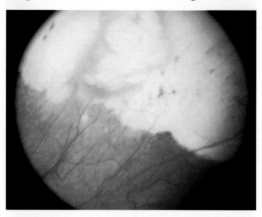

Figure 15-98. Same lesion shown in Fig. 15-97, 2 years after plaque radiotherapy. Note the surrounding atrophy of the retinal pigment epithelium and the central nodule of calcification.

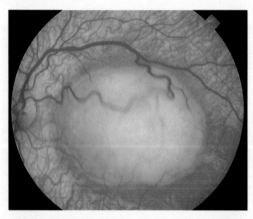

Figure 15-99. Retinoblastoma in the central macular area.

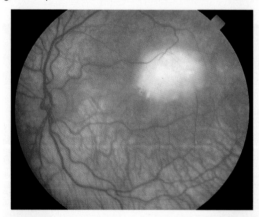

Figure 15-100. Appearance of the lesion shown in Fig. 15-99, 1 month after plaque radiotherapy, showing excellent tumor regression.

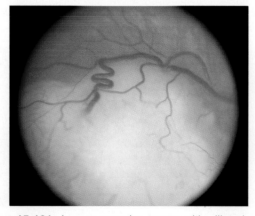

Figure 15-101. Larger macular tumor with dilated retinal blood vessels.

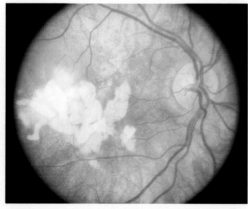

Figure 15-102. Appearance of the lesion shown in Fig. 101, 2 years after plaque radiotherapy, showing excellent tumor regression. The treated lesion has remained stable for 9 years.

Retinoblastoma—Plaque Radiotherapy

Plaque radiotherapy can bring about good regression of retinoblastoma and still preserve a good cosmetic appearance. A case example is shown.

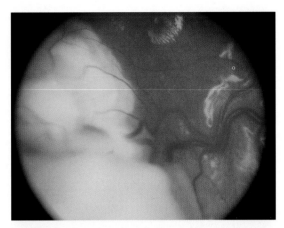

Figure 15-103. Large retinoblastoma inferotemporal to the foveal region with endophytic and exophytic components.

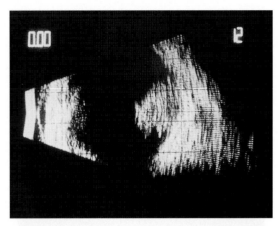

Figure 15-104. B-scan ultrasonogram showing lesion.

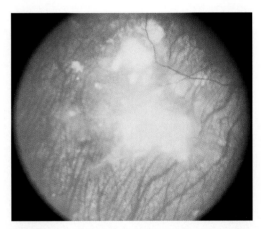

Figure 15-105. Appearance of the lesion 6 months after plaque radiotherapy showing excellent resolution.

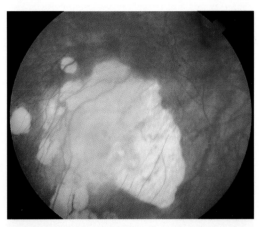

Figure 15-106. Appearance 11 years after plaque radiotherapy showing complete disappearance of tumor with no signs of recurrence.

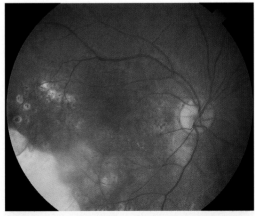

Figure 15-107. Appearance of the foveal region 11 years after treatment showing only mild alterations in the retinal pigment epithelium. Visual acuity was 6/9 (20/30).

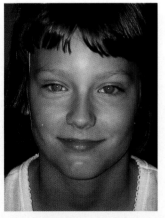

Figure 15-108. Facial appearance of the patient 6 years after treatment showing good cosmetic appearance. Compare this with the appearance of the child shown in Fig. 15-96.

Retinoblastoma—Chemothermotherapy

Chemothermotherapy involves giving intravenous carboplatin followed by treatment of the tumor with transpupillary thermotherapy using a specific protocol. The combined effect of the chemotherapy and heat treatment causes tumor destruction.

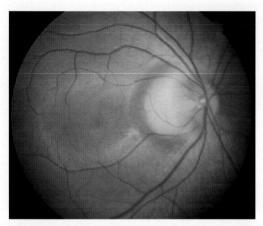

Figure 15-109. Small retinoblastoma located temporal to the optic disc in the papillomacular bundle in a child with familial retinoblastoma.

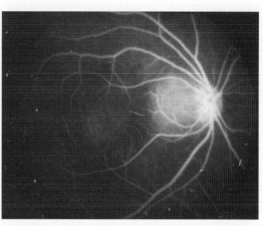

Figure 15-110. Fluorescein angiogram showing tumor vascularity.

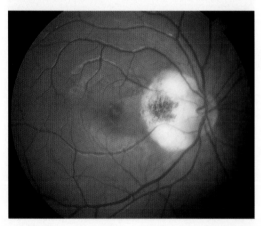

Figure 15-111. Appearance after chemothermotherapy showing complete tumor destruction and preservation of the fovea.

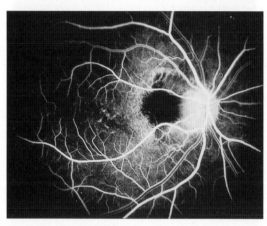

Figure 15-112. Fluorescein angiogram after treatment showing hypofluorescence of the lesion, suggesting that the tumor is no longer vascularized.

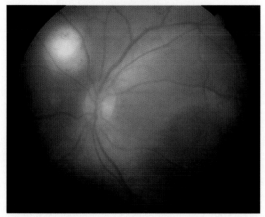

Figure 15-113. Small retinoblastoma superior to the optic disc in the opposite eye of the same patient immediately after chemothermotherapy.

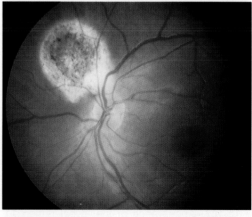

Figure 15-114. Appearance of the lesion shown in Fig. 15-113 several months after chemothermotherapy.

Retinoblastoma—Chemoreduction

Chemotherapy traditionally has been used to treat retinoblastoma with optic nerve extension, orbital invasion, and distant metastasis. Chemoreduction, using a combination of carboplatin, vincristine, and etoposide, is a more recently employed method in which chemotherapy is given in hopes of either controlling the tumor(s) or reducing tumor size so that a more conservative method of treatment can be used. In addition, secondary retinal detachment shows dramatic resolution after chemotherapy. In some instances, very large tumors with extensive secondary retinal detachment show a dramatic initial response to chemoreduction. However, recurrence or persistence of vitreal or subretinal seeds is a frequent problem that necessitates further treatment and sometimes enucleation. Very advanced unilateral tumors generally are managed best by enucleation rather than attempts at chemoreduction.

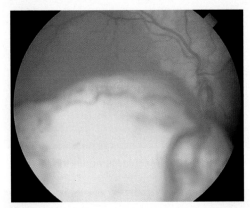

Figure 15-115. Retinoblastoma located inferior to the optic disc and foveal area. Chemoreduction was given.

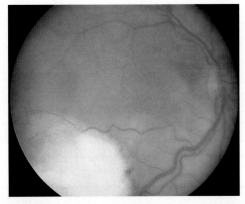

Figure 15-116. Same lesion shown in Fig. 15-115, 3 weeks later, showing shrinkage and calcification of the tumor.

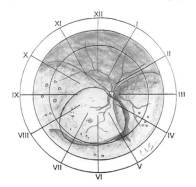

Figure 15-117. Fundus drawing of the lesion shown in Fig. 15-115 showing tumor (yellow) and secondary retinal detachment (blue).

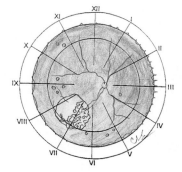

Figure 15-118. Fundus drawing showing appearance 3 weeks after chemoreduction showing decrease in tumor size and disappearance of the retinal detachment.

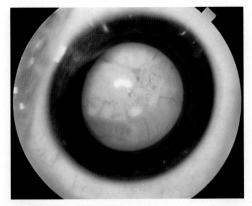

Figure 15-119. Photograph of the left eye in a patient with bilateral advanced retinoblastoma.

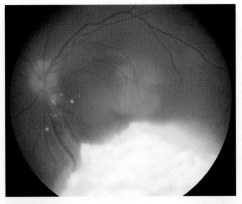

Figure 15-120. Fundus photograph of the eye shown in Fig. 15-119 showing dramatic response to chemoreduction. Plaque radiotherapy was subsequently used, but the patient had severe visual loss after 2 years.

Retinoblastoma—Combined Chemoreduction and Chemothermotherapy

In some cases, a combination of chemoreduction and chemothermotherapy can be used in order to achieve tumor control. An example is shown of bilateral macular retinoblastoma treated by such an approach.

Figs. 15-121 through 15-126 from Shields JA, Shields CL, De Potter P, Needle M. Bilateral macular retinoblastoma managed by chemoreduction and chemothermotherapy. *Arch Ophthalmol* 1996;114:1426–1427.

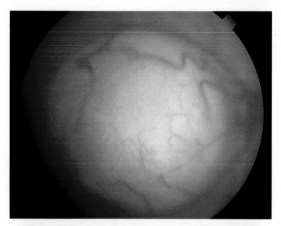

Figure 15-121. Macular tumor in the right eye.

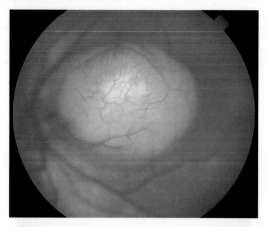

Figure 15-122. Macular tumor in the left eye.

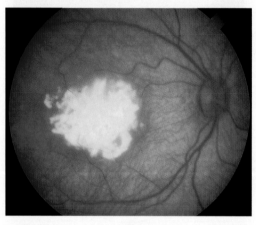

Figure 15-123. Appearance of the right eye after chemoreduction.

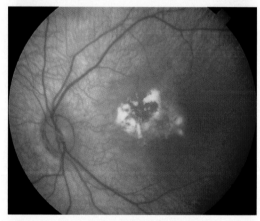

Figure 15-124. Appearance of the left eye after chemoreduction. Because such tumors frequently recur after chemoreduction alone, additional chemothermotherapy was deemed necessary.

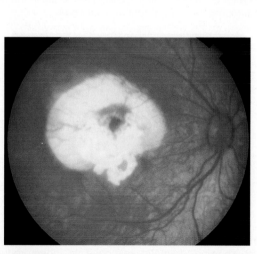

Figure 15-125. Appearance of the right eye after chemoreduction and chemothermotherapy.

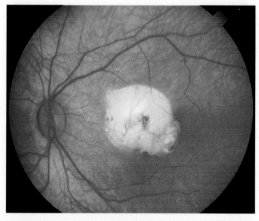

Figure 15-126. Appearance of the left eye after chemoreduction and chemothermotherapy.

Retinoblastoma—Enucleation

Enucleation generally is preferred for most cases of advanced unilateral retinoblastoma and for many cases of bilateral retinoblastoma in which there is no hope for salvageable vision in the affected eye. In performing enucleation, it is important to obtain a long section of optic nerve, because the main route of extension of the tumor is via the optic nerve to the central nervous system. In addition, it often is desirable to harvest fresh tumor tissue for genetic analysis and other studies.

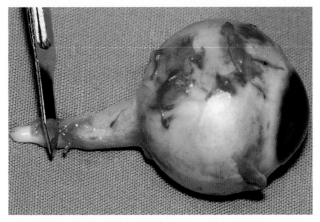

Figure 15-127. The eye has been removed with a long section of optic nerve. The end of the optic nerve being sectioned with a blade will be submitted separately for histopathologic study.

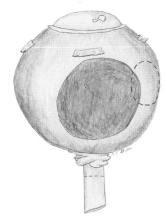

Figure 15-128. Diagram showing base of the tumor (*shadow*) and the planned area for scleral trephine opening (*dotted circle*).

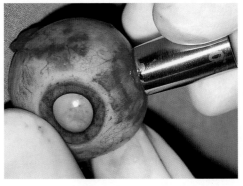

Figure 15-129. Corneal trephine (8-mm diameter) being used to make a circular area in the sclera near the equator and straddling the margin of the tumor as shown in the *dotted circle* in Fig. 15-128.

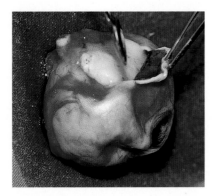

Figure 15-130. The opening has been made and fresh white tumor tissue is being harvested.

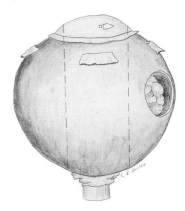

Figure 15-131. The tissue has been harvested and the globe has been fixed. The pathologist draws two parallel dotted lines so that the main part of the tumor will be in the major calotte and the scleral window will be in the minor calotte.

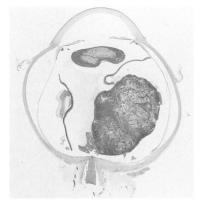

Figure 15-132. Histopathologic section showing that the specimen is still well oriented in spite of opening the globe prior to fixation.

CHAPTER 16

Lesions Simulating Retinoblastoma

LESIONS SIMULATING RETINOBLASTOMA

There are a number of conditions that can simulate retinoblastoma either by causing a small white fundus lesion or by causing leukocoria. Many simulating lesions are other tumors, such as astrocytic hamartoma, medulloepithelioma, and combined hamartoma, and they are covered in other chapters. This chapter describes some non-neoplastic conditions that can simulate retinoblastoma.

In a series of 500 consecutive patients referred with the diagnosis of possible retinoblastoma, 288 proved to have retinoblastoma on subsequent evaluation and 212 proved to have simulating lesions. The three conditions that most closely simulated retinoblastoma were persistent hyperplastic primary vitreous (28%), Coats' disease (16%), and ocular toxocariasis (16%). Other nonneoplastic conditions included retinopathy of prematurity, dominant exudative vitreoretinopathy, endogenous endophthalmitis, congenital cataract, congenital toxoplasmosis, chorioretinal coloboma, myelinated nerve fibers, and scar tissue secondary to surgical trauma. The specific clinical features that help to differentiate these conditions are discussed in detail in the literature (1–7).

SELECTED REFERENCES

1. Shields JA, Shields CL. *Intraocular tumors. A text and atlas.* Philadelphia: WB Saunders, 1992:341–362.
2. Shields JA, Parsons HM, Shields CL, Shah P. Lesions simulating retinoblastoma. *J Pediatr Ophthalmol Strabismus* 1991;28:338–340.
3. Shields JA, Shields CL, Parsons HM. Review: differential diagnosis of retinoblastoma. *Retina* 1991;11: 232–243.
4. Ridley ME, Shields JA, Brown GC, Tasman WS. Coats' disease. Evaluation of management. *Ophthalmology* 1982;89:1381–1387.
5. Shields JA. Ocular toxocariasis. A review. *Surv Ophthalmol* 1984;28:361–381.
6. Shields JA, Shields CL, Eagle RC Jr, Barrett J, De Potter P. Endogenous endophthalmitis simulating retinoblastoma. A report of six cases. The 1993 Seslen Lecture. *Retina* 1995;15:213–219.
7. Shields JA, Shields CL, Eagle RC Jr, De Potter P, Douglas H. Calcified intraocular abscess simulating retinoblastoma. *Am J Ophthalmol* 1992;114:227–229.

Coats' Disease

Coats' disease can simulate retinoblastoma by producing a small fundus lesion, often in the macular region, or by producing a total retinal detachment that can simulate an exophytic retinoblastoma. Unlike retinoblastoma, Coats' disease shows irregular caliber telangiectasia in the peripheral fundus and yellow intraretinal and subretinal exudation. The retinal vessels tend to course over the detachment and do not dip into it as they do in retinoblastoma.

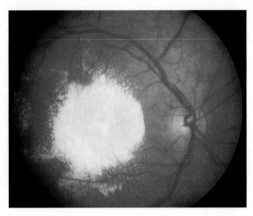

Figure 16-1. Macular exudation in Coats' disease. Such exudation is not seen with retinoblastoma, but it is very characteristic of Coats' disease.

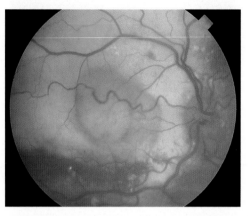

Figure 16-2. More extensive macular exudation in Coats' disease.

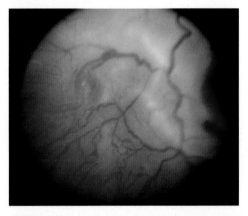

Figure 16-3. Peripheral retinal telangiectasia and retinal detachment in Coats' disease. Irregular-caliber blood vessels as shown here rarely are seen with retinoblastoma.

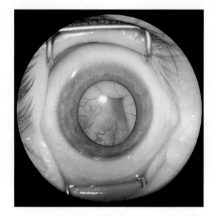

Figure 16-4. Total retinal detachment secondary to Coats' disease.

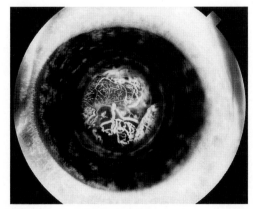

Figure 16-5. Fluorescein angiogram of Coats' disease with total retinal detachment showing the characteristic telangiectasia.

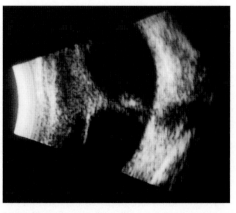

Figure 16-6. B-scan ultrasonogram of Coats' disease showing the total funnel-shaped retinal detachment.

Coats' Disease—Clinicopathologic Findings

Like retinoblastoma, Coats' disease can produce a total retinal detachment and neovascular glaucoma, and it can require enucleation of the affected eye. In some cases, enucleation is done because the possibility of retinoblastoma cannot be absolutely excluded. In the case cited here, the diagnosis of Coats' disease was evident, but enucleation was performed because of severe ocular pain secondary to neovascular glaucoma.

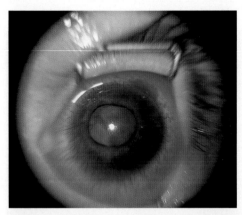

Figure 16-7. Total retinal detachment and iris neovascularization secondary to Coats' disease. The child had severe neovascular glaucoma.

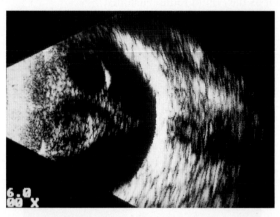

Figure 16-8. B-scan ultrasonogram showing total retinal detachment but no evidence of a mass.

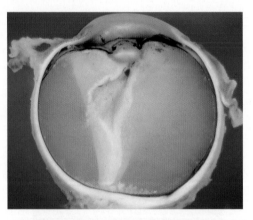

Figure 16-9. Section of enucleated eye showing total retinal detachment and yellow exudation filling the subretinal space.

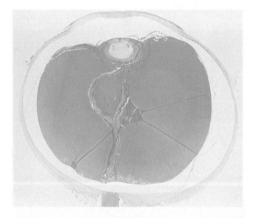

Figure 16-10. Low-magnification photograph of sectioned eye showing total retinal detachment and homogeneous eosinophilic exudation filling the subretinal space.

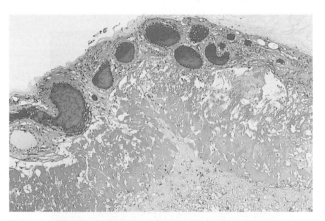

Figure 16-11. Photomicrograph of thickened detached retina showing large dilated blood vessels in the retina and marked retinal thickening due to intraretinal exudation (hematoxylin–eosin, original magnification × 50).

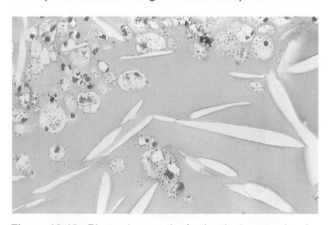

Figure 16-12. Photomicrograph of subretinal space showing eosinophilic exudation containing lipid-laden macrophages and cholesterol clefts, features typical of Coat's disease.

Persistent Hyperplastic Primary Vitreous

Persistent hyperplastic primary vitreous also can produce leukocoria and simulate retinoblastoma. In contrast to retinoblastoma, however, it generally is present at birth in a microphthalmic eye. The congenital retrolental fibrovascular tissue and secondary cataract are not seen with retinoblastoma. In contrast to retinoblastoma, it is almost always unilateral and nonfamilial. Persistent hyperplastic primary vitreous can range from mild to severe forms, the latter often resulting in a total secondary retinal detachment and blindness.

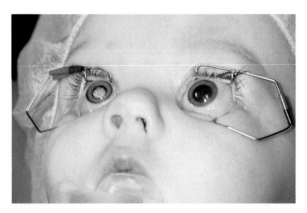

Figure 16-13. Leukocoria of the right eye in a child with persistent hyperplastic primary vitreous. Note the slight microphthalmia of the affected eye.

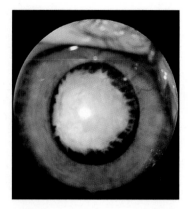

Figure 16-14. Closer view of the right eye showing dense secondary cataract and characteristic dragging of the ciliary processes into the retrolental mass.

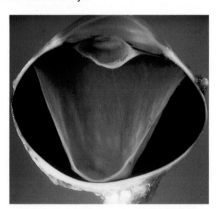

Figure 16-15. Gross appearance of sectioned eye with persistent hyperplastic primary vitreous and no retinal detachment. Note the subtle hyaloid artery passing from the optic disc region to the dense white retrolental mass. (Photograph courtesy of Armed Forces Institute of Pathology, Washington, DC.)

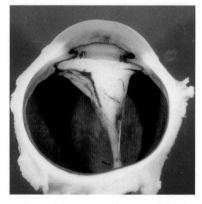

Figure 16-16. Gross appearance of sectioned eye with persistent hyperplastic primary vitreous with a total secondary retinal detachment. When such a detachment occurs with persistent hyperplastic primary vitreous, there is no hope for visual recovery.

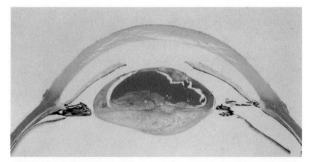

Figure 16-17. Low-magnification photomicrograph of persistent hyperplastic primary vitreous showing retrolental fibrovascular mass, secondary cataract, dragging of the ciliary processes, and anterior displacement of the retina over the pars plana (hematoxylin–eosin, original magnification × 3). (Courtesy of Armed Forces Institute of Pathology, Washington, DC.)

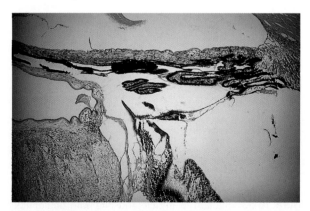

Figure 16-18. Low-magnification photomicrograph of persistent hyperplastic primary vitreous showing dragging of the ciliary processes (hematoxylin–eosin, original magnification × 10). (Courtesy of Armed Forces Institute of Pathology, Washington, DC.)

Ocular Toxocariasis

Ocular toxocariasis is due to the infestation of the eye with the second stage larva of the canine roundworm, *Toxocara canis*. It can simulate retinoblastoma by causing either a white fundus granuloma or a diffuse endophthalmitis. The clinical features, diagnosis, and management of this condition are discussed in the literature. Unlike retinoblastoma, ocular toxocariasis tends to produce more severe vitreoretinal traction.

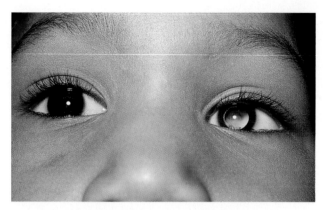

Figure 16-19. Leukocoria and esotropia of the left eye in a child with ocular toxocariasis.

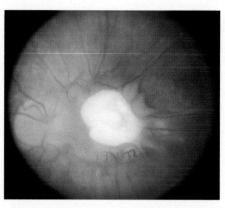

Figure 16-20. Macular granuloma secondary to ocular toxocariasis. The associated retinal traction does not tend to occur with a comparable-sized retinoblastoma.

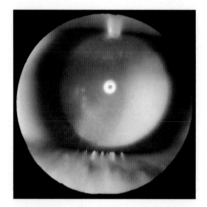

Figure 16-21. Ocular toxocariasis with a peripheral inflammatory mass. Note the fibrillary margin of the white lesion, suggesting vitreous traction and early cyclitic membrane formation. Such findings would be unlikely with retinoblastoma.

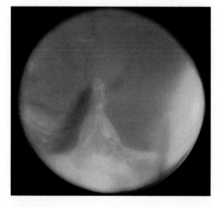

Figure 16-22. Wide-angle fundus photograph showing an inferior falciform fold secondary to a peripheral granuloma in a child with ocular toxocariasis. A falciform fold would almost never occur with untreated retinoblastoma.

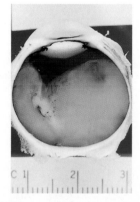

Figure 16-23. Section of enucleated eye with ocular toxocariasis. There is a total retinal detachment associated with the dense white retinal mass.

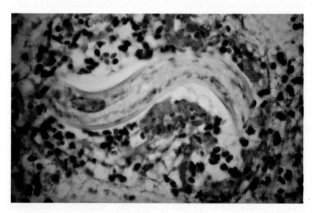

Figure 16-24. Photomicrograph through chorioretinal eosinophilic abscess showing larva of *Toxocara canis* (hematoxylin–eosin, original magnification × 250). (Courtesy of Armed Forces Institute of Pathology, Washington, DC.)

Endogenous Endophthalmitis Simulating Retinoblastoma

Prior to the advent of antibiotics, endogenous endophthalmitis was more common in children and frequently was confused clinically with retinoblastoma. Although less common today, cases of endophthalmitis frequently are referred with the diagnosis of possible retinoblastoma. Examples are cited.

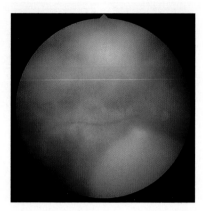

Figure 16-25. Cytomegalovirus endophthalmitis simulating endophytic retinoblastoma in an infant. Note the fluffy-white endophytic mass. The opposite eye had similar findings. Peripheral retinal signs of acute retinal necrosis suggested a viral infection rather than retinoblastoma.

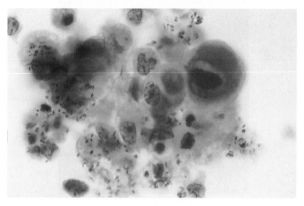

Figure 16-26. Fine-needle aspiration biopsy specimen of the lesion shown in Fig. 16-25 demonstrating large cell with inclusion body characteristic of cytomegalovirus. (Papanicolaou, original magnification × 400.)

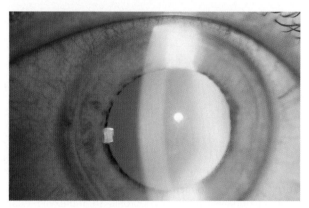

Figure 16-27. Diffuse vitreous cells secondary to streptococcal endophthalmitis following dental surgery. The child was referred with a diagnosis of diffuse retinoblastoma.

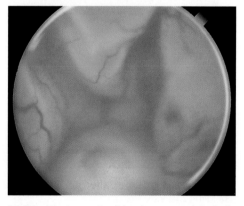

Figure 16-28. Photograph of fundus mass inferiorly associated with a total secondary retinal detachment. Although the findings were atypical, enucleation was performed because retinoblastoma could not be excluded.

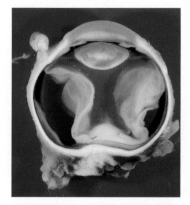

Figure 16-29. Photograph of the sectioned eye shown in Fig. 16-28 showing white mass in retina and choroidal posteriorly.

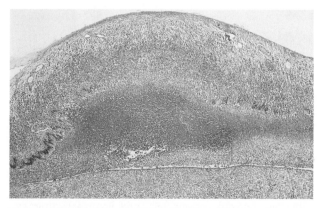

Figure 16-30. Histopathologic section through the mass shown in Figs. 16-27 and 16-28. A necrotic abscess is present (hematoxylin–eosin, original magnification × 50). Although the mass was clearly infectious, no organisms could be identified and the etiology was never determined.

Idiopathic Calcified Intraocular Abscess Simulating Retinoblastoma

Figs. 16-31 through 16-36 from Shields JA, Shields CL, Eagle RC Jr, De Potter P, Douglas CH. Calcified intraocular abscess simulating retinoblastoma. *Am J Ophthalmol* 1992;114:227–229.

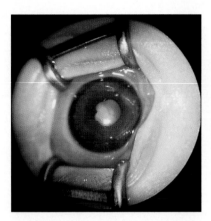

Figure 16-31. Leukocoria and posterior synechia in a newborn girl.

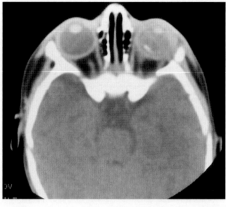

Figure 16-32. Axial computed tomogram showing diffuse intraocular mass with foci of calcification.

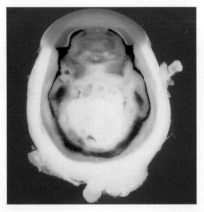

Figure 16-33. Sectioned eye after enucleation showing white mass filling the vitreous cavity.

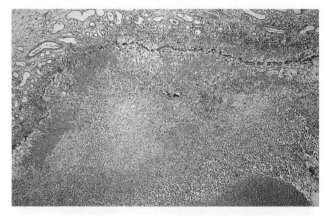

Figure 16-34. Photomicrograph of the intraocular mass showing extensive areas of necrosis (hematoxylin–eosin, original magnification × 25).

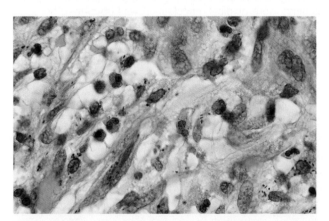

Figure 16-35. Photomicrograph of another area showing viable lymphocytes, eosinophils, and fibroblasts (hematoxylin–eosin, original magnification × 200).

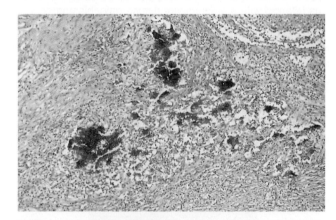

Figure 16-36. Photomicrograph showing foci of dystrophic calcification in the same lesion. These accounted for the dense foci seen with computed tomography. No organisms were demonstrated in spite of numerous studies (hematoxylin–eosin, original magnification × 75).

Miscellaneous Conditions Simulating Retinoblastoma

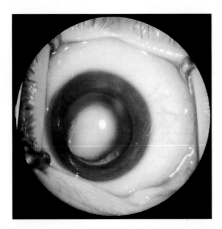

Figure 16-37. Congenital cataract of uncertain etiology simulating retinoblastoma.

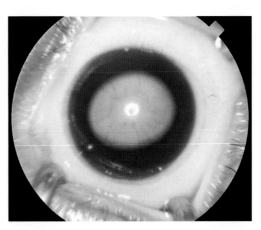

Figure 16-38. Retinopathy of prematurity. A total retinal detachment with gliotic retina immediately behind the lens is shown. Extensive gliosis is not seen in the retinal detachment associated with retinoblastoma.

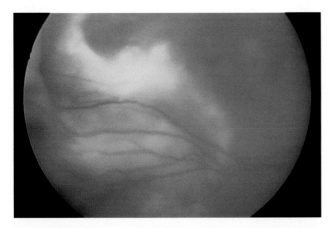

Figure 16-39. Dominant exudative vitreoretinopathy. Exudative mass in peripheral retina temporally with retinal dragging. Such retinal traction and exudation is not seen with comparable-sized retinoblastoma.

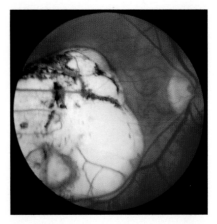

Figure 16-40. Congenital toxoplasmic retinochoroiditis. The macular lesion was large enough to produce a white pupillary reflex. Unlike retinoblastoma, this lesion appears flat with indirect ophthalmoscopy.

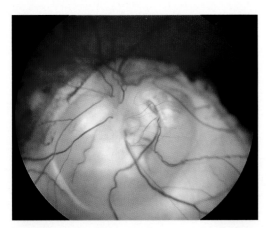

Figure 16-41. Congenital retinochoroidal coloboma. The lesion involved the inferior fundus, incorporated the optic disc, and produced a white pupillary reflex. Unlike retinoblastoma, this lesion appears depressed, rather than elevated, with indirect ophthalmoscopy.

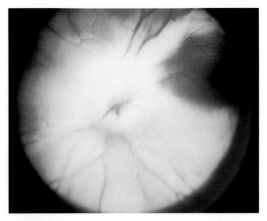

Figure 16-42. Extensive myelinated retinal nerve fibers. This was large enough to produce leukocoria.

CHAPTER 17

Vascular Tumors of the Retina and Optic Disc

RETINAL CAPILLARY HEMANGIOMA

Vascular tumors of the retina include capillary hemangioma, cavernous hemangioma, racemose hemangioma, and the acquired vasoproliferative tumor. Each of these lesions has different clinical features, systemic implications, complications, and management.

Retinal capillary hemangioma usually is diagnosed in children or young adults. It can occur as a solitary tumor without systemic disease or as a component of the von Hippel–Lindau (VHL) syndrome, an autosomal dominant condition with various combinations of cerebellar hemangioblastoma, pheochromocytoma, hypernephroma, and other systemic tumors and cysts. The genetic defect is on the short arm of chromosome 3. A patient with a retinal capillary hemangioma generally should be evaluated and followed for the VHL syndrome (1–4). A similar tumor has been seen in association with Marshall–Stickler syndrome (4). Clinically, retinal capillary hemangioma usually appears as a reddish-pink tumor in the peripheral retina or on the optic disc. It can occur as an exudative or tractional type. The exudative form is characterized by the presence of intraretinal and subretinal exudation that has an affinity for the macular region and can lead to an exudative retinal detachment, similar to that seen with Coats' disease. In contrast to Coats' disease, however, the retinal capillary hemangioma shows dilated feeding and draining blood vessels and a distinct mass. The tractional type often is associated with vitreoretinal traction and overlying vitreous fibrosis. It often is associated with a preretinal membrane, sometimes in the macular area remote from the peripheral tumor. With fluorescein angiography, retinal capillary hemangioma shows rapid filling of the mass with intense late staining, sometimes with leakage of fluorescein into the overlying vitreous. Histopathology shows a vascular tumor composed of proliferating endothelial cells and glial cells (1).

Management depends on the extent of the disease and whether it is a part of the VHL syndrome, in which cases the tumors appear at an earlier age and seem to be more aggressive. Small asymptomatic tumors can be followed cautiously for progression. Tumors with limited retinal exudation or retinal detachment can be managed by laser photocoagulation or cryotherapy. More advanced lesions may require additional retinal detachment surgery. External beam or plaque radiotherapy can be employed for resistant tumors, but its role is not clearly established.

SELECTED REFERENCES

1. Gass JDM. Retinal and optic disc hemangiomas. In: Gass JDM, ed. *Stereoscopic atlas of macular diseases,* 2nd Ed. St. Louis: CV Mosby, 1997:850–859.
2. Shields JA, Shields CL. *Intraocular tumors. A text and atlas.* Philadelphia: WB Saunders, 1992:393–419.
3. Shields JA, Shields CL. *Intraocular tumors. A text and atlas.* Philadelphia: WB Saunders, 1992:513–539.
4. Shields JA, Shields CL, Deglin E. Retinal capillary hemangioma in Marshall–Stickler syndrome. *Am J Ophthalmol* 1997;124:120–122.

Peripheral Retinal Capillary Hemangioma

Peripheral retinal capillary hemangioma is one that occurs in the sensory retina away from the optic disc. It appears as a reddish-pink intraretinal tumor with a dilated, tortuous feeding retinal artery and a similar draining vein.

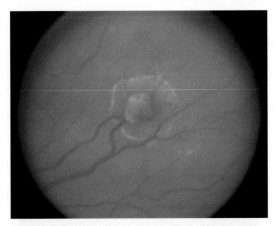

Figure 17-1. Small retinal capillary hemangioma with minimal surrounding exudative retinal detachment.

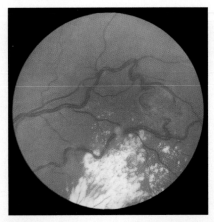

Figure 17-2. Retinal capillary hemangioma with typical intraretinal exudation.

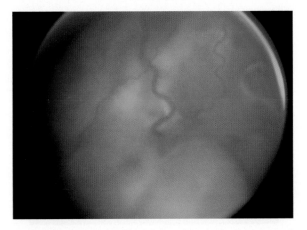

Figure 17-3. Larger inferiorly located lesion with secondary exudative retinal detachment.

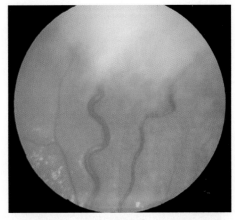

Figure 17-4. Tractional form of retinal capillary hemangioma. The tumor is obscured by overlying fibrosis in the vitreous.

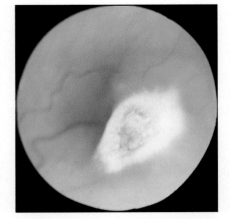

Figure 17-5. "Free-floating" hemangioma. Severe vitreous traction has blanched the tumor and pulled it into the overlying vitreous cavity above the retina.

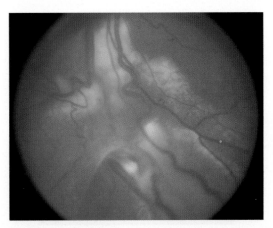

Figure 17-6. Combined exudative and tractional type of retinal capillary hemangioma.

Optic Disc (Papillary) Involvement with Retinal Capillary Hemangioma

In some instances, a retinal capillary hemangioma can lie partly or entirely over the optic disc. In such cases, the prominent feeding and draining blood vessels are less apparent. It can assume a nodular or sessile growth pattern. This form has the same relationship to VHL syndrome as the peripheral type.

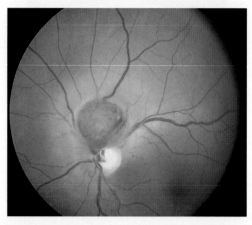

Figure 17-7. Nodular capillary hemangioma overlying superior margin of the optic disc. (Courtesy of Dr. William Hagler.)

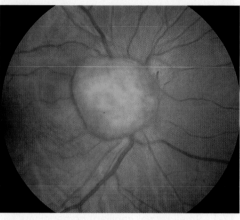

Figure 17-8. Nodular capillary hemangioma overlying the entire optic disc. (Courtesy of Dr. Fox Boswell.)

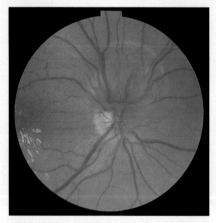

Figure 17-9. Sessile capillary hemangioma over superior margin of the optic disc. Note the larger feeding blood vessel and the intraretinal exudation in the foveal area (to the *left*).

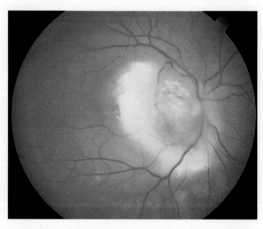

Figure 17-10. Sessile capillary hemangioma covering the optic disc and producing secondary circinate exudation.

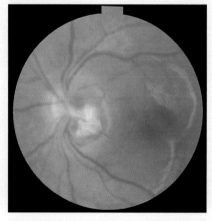

Figure 17-11. Sessile hemangioma of the optic disc in a 5-year-old child with von Hippel–Lindau syndrome.

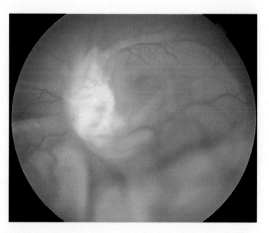

Figure 17-12. Appearance of the lesion shown in Fig. 17-11, 6 years later. The lesion has enlarged dramatically and there is a total secondary exudative retinal detachment.

Fluorescein Angiography of Retinal Capillary Hemangioma

Retinal capillary hemangioma has typical fluorescein angiographic features. It shows rapid filling in the arterial phase and intense late staining.

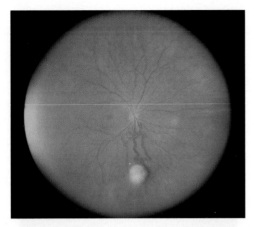

Figure 17-13. Wide-angle fundus photograph of an inferior retinal capillary hemangioma at the equator inferiorly. Note the dilated, tortuous retinal blood vessels between the optic disc and the tumor.

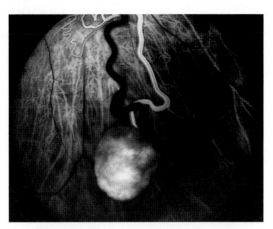

Figure 17-14. Same lesion shown in Fig. 17-13 in arterial phase showing filling of the feeding artery.

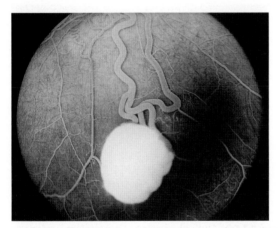

Figure 17-15. Same lesion in recirculation phase showing prominent blood vessels and hyperfluorescence of the mass.

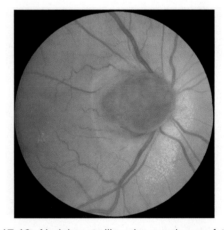

Figure 17-16. Nodular capillary hemangioma of the optic disc. (Courtesy of Dr. Richard Chenoweth.)

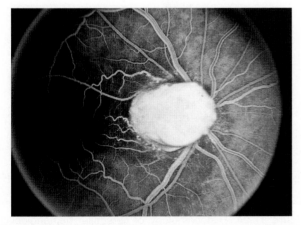

Figure 17-17. Same lesion shown in Fig. 17-16 in late venous phase showing marked hyperfluorescence of the mass.

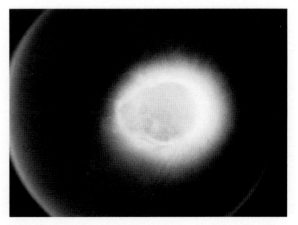

Figure 17-18. Late angiogram of the same lesion showing intense hyperfluorescence with leakage of fluorescein into the overlying vitreous.

Retinal Capillary Hemangioma—Association with von Hippel–Lindau Syndrome

The VHL syndrome is characterized by various combinations of retinal capillary hemangioma, cerebellar hemangioma, pheochromocytoma, hypernephroma, and a variety of other vascular and cystic lesions in various parts of the body. The genetic defect has been localized on the short arm of chromosome 3. This details of this syndrome are discussed in the literature.

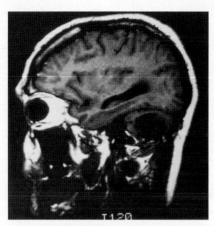

Figure 17-19. Sagittal magnetic resonance image showing cerebellar mass in a 34-year-old man. He had no retinal tumors or other manifestations of the von Hippel–Lindau syndrome.

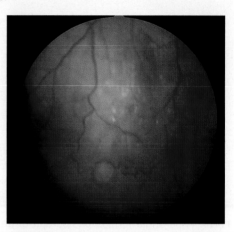

Figure 17-20. Fundus photograph of the 10-year-old son of the patient depicted in Fig. 17-19 showing small, inferiorly located retinal capillary hemangioma.

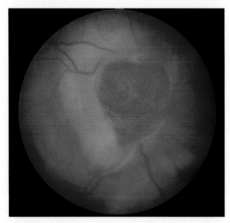

Figure 17-21. Fundus photograph of the 5-year-old son of the patient depicted in Fig. 17-19 showing red hemangioma of the optic disc.

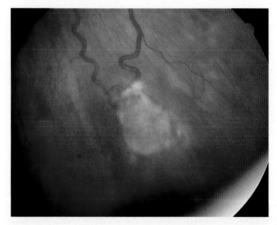

Figure 17-22. Retinal capillary hemangioma inferiorly in a 28-year-old man. The patient had cerebellar hemangioblastoma and hypernephroma. (Courtesy of Dr. Careen Lowder.)

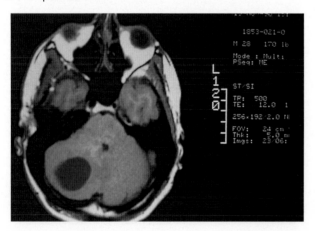

Figure 17-23. Axial magnetic resonance image of the patient depicted in Fig. 17-22 showing cerebellar mass. (Courtesy of Dr. Careen Lowder.)

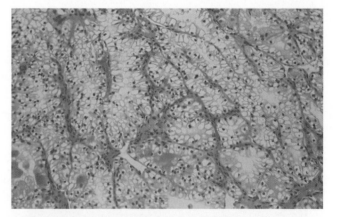

Figure 17-24. Histopathology of cerebellar hemangioblastoma from the same patient shown in Fig. 17-22 (hematoxylin–eosin, original magnification × 150). (Courtesy of Dr. Careen Lowder.)

Retinal Capillary Hemangioma—Clinicopathologic Correlation

In some cases, aggressive retinal capillary hemangioma may not be controlled and enucleation of the affected eye may be necessary because of pain, secondary glaucoma, or phthisis bulbi. An example is shown.

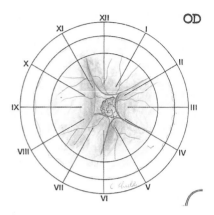

Figure 17-25. Fundus drawing of a red optic disc mass and secondary retinal detachment in a 4-year-old girl with a negative family history.

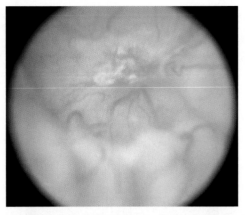

Figure 17-26. Fundus photograph of the ill-defined optic disc mass shown in Fig. 17-25. Note the retinal detachment inferiorly. After unsuccessful attempts at retinal detachment repair, the blind painful eye was enucleated.

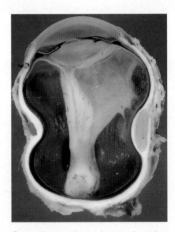

Figure 17-27. Grossly sectioned eye showing mass over the optic disc, total retinal detachment, and silicone encircling band from the retinal detachment repair.

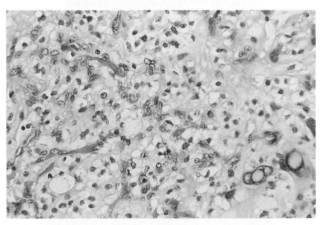

Figure 17-28. Histopathology of tumor showing vascular mass composed of capillary-caliber vessels and intervascular stromal cells with foamy cytoplasm.

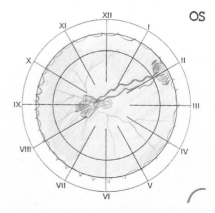

Figure 17-29. The patient's opposite eye was entirely normal until 3 years after the initial diagnosis, at which time a peripheral hemangioma developed and preretinal macular fibrosis occurred, requiring surgical peeling of the preretinal membrane. The patient continues to have limited vision in the remaining eye.

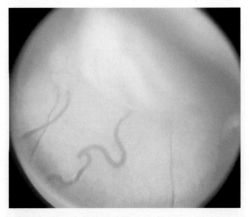

Figure 17-30. Peripheral fundus photograph of the eye shown in Fig. 17-29 showing dilated retinal blood vessels and retinovitreal fibrous tissue over the peripheral vascular tumor.

Retinal Capillary Hemangioma in Older Patients and in a Patient with Marshall–Stickler Syndrome

Retinal capillary hemangioma can occur as a sporadic lesion or as a part of VHL syndrome. It usually is diagnosed in the first 2 decades of life, particularly in patients with the VHL genetic abnormality. In some cases, it can occur in older individuals with no personal or familial evidence of VHL syndrome. A similar retinal tumor also has been observed in association with Marshall–Stickler syndrome, an autosomal dominant condition characterized by typical facies, arthropathy, cataracts, myopia, and retinal detachment.

Figs. 17-35 and 17-36 from Shields JA, Shields CL, Deglin E. Retinal capillary hemangioma in Marshall–Stickler syndrome. *Am J Ophthalmol* 1997;124:120–122.

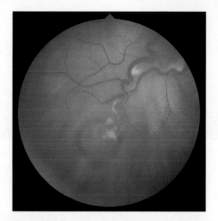

Figure 17-31. Solitary retinal capillary hemangioma in a 65-year-old woman.

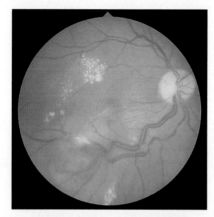

Figure 17-32. Solitary retinal capillary hemangioma in a 62-year-old man.

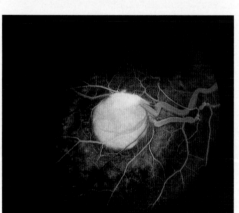

Figure 17-33. Fluorescein angiogram of the lesion shown in Fig. 17-32 demonstrating typical features of a retinal capillary hemangioma.

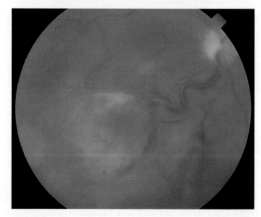

Figure 17-34. Fundus photograph of the lesion shown in Fig. 17-32, after 9 years, revealing enlargement of the lesion. It was treated with plaque radiotherapy.

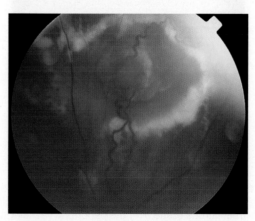

Figure 17-35. Superior retinal capillary hemangioma in a 31-year-old man with Marshall–Stickler syndrome.

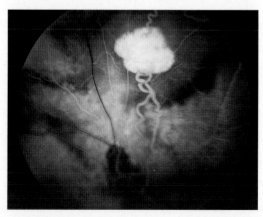

Figure 17-36. Fluorescein angiogram of the lesion shown in Fig. 17-35 depicting the hyperfluorescent mass and dilated feeding artery and draining vein.

Retinal Capillary Hemangioma—Management by Laser Photocoagulation

If small capillary hemangiomas can be controlled with laser photocoagulation, the complications of exudative maculopathy and retinal detachment can be reversed or prevented. It usually requires from one to three laser treatments about 2 to 3 months apart to achieve satisfactory results. The technique of laser photocoagulation is reported in the literature.

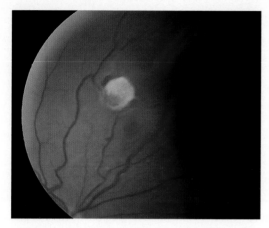

Figure 17-37. Progressively growing small retinal capillary hemangioma in a 42-year-old man.

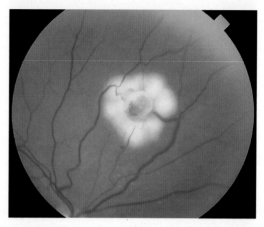

Figure 17-38. Appearance of the lesion immediately after photocoagulation.

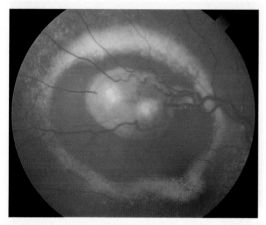

Figure 17-39. Capillary hemangioma superotemporal to the foveal region in a 5-year-old boy. Note the circinate exudation that extended into the fovea, causing a visual decrease to 6/30 (20/100).

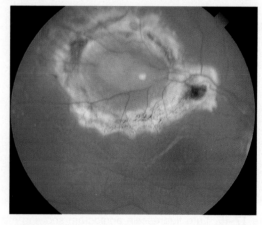

Figure 17-40. Appearance of the lesion after laser photocoagulation showing resolution of the exudation. Visual acuity returned to 6/9.

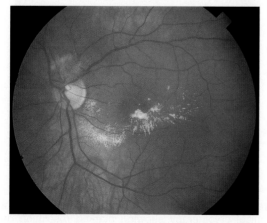

Figure 17-41. Small capillary hemangioma on superior margin of the optic disc with foveal exudation. The tumor was treated with surface laser photocoagulation.

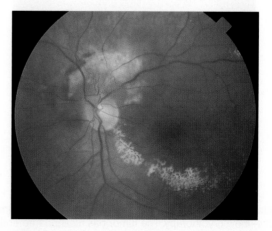

Figure 17-42. Appearance 3 years later showing partial resolution of the foveal exudation. Visual acuity improved. There is still some circinate exudation inferiorly.

Retinal Capillary Hemangioma—Management by Cryotherapy

Cryotherapy can be employed for somewhat larger peripherally located retinal capillary hemangiomas. A triple freeze–thaw technique generally is employed, waiting at least 2 to 3 months before giving additional treatment, if necessary.

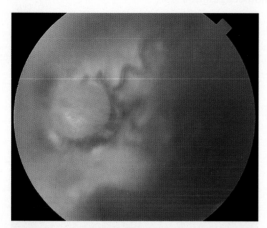

Figure 17-43. Pedunculated capillary hemangioma near the temporal equator in the right eye.

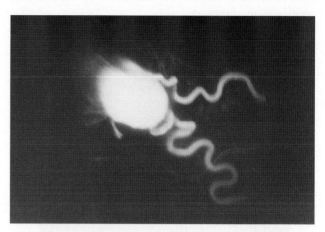

Figure 17-44. Fluorescein angiogram in venous phase.

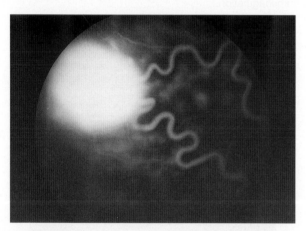

Figure 17-45. Late fluorescein angiogram showing marked hyperfluorescence of the tumor and leakage of dye into the overlying vitreous.

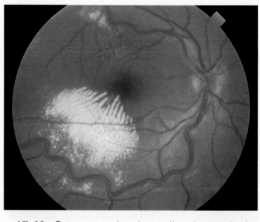

Figure 17-46. Same eye showing yellow intraretinal exudation in the foveal region.

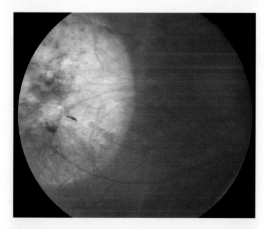

Figure 17-47. Appearance of peripheral tumor after double freeze–thaw cryotherapy. The tumor has disappeared entirely.

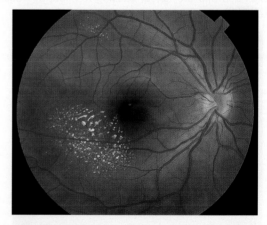

Figure 17-48. Appearance of the macular area 10 months after initial cryotherapy showing marked resolution of the macular exudation.

Retinal Capillary Hemangioma—Management by Cryotherapy

Following successful treatment of a retinal capillary hemangioma, the size and configuration of the retinal blood vessels may return to normal.

Figs. 17-49 through 17-54 from Shields JA. Response of retinal capillary hemangioma to cryotherapy. *Arch Ophthalmol* 1993;111:551.

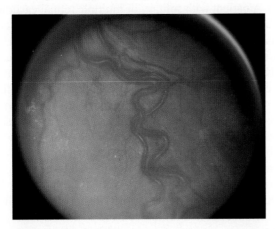

Figure 17-49. Dilated tortuous retinal blood vessels inferiorly in a 13-year-old girl.

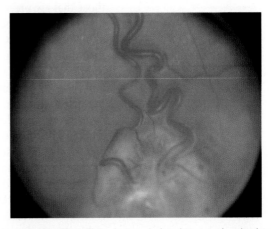

Figure 17-50. The dilated vessels lead to a red retinal tumor inferiorly at the equator.

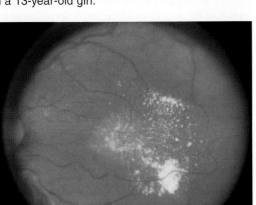

Figure 17-51. Macular exudation in the same patient. Visual acuity was 6/60 (20/200).

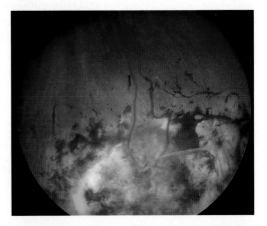

Figure 17-52. Area shown in Fig. 17-50 showing disappearance of tumor after cryotherapy.

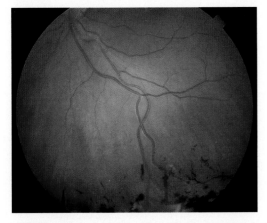

Figure 17-53. Area shown in Fig. 17-49 showing that the retinal vessels have returned to normal size and distribution after cryotherapy of the tumor.

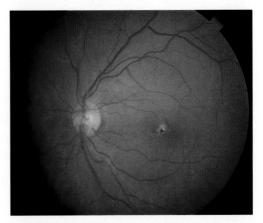

Figure 17-54. Macular area after destruction of the tumor with cryotherapy. Note that the macular exudation seen in Fig. 17-51 has disappeared and mild retinal pigment epithelial alteration is present. Vision returned to 6/6 (20/20) and has remained normal for 23 years since treatment.

RETINAL CAVERNOUS HEMANGIOMA

Retinal cavernous hemangioma is a benign vascular tumor that usually is diagnosed in children or young adults. It can occur as an isolated solitary tumor or as a component of an oculoneurocutaneous syndrome that has an autosomal dominant hereditary pattern. It consists of intracranial and cutaneous vascular malformations similar to those that are present in the retina. A patient with solitary or multiple retinal cavernous hemangiomas generally should be evaluated and followed for such related vascular anomalies (1–4). Clinically, retinal cavernous hemangioma usually appears as a reddish-blue sessile tumor in the peripheral retina on or near the optic disc. In contrast to the retinal capillary hemangioma, it does not produce significant retinal exudation, and it has its epicenter along the course of a retinal vein without a dilated retinal feeding artery. It often is associated with white fibroglial tissue that may occur spontaneously or secondary to small hemorrhages near the tumor surface. With fluorescein angiography, retinal cavernous hemangioma has a very typical, if not pathognomonic, pattern. In the vascular filling phases, the tumor remains mostly hypofluorescent. In the late venous phase, the saccular aneurysms gradually fill with fluorescein. Eventually, the upper half of the vascular spaces fills with fluorescein while the lower half remains hypofluorescent due to the presence of blood inferiorly. Histopathology shows a vascular tumor composed of dilated, congested retinal veins (1).

Most retinal cavernous hemangiomas require no treatment. The main complication is vitreous hemorrhage, which appears to be relatively uncommon. In cases with extensive vitreous hemorrhage, removal of the blood by vitrectomy techniques may be acceptable. The role of laser or cryotherapy to treat the tumor is not clearly established, but they can be attempted in special cases.

SELECTED REFERENCES

1. Gass JDM. Cavernous hemangioma of the retina. A neuro-oculocutaneous syndrome. *Am J Ophthalmol* 1971;71:799–814.
2. Shields JA, Shields CL. *Intraocular tumors. A text and atlas.* Philadelphia: WB Saunders, 1992:393–419.
3. Shields JA, Shields CL. *Intraocular tumors. A text and atlas.* Philadelphia: WB Saunders, 1992:513–539.
4. Goldberg RE, Pheasant TR, Shields JA. Cavernous hemangioma of the retina. A four-generation pedigree with neuro-oculocutaneous involvement and an example of bilateral retinal involvement. *Arch Ophthalmol* 1979;97:2321–2324.

Retinal Cavernous Hemangioma—Clinical Variations

The clinical appearance of retinal cavernous hemangioma can vary considerably from case to case. It can range from a small subtle cluster of aneurysms to a more massive blue-red tumor. Fibroglial tissue in the larger lesions can cause considerable dragging of the retina.

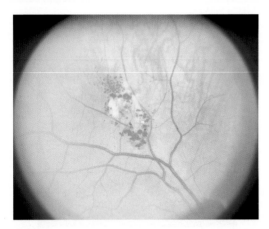

Figure 17-55. Small sessile retinal cavernous hemangioma with mild fibroglial tissue.

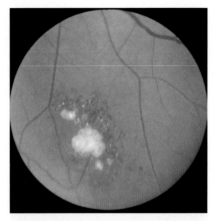

Figure 17-56. Small sessile retinal cavernous hemangioma with moderate fibroglial tissue.

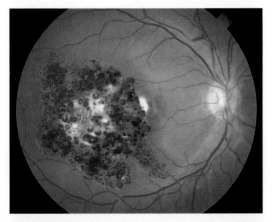

Figure 17-57. Retinal cavernous hemangioma centered in the macular area.

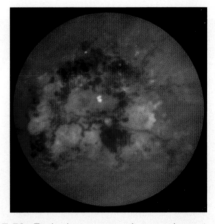

Figure 17-58. Retinal cavernous hemangioma temporal to the macular area.

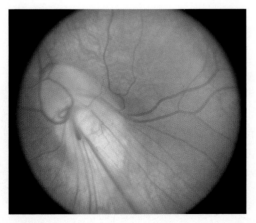

Figure 17-59. Retinal dragging secondary to retinal cavernous hemangioma. Posterior pole showing retinal fold extending inferotemporally from the optic disc.

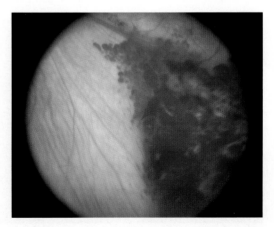

Figure 17-60. Large peripheral retinal cavernous hemangioma in same eye shown in Fig. 17-59. The glial tissue on the cavernous hemangioma accounted for the retinal dragging.

Retinal Cavernous Hemangioma—Clinical Variations, Ultrasonography, and Histopathology

Larger retinal cavernous hemangiomas can resemble a choroidal melanoma. Examples are cited that prompted referral because of suspected choroidal melanoma. However, the characteristic clinical and angiographic features should help to differentiate it from melanoma.

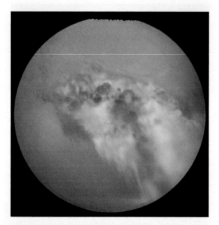

Figure 17-61. Large retinal cavernous hemangioma with fibroglial tissue on the surface.

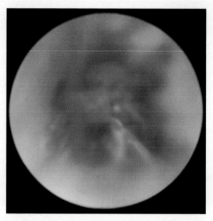

Figure 17-62. Large peripheral retinal cavernous hemangioma that simulated a mushroom-shaped melanoma with extensive vitreous hemorrhage.

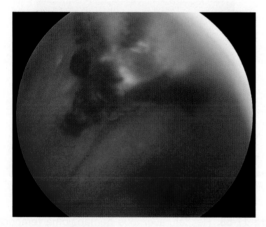

Figure 17-63. Large superior retinal cavernous hemangioma.

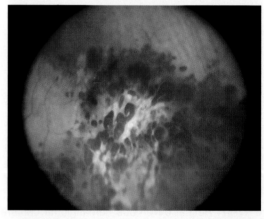

Figure 17-64. Large temporal retinal cavernous hemangioma.

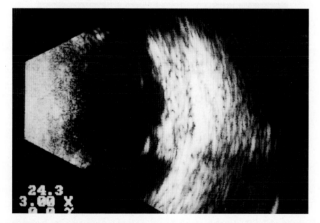

Figure 17-65. B-scan ultrasonogram of large retinal cavernous hemangioma shown in Fig. 17-60 showing the irregular mass with acoustic solidity.

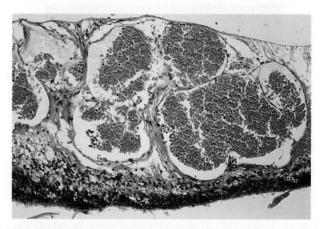

Figure 17-66. Histopathology of retinal cavernous hemangioma showing large, dilated, thin-walled cavernous vascular channels (hematoxylin–eosin, original magnification × 30). (Courtesy of Dr. Ramon Font.)

Retinal Cavernous Hemangioma—Fluorescein Angiography

Fluorescein angiography shows a highly characteristic pattern in cases of retinal cavernous hemangioma. The lesion generally shows hypofluorescence in the arterial filling phases and gradual filling of the aneurysms with fluorescein in the late venous and recirculation phases. This is explained by the fact that the lesion lies on the venous side of the circulation and has a slow, almost stagnant, flow of blood.

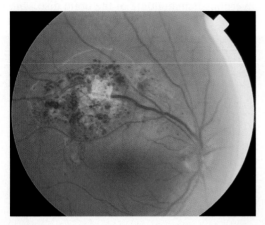

Figure 17-67. Retinal cavernous hemangioma along the superotemporal retinal vascular arcade. (Courtesy of Drs. William Benson and Gary Brown.)

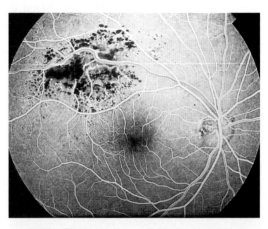

Figure 17-68. Fluorescein angiogram in laminar venous phase showing general hypofluorescence of the mass.

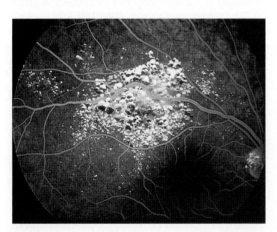

Figure 17-69. Late angiogram showing typical hyperfluorescence of the superior aspect and hypofluorescence of the inferior aspect of the aneurysms.

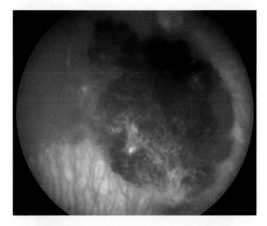

Figure 17-70. Large globular retinal cavernous hemangioma that resembles a retinal hemorrhage.

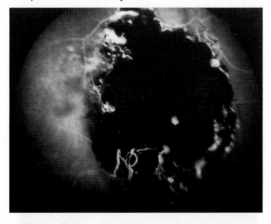

Figure 17-71. Early angiogram showing hypofluorescence of the lesion.

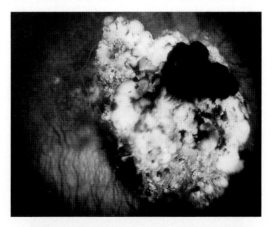

Figure 17-72. Late angiogram showing hyperfluorescence of the aneurysms, which is quite different from the persistent hypofluorescence that would be seen with a hemorrhage alone.

Juxtapapillary Retinal Cavernous Hemangioma

Like retinal capillary hemangioma, retinal cavernous hemangioma also occasionally can be located on or adjacent to the optic disc.

Fig. 17-73 courtesy of Dr. Kenneth Moffat. From Moffat KP, Lee MS, Ghosh M. Retinal cavernous hemangioma. *Can J Ophthalmol* 1988;23:133–136.

Figs. 17-76 through 17-78 courtesy of Dr. Jerry Drummond. From Drummond JW, Hall DL, Steen WH Jr, Lusk JE. Cavernous hemangioma of the optic disc. *Ann Ophthalmol* 1980;12:1017–1018.

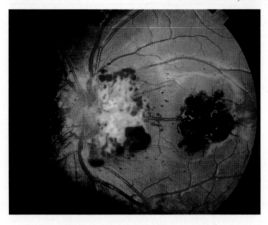

Figure 17-73. Retinal cavernous hemangioma located on the optic disc. Note the second similar tumor in the foveal region.

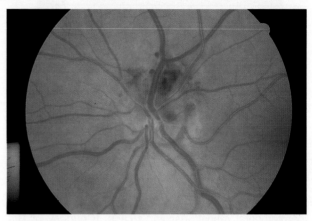

Figure 17-74. Retinal cavernous hemangioma on the optic disc simulating a melanocytoma. Fluorescein angiography revealed the cavernous vascular channels that characterize cavernous hemangioma.

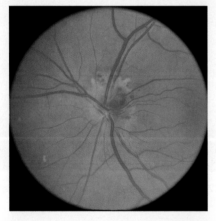

Figure 17-75. Small retinal cavernous hemangioma on the optic disc with moderate amount of fibroglial tissue.

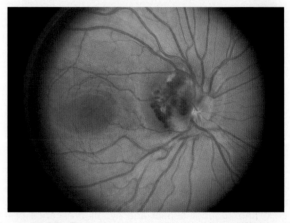

Figure 17-76. Retinal cavernous hemangioma affecting the temporal half of the optic disc.

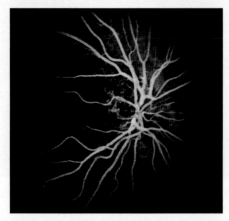

Figure 17-77. Fluorescein angiogram in vascular filling phase showing hypofluorescence of the lesion.

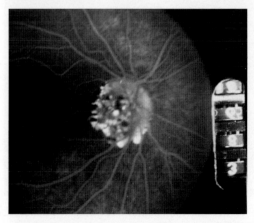

Figure 17-78. Late phase angiogram showing characteristic hyperfluorescence of the aneurysms.

Retinal Cavernous Hemangioma Associated with Central Nervous System and Cutaneous Vascular Anomalies

Retinal cavernous hemangiomatosis is often a part of a familial oculoneurocutaneous syndrome with similar vascular lesions in the central nervous system and the skin.

Figs. 17-79 through 17-84 from Goldberg RE, Pheasant TR, Shields JA. Cavernous hemangioma of the retina. A four-generation pedigree with neuro-oculocutaneous involvement and an example of bilateral retinal involvement. *Arch Ophthalmol* 1979;97:2321–2324.

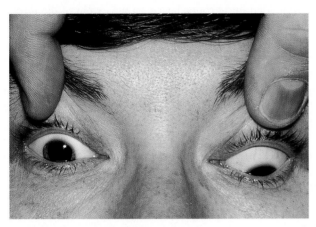

Figure 17-79. Middle-aged woman presented with right oculomotor nerve palsy. Note failure of infraduction of the right eye. In view of the familial findings described following, it was believed that the nerve palsy was secondary to hemorrhage from a small intracranial vascular anomaly.

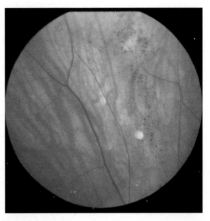

Figure 17-80. Superior fundus of the patient shown in Fig. 17-79 demonstrating very subtle retinal aneurysms.

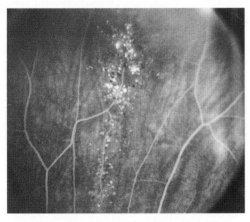

Figure 17-81. Late fluorescein angiogram of the eye shown in Fig. 17-80 demonstrating typical venous aneurysms.

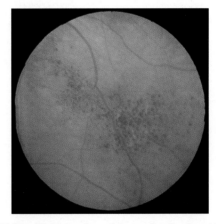

Figure 17-82. Right fundus of the patient's daughter showing subtle retinal cavernous hemangioma.

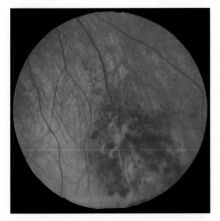

Figure 17-83. Left fundus of the patient's daughter showing more conspicuous retinal cavernous hemangioma.

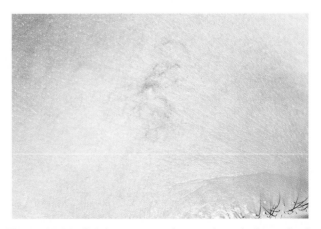

Figure 17-84. Subtle cutaneous hemangioma in the patient's daughter.

RETINAL RACEMOSE HEMANGIOMA

Retinal racemose (cirsoid) hemangioma is a benign retinal arteriovenous communication that can occur as an isolated solitary lesion or as a component of the Wyburn–Mason syndrome (1–6). A patient with retinal racemose hemangiomas generally should be evaluated and followed for similar arteriovenous communications in the midbrain, mandible, maxilla, orbit, and other predisposed areas (1,2). Retinal racemose hemangioma has been divided into groups based on the extent of the retinal involvement (1,3,4). It is characterized clinically by a dilated retinal artery that communicates directly with a dilated retinal vein, usually without an intervening capillary bed. It can range from a simple arteriovenous communication to a more complex mass of vascular channels. The lesion can show a changing pattern if followed for years (5). Fluorescein angiography demonstrates the arteriovenous communication with rapid transit and no leakage of fluorescein. There is little available information on the histopathology, but it probably consists of a mass of dilated vascular channels (1).

Most retinal racemose hemangiomas require no treatment. Rather rare complications include vitreous hemorrhage and branch retinal vein obstruction, both of which should be managed like other cases of vitreous hemorrhage and vascular obstruction, based on the clinical situation (6,7).

SELECTED REFERENCES

1. Gass JDM. *Stereoscopic atlas of macular diseases*, 2nd ed. St. Louis: CV Mosby, 1997:440–441.
2. Shields JA, Shields CL. *Intraocular tumors. A text and atlas.* Philadelphia: WB Saunders, 1992:393–419.
3. Shields JA, Shields CL. *Intraocular tumors. A text and atlas.* Philadelphia: WB Saunders, 1992:513–539.
4. Archer DB, Deutman A, Ernest JT, et al. Arteriovenous communications of the retina. *Am J Ophthalmol* 1973;75:224–241.
5. Augsburger JJ, Goldberg RE, Shields JA, Mulberger RD, Magargal LE. Changing appearance of retinal arteriovenous malformation. *Graefes Klin Exp Ophthalmol* 1980;215:65–70.
6. Mansour AM, Wells CG, Jampol LM, Kalina RE. Ocular complications of arteriovenous communications of the retina. *Arch Ophthalmol* 1989;107:232–236.
7. Shah GK, Shields JA, Lanning R. Branch retinal vein obstruction secondary to retinal arteriovenous communication. *Am J Ophthalmol* 1998;126:446–448.

Retinal Racemose Hemangioma—Clinical Features

Retinal racemose hemangioma (arteriovenous communication) can range from a simple communication to a more complex array of intertwining blood vessels.

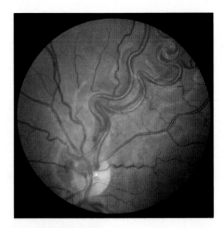

Figure 17-85. Dilated retinal artery and vein superior to the optic disc in a young child.

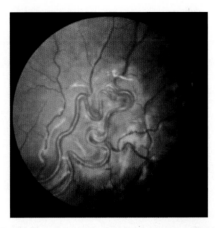

Figure 17-86. Fundus photograph of an area slightly peripheral to the area shown in Fig. 17-85 demonstrating the arteriovenous communication.

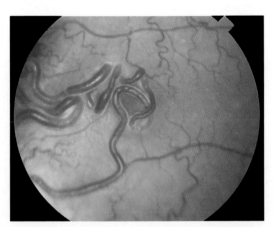

Figure 17-87. Slightly more complex retinal racemose hemangioma.

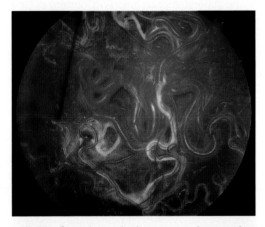

Figure 17-88. Complex retinal racemose hemangioma with a sclerotic white appearance to some of the retinal vessels. (Courtesy of Dr. Robert Kalina.)

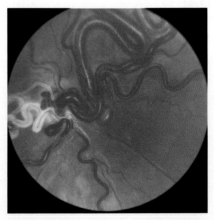

Figure 17-89. Complex racemose hemangioma in a 10-year-old girl with Wyburn–Mason syndrome. She subsequently was found have a similar complex vascular anomaly in the maxilla after having prolonged bleeding from dental treatment. A few years later, she developed hemorrhage from a similar lesion in the midbrain.

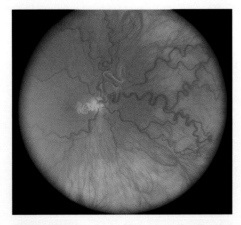

Figure 17-90. Wide-angle fundus photograph of the lesion shown in Fig. 17-89 demonstrating the full extent of the vascular anomaly.

Retinal Racemose Hemangioma—Fluorescein Angiography

In most instances, the blood vessels in a retinal racemose hemangioma fill rapidly with fluorescein but do not tend to leak the dye.

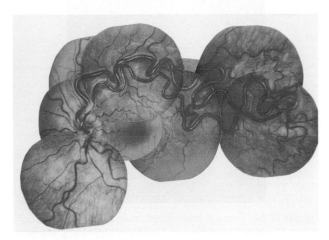

Figure 17-91. Montage of a large arteriovenous communication in the superotemporal fundus. (Courtesy of Dr. Robert Kalina.)

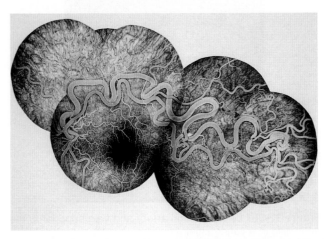

Figure 17-92. Montage of the fluorescein angiogram of the patient shown in Fig. 17-91.

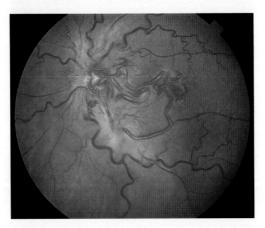

Figure 17-93. Retinal racemose hemangioma in the macular area of a 35-year-old man.

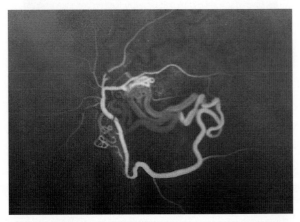

Figure 17-94. Fluorescein angiogram in arterial phase of the lesion shown in Fig. 17-93.

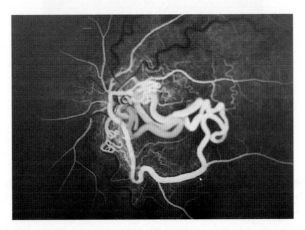

Figure 17-95. Fluorescein angiogram in early venous phase of the lesion shown in Fig. 17-93.

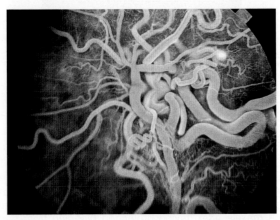

Figure 17-96. Close-up view of the vessels shown in Fig. 17-95 demonstrating the complex nature of the vascular lesion.

Retinal Racemose Hemangioma Complicated by Branch Retinal Vein Obstruction

In rare instances, retinal racemose hemangioma can be complicated by a branch retinal vein obstruction. The precise mechanism is unclear.

Figs. 17-97 through 17-102 from Shah GK, Shields JA, Lanning R. Branch retinal vein obstruction secondary to retinal arteriovenous communication. *Am J Ophthalmol* 1998;126:446–448.

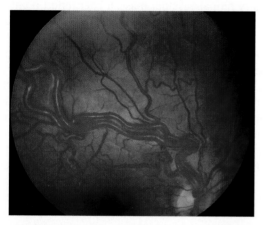

Figure 17-97. Superotemporal enlarged blood vessels in the right eye of a 12-year-old girl with 20/30 vision.

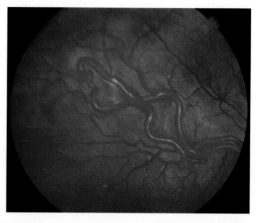

Figure 17-98. More peripheral view showing arteriovenous communication.

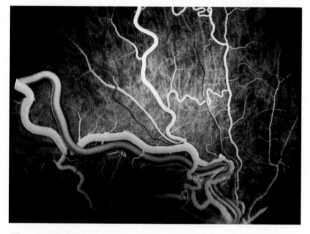

Figure 17-99. Fluorescein angiogram in venous phase.

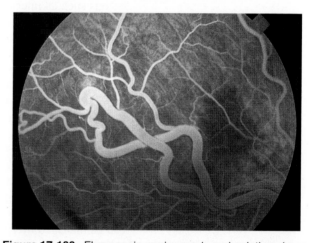

Figure 17-100. Fluorescein angiogram in recirculation phase.

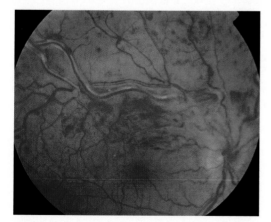

Figure 17-101. Appearance 9 years later when the patient developed sudden worsening of vision in the affected right eye. Note the hemorrhagic retinopathy typical of branch vein obstruction along the course of the vascular anomaly.

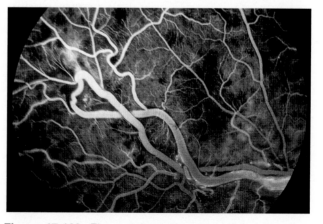

Figure 17-102. Fluorescein angiogram showing hypofluorescence of the retinal hemorrhages in the distribution of the vascular anomaly.

VASOPROLIFERATIVE TUMOR OF THE OCULAR FUNDUS (ACQUIRED RETINAL HEMANGIOMA)

Retinal vasoproliferative tumor is a term applied to a vascularized fundus lesion that has received a good deal of attention in the recent literature. One of the earlier reports used the term presumed acquired retinal hemangioma to characterize this condition and discussed those features that differentiate it from retinal capillary hemangioma, choroidal melanoma, and other fundus lesions (1). Because of the possibility that this condition is not necessarily a primary retinal vascular mass, a later report pointed out that the term vasoproliferative tumor of the ocular fundus (VPTOF) may be preferable (2).

The ophthalmoscopic features of VPTOF vary from case to case but, in general, the lesion appears as an elevated reddish-pink mass that has a retinal feeding artery and draining vein. These vessels are slightly enlarged but are not so dilated and tortuous as those seen with the retinal capillary hemangioma associated with VHL syndrome. The VPTOF characteristically produces exudation that usually extends from the peripheral lesion toward the posterior pole. The exudation is usually continuous with the mass and is not usually in the macular area remote from the tumor, as seen with retinal capillary hemangioma. However, preretinal macular gliosis can occur remote from the lesion.

VPTOF can occur as a primary or as a secondary lesion (2). The primary type generally is a unilateral, solitary lesion in the fundus inferotemporally. About half of affected patients have systemic hypertension, but no other specific abnormalities have been identified. The secondary type occurs in eyes that have certain predisposing lesions such as intermediate uveitis, retinal pigmentary dystrophy ("retinitis pigmentosa") (3), ocular toxocariasis, Coats' disease, chronic retinal detachment, and other entities associated with ocular trauma or inflammation. We have observed it bilaterally often in young adult women who have diffuse intraretinal exudation and retinal detachment similar to that seen with Coats' disease. There is little information available on this histopathology of VPTOF. It is speculated that it is a reactive mass containing blood vessels that may derive from the sensory retina and possibly from glial cells or retinal pigment epithelial cells. Some may have a combination of these different cells.

Management varies from case to case. Asymptomatic lesions may be observed and may be stable for years or even regress spontaneously. Those with progressive exudation or vitreous hemorrhage may be managed by cryotherapy, which sometimes can induce dramatic tumor regression. Smaller lesions without extensive exudation or retinal detachment can be treated with laser photocoagulation. Cases that do not respond can be managed by episcleral plaque brachytherapy.

SELECTED REFERENCES

1. Shields JA, Decker WL, Sanborn GE, Augsburger JJ, Goldberg RE. Presumed acquired retinal hemangiomas. *Ophthalmology* 1983;90:1292–1300.
2. Shields CL, Shields JA, Barrett J, De Potter P. Vasoproliferative tumors of the ocular fundus. Classification and clinical manifestations in 103 patients. *Arch Ophthalmol* 1995;113:615–623.
3. Medlock R, Shields JA, Shields CL, Yarian D, Beyrer C. Retinal hemangioma-like lesions in eyes with retinitis pigmentosa. *Retina* 1991;10:274–277.

Vasoproliferative Tumor of the Ocular Fundus—Primary Type—Clinical Features

The primary type of VPTOF usually is located in the inferior aspect of the fundus between the equator and the ora serrata.

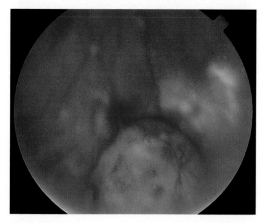

Figure 17-103. Characteristic vasoproliferative tumor of the ocular fundus inferiorly in a 65-year-old man showing pink-yellow lesion with adjacent intraretinal exudation.

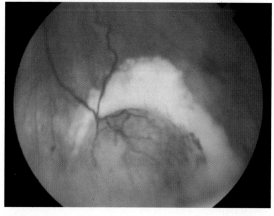

Figure 17-104. Characteristic vasoproliferative tumor of the ocular fundus inferiorly with adjacent circinate exudation in a 40-year-old man.

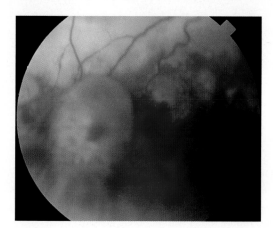

Figure 17-105. Vasoproliferative tumor of the ocular fundus inferiorly with adjacent intraretinal hemorrhage in a 30-year-old woman.

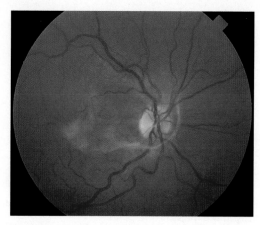

Figure 17-106. Posterior pole of the same eye shown in Fig. 17-105 demonstrating the preretinal macular gliosis that frequently occurs with this condition.

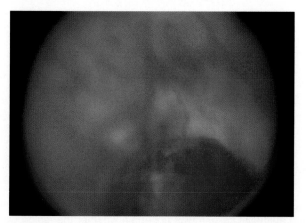

Figure 17-107. Pretreatment appearance of relatively large vasoproliferative tumor of the ocular fundus inferiorly in a 46-year-old man.

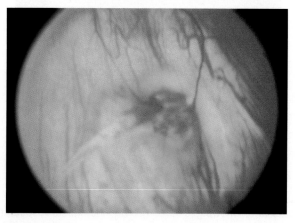

Figure 17-108. Appearance of the same lesion shown in Fig. 17-107 demonstrating marked regression of the mass after double freeze–thaw cryotherapy.

Vasoproliferative Tumor of the Ocular Fundus—Clinicopathologic Correlation

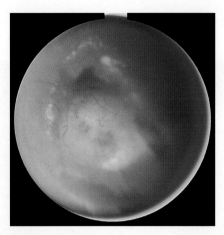

Figure 17-109. Vasoproliferative tumor of the ocular fundus near the equator inferiorly, with exudation and proliferation of the retinal pigment epithelium.

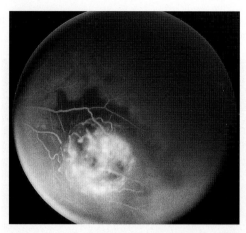

Figure 17-110. Fluorescein angiogram in recirculation phase showing hyperfluorescence of the mass.

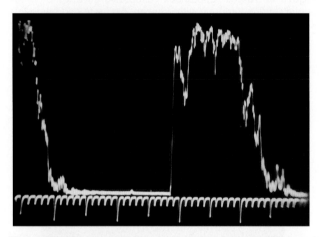

Figure 17-111. A-scan ultrasonogram showing high internal reflectivity in the mass.

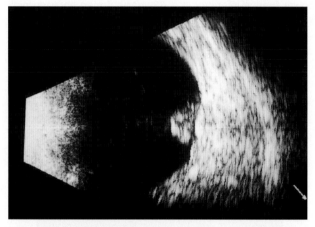

Figure 17-112. B-scan ultrasonogram showing dome-shaped retinal mass with acoustic solidity.

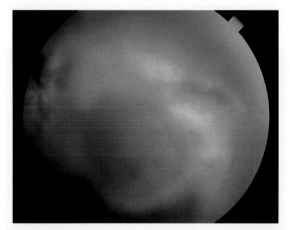

Figure 17-113. Clinical appearance of the lesion about 2 years later showing definite growth, increased vascularity, and hemorrhage, in spite of attempts at cryotherapy. The blind eye became painful and was enucleated.

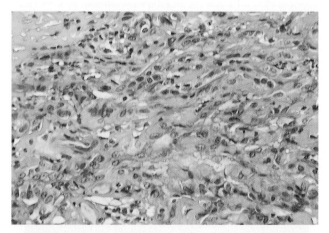

Figure 17-114. Histopathology showing benign spindle cells and epithelial cells. It was uncertain whether the lesion was primarily a vascular mass. The proliferated retinal pigment epithelial cells raised also the possibility of a primary tumor of the pigment epithelium.

Vasoproliferative Tumor of the Ocular Fundus—Secondary Type

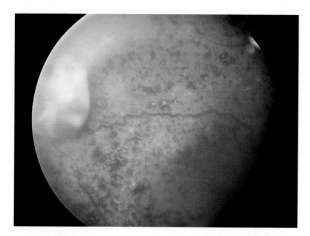

Figure 17-115. Vasoproliferative tumor of the ocular fundus in a patient with familial pigmentary dystrophy of the retina ("retinitis pigmentosa").

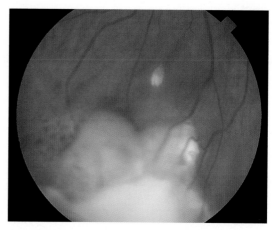

Figure 17-116. Inferior secondary vasoproliferative tumor of the ocular fundus arising from a presumed toxocara granuloma.

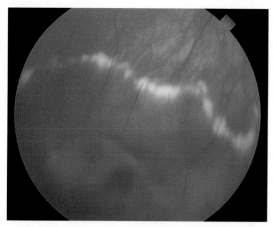

Figure 17-117. Peripheral vasoproliferative tumor of the ocular fundus in a patient who had a typical scar of retinal toxoplasmosis in the posterior pole.

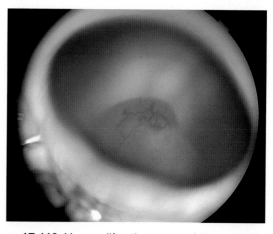

Figure 17-118. Vasoproliferative tumor of the ocular fundus in a patient with Coats' disease.

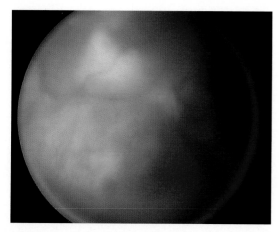

Figure 17-119. Right eye of a 23-year-old woman with the diffuse bilateral type of vasoproliferative tumor of the ocular fundus.

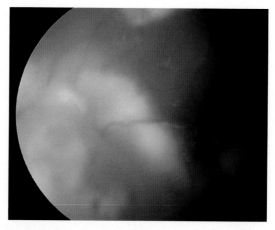

Figure 17-120. Left eye of the same patient shown in Fig. 17-119. The patient had irregular, inferiorly located vascular masses and diffuse intraretinal exudation similar to that seen with Coats' disease.

CHAPTER 18

Glial Tumors of the Retina and Optic Disc

REACTIVE GLIOSIS OF THE RETINA

Lesions that originate from the glial cells of the retina include reactive gliosis, astrocytic hamartoma, and acquired retinal astrocytoma (1).

Reactive gliosis may not be a true neoplasm but rather a secondary proliferation of glial cells that can assume tumorous proportions, in which case it is sometimes called massive gliosis of the retina. It occurs most often in eyes with chronic inflammation, prior ocular trauma, Coats' disease, retinal capillary hemangioma, or congenital malformations. In such cases, the entity usually is not diagnosed clinically, but is diagnosed histopathologically after enucleation of the blind uncomfortable eye (1–3).

Reactive gliosis occasionally can occur as an isolated lesion with no apparent predisposing factors. In such a case, it may be difficult or impossible to differentiate the lesion clinically and histopathologically from acquired astrocytoma, to be discussed subsequently. Such a smaller lesion can be visualized ophthalmoscopically as a circumscribed fundus mass that may be similar, if not identical, to the vasoproliferative vascular tumor described in the prior section.

Histopathologically, reactive gliosis consists of a mass of closely arranged, well-differentiated astrocytes. Marked vascularity frequently is present, raising the possibility that some cases may represent a primary vascular tumor with secondary gliosis. Dystrophic calcification and even bone formation may be present in some cases. No specific treatment is warranted for advanced lesions. A localized, progressive lesion in an eye with visual potential can be managed with laser photocoagulation or cryotherapy.

SELECTED REFERENCES

1. Shields JA, Shields CL. *Intraocular tumors. A text and atlas.* Philadelphia: WB Saunders, 1992:421–435.
2. Yanoff M, Zimmerman LE, Davis RL. Massive gliosis of the retina. *Int Ophthalmol Clin* 1971;11:211–229.
3. Nowinski T, Shields JA, Augsburger JJ, Devenuto JJ. Exophthalmos secondary to massive intraocular gliosis in a patient with a colobomatous cyst. *Am J Ophthalmol* 1984;97:641–643.

Reactive Gliosis of the Retina

Reactive gliosis of the retina can assume a variety of clinical and histopathologic appearances.

Figs. 18-5 and 18-6 from Nowinski T, Shields JA, Augsburger JJ, Devenuto JJ. Exophthalmos secondary to massive intraocular gliosis in a patient with a colobomatous cyst. *Am J Ophthalmol* 1984;97:641–643.

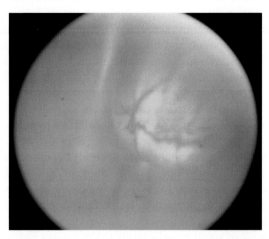

Figure 18-1. Elevated fundus mass in a 63-year-old woman. Note the similarity to the vasoproliferative tumor described in the previous section. The affected eye was obtained postmortem after the patient died of an unrelated cause. (Courtesy of Dr. Daniel Albert.)

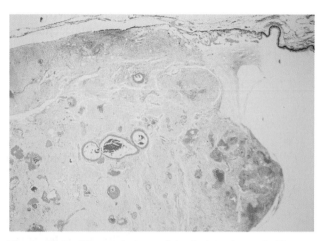

Figure 18-2. Histopathology of the lesion shown in Fig. 18-1. It consisted of well-differentiated glial cells with prominent vascularity and was diagnosed as massive gliosis. (Courtesy of Dr. Daniel Albert.)

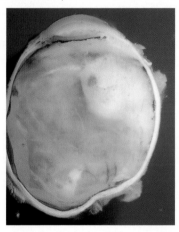

Figure 18-3. Mass of reactive gliosis found in an eye enucleated for chronic discomfort many years after surgery for congenital cataract followed by numerous complications.

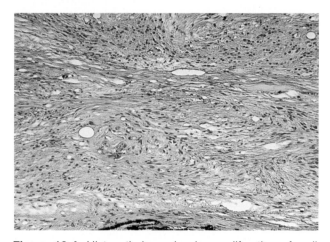

Figure 18-4. Histopathology showing proliferation of well-differentiated glial cells (hematoxylin–eosin, original magnification × 150).

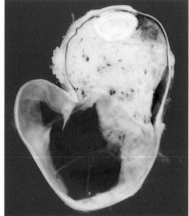

Figure 18-5. Massive retinal gliosis in an eye with congenital microphthalmia and colobomatous cyst. The eye was enucleated because of pain and progressive proptosis.

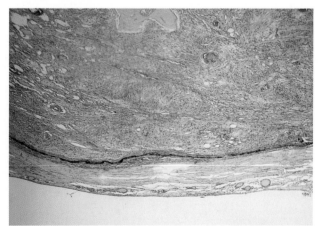

Figure 18-6. Histopathology showing massive intraocular gliosis. The sclera is toward the *bottom* of the photograph (hematoxylin–eosin, original magnification × 75).

ASTROCYTIC HAMARTOMA

Astrocytic hamartoma is a retinal tumor that is composed of benign glial cells, predominantly astrocytes (1). It is believed to be congenital in most cases, but it can become clinically apparent some time after birth. It frequently is associated with tuberous sclerosis, a syndrome that includes various combinations of intracranial astrocytoma, cutaneous angiofibromas ("adenoma sebaceum"), depigmented macules, cardiac rhabdomyoma, renal angiomyolipoma, and other hamartomas (2,3). In those cases that are part of tuberous sclerosis, various genetic alterations have been identified on chromosomes 9 and 16. Some patients have only the retinal tumor without additional findings of tuberous sclerosis (1–4).

Ophthalmoscopically, retinal astrocytic hamartoma can show considerable variation from case to case. The two most common variations are the noncalcified tumor, which appears as a gray-yellow, sessile lesion in the inner aspect of the sensory retina, and the calcified tumor, which is composed of glistening yellow spherules of calcification. In contrast to retinoblastoma, astrocytic hamartoma usually does not develop large, dilated, tortuous retinal feeding and draining blood vessels. Some cases are partly calcified. Occasionally, the tumor appears as a deep retinal lesion that usually is noncalcified and can resemble subretinal fibrosis. Fluorescein angiography of the typical lesion shows a characteristic network of small blood vessels in the venous phase with fairly intense late staining. In the case of a calcified lesion, ultrasonography shows a calcified plaque as might be seen with choroidal osteoma or calcified retinoblastoma. Fine-needle aspiration can be employed to make the diagnosis in atypical cases. Histopathologically, astrocytic hamartoma usually is composed of well-differentiated glial cells. A giant cell variant is not infrequent (5). In some instances, the tumor is locally invasive and has more poorly differentiated cells.

Although astrocytic hamartoma is usually a relatively stable lesion, it can show progressive growth and exhibit locally malignant behavior. Such lesions may continue to grow until the affected eye is destroyed.

SELECTED REFERENCES

1. Shields JA, Shields CL. *Intraocular tumors. A text and atlas.* Philadelphia: WB Saunders, 1992:421–435.
2. Shields JA, Shields CL. *Intraocular tumors. A text and atlas.* Philadelphia: WB Saunders, 1992:513–539.
3. Nyboer JH, Robertson DM, Gomez MR. Retinal lesions in tuberous sclerosis. *Arch Ophthalmol* 1976;94: 1277–1280.
4. Shields JA, Shields CL. The systemic hamartomatoses ("phakomatoses"). In: Nelson LA, ed. *Neslon: Harley's pediatric ophthalmology,* 4th ed. Philadelphia: WB Saunders, 1998:410–422.
5. Margo CE, Barletta JP, Staman JA. Giant cell astrocytoma of the retina in tuberous sclerosis. *Retina* 1993; 13:155–159.

Noncalcified Retinal Astrocytic Hamartoma—Clinical and Pathologic Features

Retinal astrocytic hamartoma often is noncalcified. In such cases that lack the typical calcification, the diagnosis can be more difficult and the lesion can be confused with an early retinoblastoma, myelinated nerve fibers, or other conditions. Close examination for extraocular signs of tuberous sclerosis can facilitate the diagnosis.

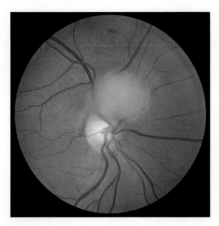

Figure 18-7. Typical noncalcified astrocytic hamartoma adjacent to the optic disc in a 43-year-old woman with tuberous sclerosis.

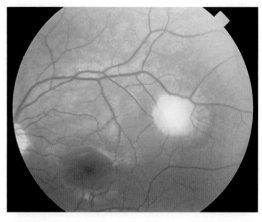

Figure 18-8. Typical noncalcified astrocytic hamartoma temporal to the foveal area.

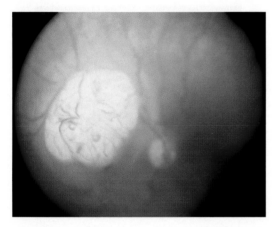

Figure 18-9. Noncalcified astrocytic hamartoma showing characteristic fine blood vessels in the tumor.

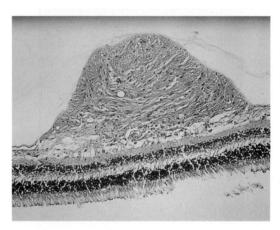

Figure 18-10. Histopathology of noncalcified astrocytic hamartoma showing mass of closely packed spindle cells arising in the inner portion of the sensory retina (hematoxylin–eosin, original magnification × 20). (Courtesy of Armed Forces Institute of Pathology, Washington, DC.)

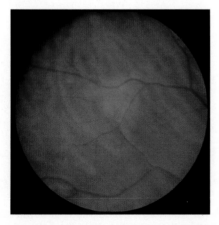

Figure 18-11. Very subtle sessile noncalcified astrocytic hamartoma in the right eye of a 12-year-old girl. The diagnosis was uncertain until the opposite eye was examined.

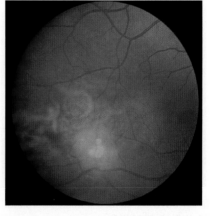

Figure 18-12. Fundus in the opposite eye of the patient shown in Fig. 18-11 depicting a typical astrocytic hamartoma that is partially calcified. Closer cutaneous examination revealed subtle adenoma sebaceum that was overlooked until fundus findings prompted closer scrutiny.

Calcified Retinal Astrocytic Hamartoma–Clinical and Pathologic Features

Retinal astrocytic hamartoma can be calcified from birth or it gradually may become calcified after birth. It sometimes may be confused with calcified retinoblastoma, but it has a glistening yellow calcification as compared to the dull, chalky-white calcification seen with retinoblastoma.

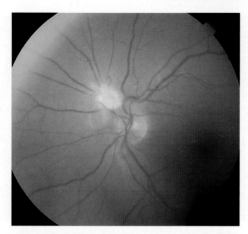

Figure 18-13. Small calcified astrocytic hamartoma superonasal to the optic disc.

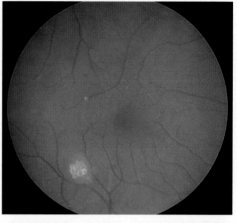

Figure 18-14. Small calcified astrocytic hamartoma inferotemporal to the fovea.

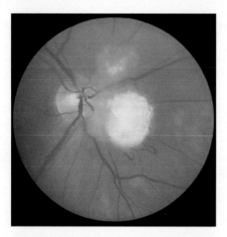

Figure 18-15. Typical calcified astrocytic hamartoma nasal to the optic disc. Note the sessile, noncalcified component of the tumor superior to the more evident calcified lesion.

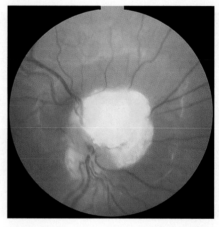

Figure 18-16. More elevated astrocytic hamartoma adjacent to the optic disc.

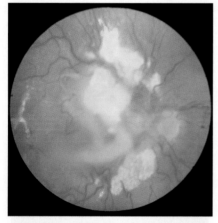

Figure 18-17. Atypical diffuse multifocal retinal astrocytic hamartoma with calcification.

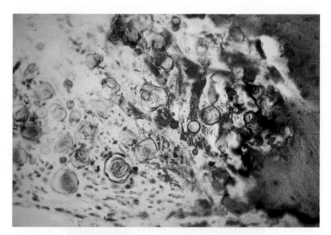

Figure 18-18. Pathology of a calcified astrocytic hamartoma that occurred on the optic disc. Note the astrocytic tumor (to the *left*), dense calcification (to the *right*) and the basophilic whorls (psammoma bodies) (hematoxylin-eosin, original magnification × 20). (Courtesy of Armed Forces Institute of Pathology, Washington, DC.)

Tuberous Sclerosis

Tuberous sclerosis (Bourneville's disease) is the syndrome most often associated with retinal astrocytic hamartoma. It has several ocular, cutaneous, neurologic, and systemic manifestations, including various combinations of low-grade intracranial astrocytoma, cutaneous angiofibromas ("adenoma sebaceum"), depigmented macules, cardiac rhabdomyoma, renal angiomyolipoma, and other hamartomas. Some examples are shown.

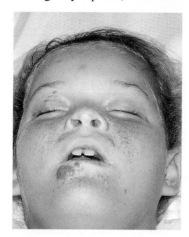

Figure 18-19. Facial angiofibromas ("sebaceous adenoma"). Although this child has involvement in the typical malar region bilaterally, there is also a larger lesion below the lip.

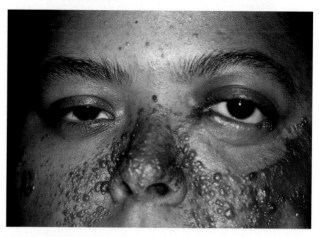

Figure 18-20. More severe facial angiofibromas in the typical butterfly distribution in the malar region.

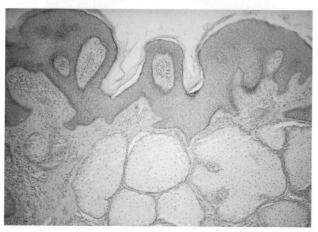

Figure 18-21. Histopathology of angiofibroma showing diffuse spindle cells in the dermis. Note the prominent component of sebaceous glands. This secondary proliferation of sebaceous glands has led to the misnomer "adenoma sebaceum."

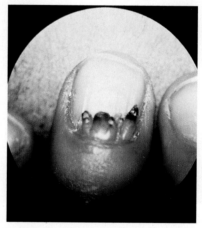

Figure 18-22. Periungal angiofibromas of the fingernail, a characteristic feature of tuberous sclerosis.

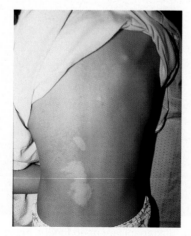

Figure 18-23. Large depigmented macule (ash-leaf sign) on the lower back of a child with tuberous sclerosis.

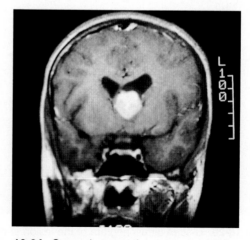

Figure 18-24. Coronal magnetic resonance image of the same patient shown in Fig. 18-23 depicting an intracranial paraventricular astrocytoma.

275

Atypical Variations of Retinal Astrocytic Hamartoma in Tuberous Sclerosis

Not all cases of retinal astrocytic hamartoma assume one of the two classic patterns described previously. Some can occur in the deep retina, some can show extensive secondary gliosis, and some can show progressive growth and exudation.

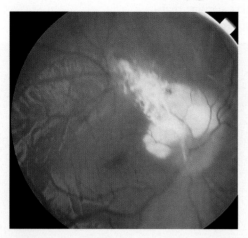

Figure 18-25. Noncalcified juxtapapillary deep fundus lesion that has secondary gliosis on the margin.

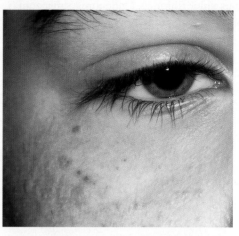

Figure 18-26. Facial photograph of the young patient shown in Fig. 18-25 revealing the facial angiofibromas characteristic of tuberous sclerosis.

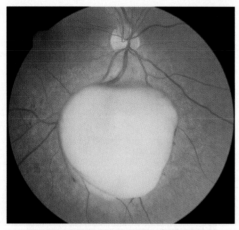

Figure 18-27. Abruptly elevated, pedunculated retinal astrocytic hamartoma adjacent to the optic disc. (Courtesy of Dr. Sergio Cunha.)

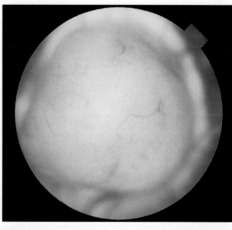

Figure 18-28. Appearance of the lesion shown in Fig. 18-27 about 2 years later demonstrating enlargement of the mass and accumulation of circinate intraretinal exudation. (Courtesy of Dr. Sergio Cunha.)

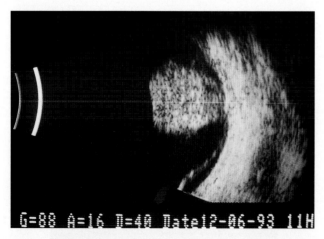

Figure 18-29. B-scan ultrasonogram of the lesion shown in Fig. 18-27 showing the pedunculated tumor with acoustic solidity. (Courtesy of Dr. Sergio Cunha.)

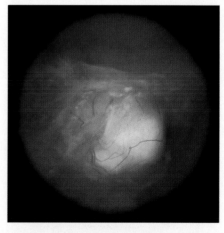

Figure 18-30. Juxtapapillary deep fundus mass with overlying retinal gliosis in a young girl with tuberous sclerosis. The presumptive diagnosis is atypical astrocytic hamartoma.

Aggressive Astrocytic Hamartoma in a Patient with Tuberous Sclerosis

Although astrocytic hamartoma associated with tuberous sclerosis is usually a benign, relatively stationary lesion, it rarely can show progressive growth and evolve into a low-grade malignancy. A clinicopathologic correlation of such a case is depicted.

Figs. 18-31 through 18-36 from Gunduz K, Eagle RC Jr, Shields JA, Shields CL, Augsburger JJ. Invasive giant cell astrocytoma of the retina in a patient with tuberous sclerosis. *Ophthalmology (in press)*.

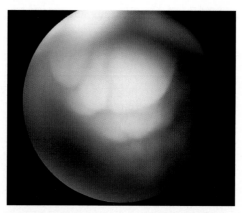

Figure 18-31. White mass in the right eye in an infant girl. On the basis of the findings in this eye, retinoblastoma initially was suspected.

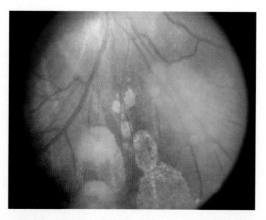

Figure 18-32. Sessile, diffuse astrocytic hamartomas in the left eye of the same patient.

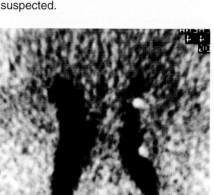

Figure 18-33. Coronal computed tomogram of the head showing two paraventricular calcified astrocytomas typical of tuberous sclerosis. Based on the ocular and cranial findings, a diagnosis of tuberous sclerosis was made. No treatment was given to either eye.

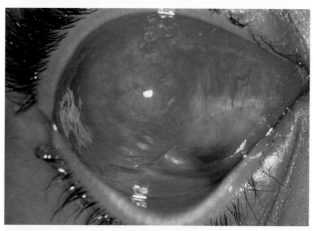

Figure 18-34. Appearance of the right eye at age 10 years. The mass shown in Fig. 18-31 had progressed to fill the entire globe and extend extrasclerally.

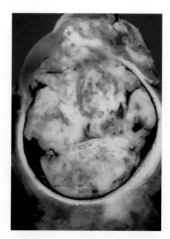

Figure 18-35. Section of enucleated eye showing mass filling the vitreous cavity and extending through the cornea and sclera anteriorly.

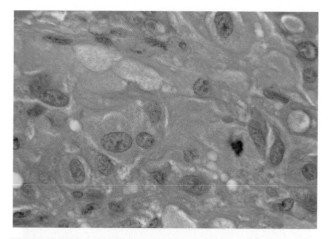

Figure 18-36. Histopathology showing large astrocytes with atypical nuclei and abundant cytoplasm (hematoxylin–eosin, original magnification × 100).

Retinal Astrocytic Hamartoma—Fluorescein Angiography

Fluorescein angiography shows rather typical features with astrocytic hamartoma. In the vascular filling phases, the tumors shows a network of fine blood vessels, and in the late angiograms there is fairly intense late staining of the mass.

Figs. 18-40 through 18-42 courtesy of Dr. James Staman. From Margo CE, Barletta JP, Staman JA. Giant cell astrocytoma of the retina in tuberous sclerosis. *Retina* 1993; 13:155–159.

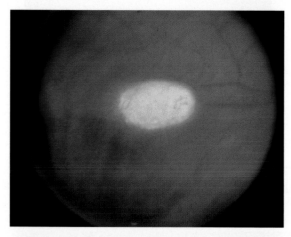

Figure 18-37. Calcified astrocytic hamartoma.

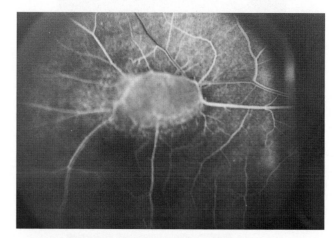

Figure 18-38. Fluorescein angiogram of the lesion shown in Fig. 18-37 demonstrating mild hyperfluorescence of the lesion.

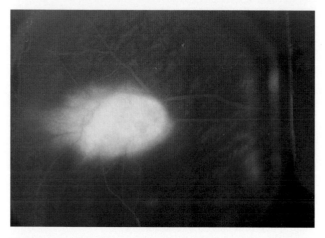

Figure 18-39. Late angiogram showing relatively intense hyperfluorescence of the lesion.

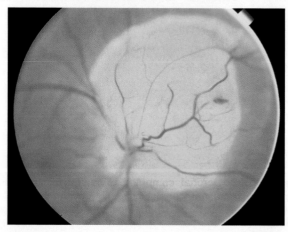

Figure 18-40. Larger noncalcified astrocytic hamartoma located superior to the optic disc.

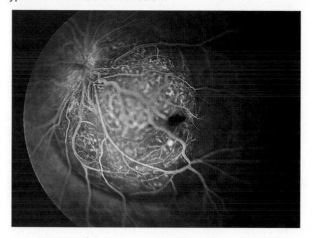

Figure 18-41. Fluorescein angiogram of the lesion shown in Fig. 18-40 in the venous phase showing the characteristic reticular pattern of fine blood vessels in the tumor.

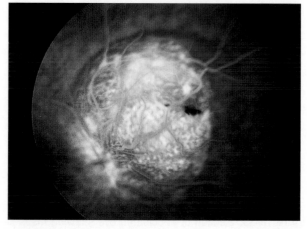

Figure 18-42. Recirculation phase showing moderately intense late staining of the lesion. The eye was enucleated elsewhere and the lesion was confirmed to be a giant-cell astrocytoma.

Atypical Retinal Astrocytic Hamartoma Diagnosed by Fine-needle Aspiration Biopsy

Fine-needle aspiration biopsy generally is not recommended in the diagnosis of astrocytic hamartoma. However, in atypical cases it may prove to be a valuable diagnostic method. A case is cited.

Figs. 18-43 through 18-48 from Shields JA, Shields CL, Ehya H, Buckley E, De Potter P. Atypical retinal astrocytic hamartoma diagnosed by fine needle biopsy. *Ophthalmology* 1996;103:949–952.

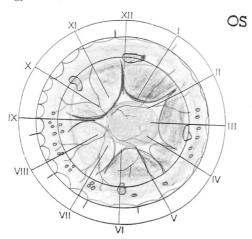

Figure 18-43. Drawing showing a yellow macular tumor in a baby boy with a secondary bullous retinal detachment (shown in blue) and peripheral alterations in the retinal pigment epithelium.

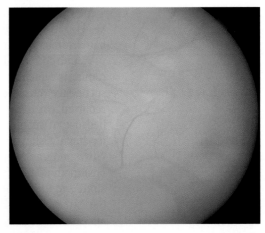

Figure 18-44. Fundus photograph of poorly defined light-yellow lesion in the macular area.

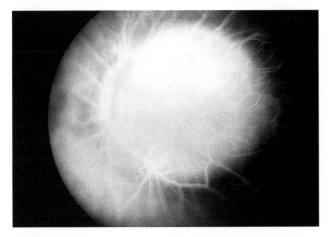

Figure 18-45. Late fluorescein angiogram showing hyperfluorescence of the mass.

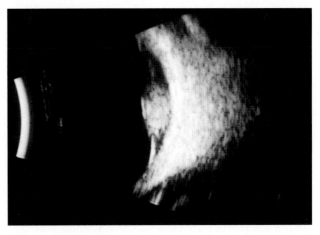

Figure 18-46. B-scan ultrasonogram showing retinal mass in the posterior pole with acoustic solidity and a secondary retinal detachment.

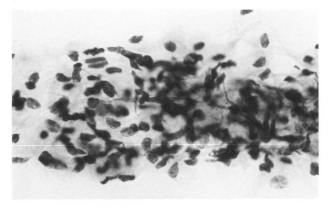

Figure 18-47. Cytology of fine-needle aspiration biopsy specimen showing characteristic spindle cells (Papanicolaou, original magnification × 150).

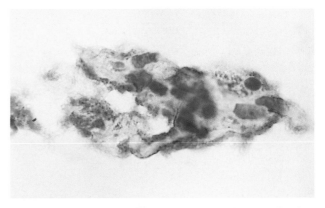

Figure 18-48. Immunohistochemical stain for glial–fibrillary acidic protein showing characteristic staining for glial cells (original magnification × 150).

ACQUIRED RETINAL ASTROCYTOMA

Retinal astrocytic hamartoma accounts for the great majority of glial tumors of the sensory retina. In most instances, it is associated with other signs of tuberous sclerosis. The typical case that is unassociated with clinically evident tuberous sclerosis may represent a forme fruste of tuberous sclerosis in which only the ocular features are manifest. Occasionally, however, the retina can spawn an acquired astrocytoma in somewhat older individuals who have no clinical manifestations of tuberous sclerosis (1–4). Most such tumors appear to be different from the classic congenital astrocytic hamartoma, although there may be some overlap between the two conditions.

Acquired retinal astrocytoma appears as a solitary mass that arises in the sensory retina. It typically is yellow and has abundant vascularity. Intraretinal exudation and secondary retinal detachment usually occur as the tumor gradually enlarges. In most reported cases, the affected eye has been enucleated because of complications or because of suspicion that the lesion is a melanoma. Fluorescein angiography characteristically shows fine blood vessels in the tumor and rather intense late staining. Ultrasonography shows a noncalcified retinal mass with high internal reflectivity. Histopathologically, acquired retinal astrocytoma is composed of mature glial cells, similar to the astrocytic hamartoma. However, the acquired tumors do not tend to have the extensive calcification that characterizes many astrocytic hamartomas. No management is clearly established, because most proven cases have been managed by enucleation. It is possible that if the tumor can be diagnosed earlier, laser photocoagulation, cryotherapy, or radiotherapy could control the tumor and prevent its complications.

SELECTED REFERENCES

1. Shields JA, Shields CL. *Intraocular tumors. A text and atlas.* Philadelphia: WB Saunders, 1992:421–435.
2. Ramsay RC, Kinyoun JL, Hill CW, et al. Retinal astrocytoma. *Am J Ophthalmol* 1979;88:32–36.
3. Reeser FH, Aaberg TM, Van Horn DL. Astrocytic hamartoma of the retina not associated with tuberous sclerosis. *Am J Ophthalmol* 1978;86:688–698.
4. Bornfeld N, Messmer EP, Theodossiadis G, et al. Giant cell astrocytoma of the retina. Clinicopathologic report of a case not associated with Bourneville's disease. *Retina* 1987:7:183–189.

Acquired Retinal Astrocytoma—Clincopathologic Correlation

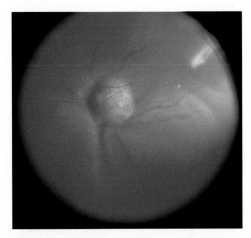

Figure 18-49. Wide-angle photograph showing amelanotic mass adjacent to the optic disc associated with a total retinal detachment in a 35-year-old woman.

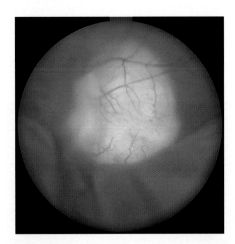

Figure 18-50. Closer view of the lesion shown in Fig. 18-49 depicting the yellow tumor with associated retinal blood vessels.

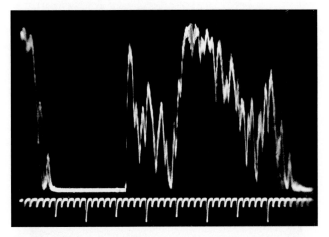

Figure 18-51. A-scan ultrasonogram showing medium internal reflectivity in the mass.

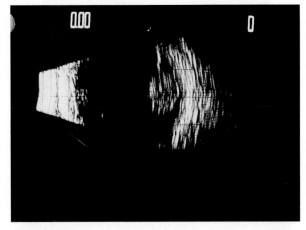

Figure 18-52. B-scan ultrasonogram showing acoustic solidity of the lesion.

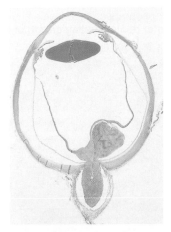

Figure 18-53. Low-magnification photomicrograph of the lesion after enucleation showing the eosinophilic mass arising from the sensory retina adjacent to the optic nerve.

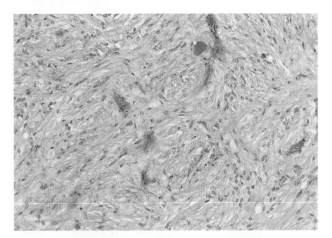

Figure 18-54. Photomicrograph of the lesion showing well-differentiated astrocytes (hematoxylin–eosin, original magnification × 50).

Acquired Retinal Astrocytoma—Clincopathologic Correlations

The lesions depicted here occurred in patients without evidence of tuberous sclerosis and presumably are examples of acquired retinal astrocytoma. Histopathology revealed a benign glial tumor in both instances.

Figs. 18-55 and 18-56 courtesy of Dr. Robert Ramsay. From Ramsay RC, Kinyoun JL, Hill CW, et al. Retinal astrocytoma. *Am J Ophthalmol* 1979;88:32–33.

Figs. 18-57 through 18-60 courtesy of Dr. Thomas Aaberg Sr. From Reeser FH, Aaberg TM, Van Horn DL. Astrocytic hamartoma of the retina not associated with tuberous sclerosis. *Am J Ophthalmol* 1978;86:688–698.

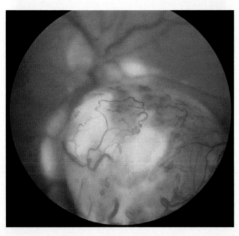

Figure 18-55. Fundus photograph of pedunculated retinal lesion inferior to the optic disc.

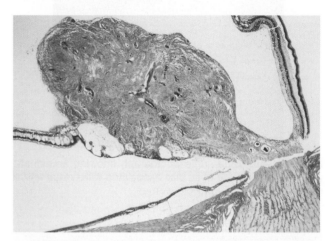

Figure 18-56. Low-magnification photomicrograph of the lesion shown in Fig. 18-55 after enucleation done elsewhere. Note the eosinophilic lesion arising from the sensory retina.

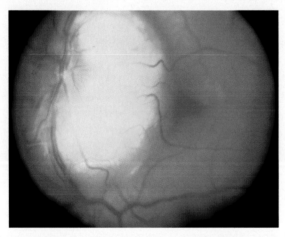

Figure 18-57. Yellow-white fundus lesion arising temporal to the optic disc.

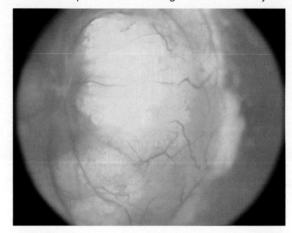

Figure 18-58. Appearance of the lesion shown in Fig. 18-57 about 2 years later demonstrating growth of the lesion.

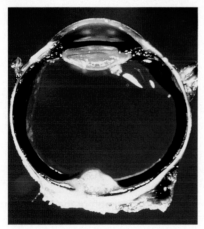

Figure 18-59. Gross photograph of enucleated eye seen in Fig. 18-58 showing white mass in the posterior pole.

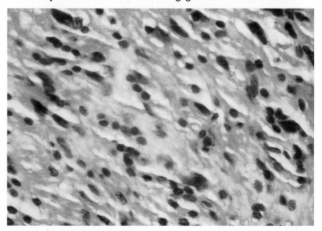

Figure 18-60. Photomicrograph of the lesion shown in Fig. 18-59 revealing the closely compact glial cells.

Presumed Acquired Retinal Astrocytomas

The lesions depicted here occurred in patients without evidence of tuberous sclerosis and presumably are examples of acquired retinal astrocytoma.

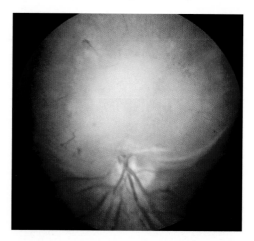

Figure 18-61. White lesion superior to the optic disc.

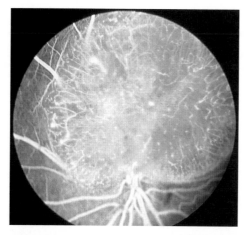

Figure 18-62. Early fluorescein angiogram of the lesion shown in Fig. 18-61 demonstrating the fine vascularity of the lesion.

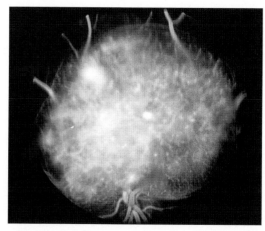

Figure 18-63. Fluorescein angiogram in recirculation phase of the lesion shown in Fig. 18-61 showing more intense hyperfluorescence of the lesion.

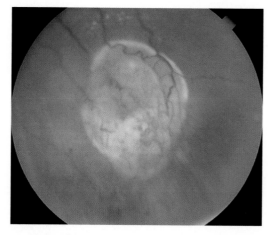

Figure 18-64. Solitary retinal tumor in a 34-year-old man.

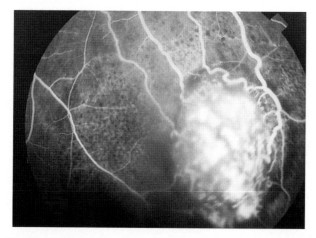

Figure 18-65. Fluorescein angiogram in venous phase of the lesion shown in Fig. 18-64 revealing early hyperfluorescence of the lesion.

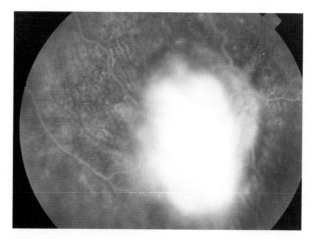

Figure 18-66. Late fluorescein angiogram of the lesion shown in Fig. 18-64 showing intense late staining and slight leakage of fluorescein into the overlying vitreous.

Miscellaneous Intraocular Tumors

CHAPTER 19

Tumors and Related Lesions of the Retinal Pigment Epithelium

CONGENITAL HYPERTROPHY AND REACTIVE HYPERPLASIA OF THE RETINAL PIGMENT EPITHELIUM

Congenital hypertrophy of the retinal pigment epithelium (CHRPE) can be solitary or multifocal. Solitary CHRPE is a presumed congenital lesion that appears clinically as a well-demarcated flat fundus plaque that can range from a black homogeneous lesion to a completely depigmented lesion (1–4). It is characterized in many instances by typical depigmented central lacunae and a marginal halo of depigmentation. Larger lesions can simulate choroidal melanoma, particularly those in the peripheral fundus. Multifocal CHRPE, also known as congenital grouped pigmentation or "bear tracks," is characterized by multiple small gray to black plaques, each of which is remarkably similar to the solitary form of CHRPE (5,6). In some instances, solitary or multifocal CHRPE is completely depigmented, a condition termed "polar bear tracks" (2).

Fluorescein angiography of CHRPE shows persistent hypofluorescence of the pigmented areas and transmission of choroidal fluorescence through the depigmented areas. Histopathologically, the retinal pigment epithelium (RPE) cells are taller and more densely packed with spherical melanosomes as compared to normal RPE.

A somewhat similar condition with multiple irregular plaques of RPE hypertrophy and hyperplasia has been associated with familial adenomatous polyposis and Gardner's syndrome, in which affected patients have a strong predisposition to familial colon cancer (7). This is characterized by multiple, bilateral lesions, the margins of which are more irregular than the typical forms of CHRPE described previously. The typical forms of CHRPE are not associated with a higher incidence of colon cancer (8).

The RPE has a marked propensity to undergo reactive hyperplasia as a result of ocular insults such as inflammation or trauma. A congenital form of presumed hyperplasia sometimes can occur in the macular area as a focal lesion. More often, it appears as one or more irregular, haphazard lesions. Such RPE proliferation can simulate choroidal or ciliary body melanoma (9).

SELECTED REFERENCES

1. Shields JA, Shields CL. *Intraocular tumors. A text and atlas.* Philadelphia: WB Saunders, 1992:43–60.
2. Gass JDM. Focal congenital anomalies of the retinal pigment epithelium. *Eye* 1989;3:1–18.
3. Purcell JJ, Shields JA. Hypertrophy with hyperpigmentation of the retinal pigment epithelium. *Arch Ophthalmol* 1975;93:1122–1126.
4. Lloyd WC III, Eagle RC Jr, Shields JA, Kwa DM, Arbizo VV. Congenital hypertrophy of the retinal pigment epithelium: electron microscopic and morphometric observations. *Ophthalmology* 1990;97:1052–1060.
5. Shields JA, T'so MOM. Congenital group pigmentation of the retina. Histopathologic description and report of a case. *Arch Ophthalmol* 1975;92:1153–1155.
6. Regillo CD, Eagle RC Jr, Shields JA, Shields CL, Arbizo VV. Histopathologic findings in congenital grouped pigmentation of the retina. *Ophthalmology* 1993;100:400–405.
7. Traboulsi EI, Maumenee IH, Krush AJ, et al. Pigmented ocular fundus lesions in the inherited gastrointestinal polyposis syndromes and in hereditary nonpolyposis colorectal cancer. *Ophthalmology* 1988;95:964–969.
8. Shields JA, Shields CL, Shah P, Pastore D, Imperiale SM Jr. Lack of association between typical congenital hypertrophy of the retinal pigment epithelium and Gardner's syndrome. *Ophthalmology* 1992;99:1705–1713.
9. Shields JA, Green WR, McDonald PR. Uveal pseudomelanoma due to post-traumatic pigmentary migration. *Arch Ophthalmol* 1973;89:519–522.

Solitary Congenital Hypertrophy of the Retinal Pigment Epithelium—Clinical Variations

Solitary CHRPE can show considerable variation in color, size, and shape.

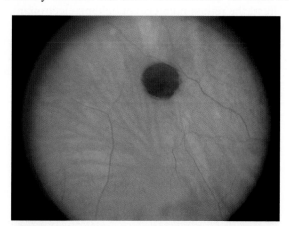

Figure 19-1. Small solitary congenital hypertrophy of the retinal pigment epithelium with a homogeneous black color in a 54-year-old man.

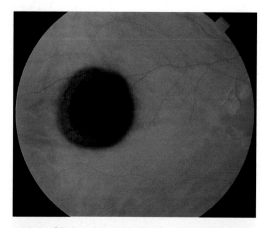

Figure 19-2. Slightly larger solitary congenital hypertrophy of the retinal pigment epithelium in a 17-year-old man. Note the black central portion and the slightly less pigmented peripheral area.

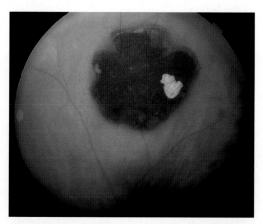

Figure 19-3. Solitary congenital hypertrophy of the retinal pigment epithelium showing a depigmented lacuna and marginal light halo in a 28-year-old man. Note that the margin is slightly irregular but smooth.

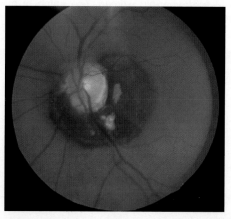

Figure 19-4. Juxtapapillary solitary congenital hypertrophy of the retinal pigment epithelium in a 40-year-old man showing features similar to the more peripheral lesion shown in Fig. 19-3.

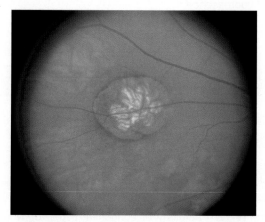

Figure 19-5. Solitary congenital hypertrophy of the retinal pigment epithelium that has a central irregular area of depigmentation in a 22-year-old woman.

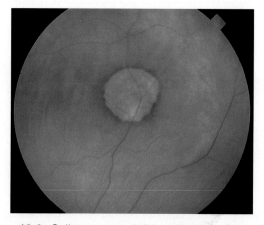

Figure 19-6. Solitary congenital hypertrophy of the retinal pigment epithelium that is homogeneously depigmented (polar bear track) in a 38-year-old woman.

Solitary Congenital Hypertrophy of the Retinal Pigment Epithelium—Fluorescein Angiography and Histopathology

Figs. 19-11 and 19-12 from Lloyd WC III, Eagle RC Jr, Shields JA, Kwa DM, Arbizo VV. Congenital hypertrophy of the retinal pigment epithelium: electron microscopic and morphometric observations. *Ophthalmology* 1990;97:1052–1060.

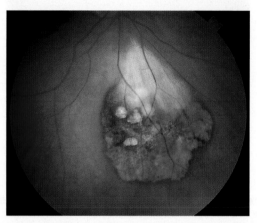

Figure 19-7. Solitary congenital hypertrophy of the retinal pigment epithelium showing characteristic depigmented lacunae in a 46-year-old woman. The patch of myelinated retinal nerve fibers over the lesion is probably coincidental.

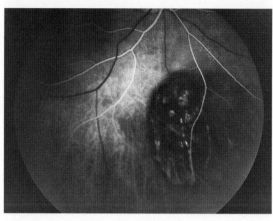

Figure 19-8. Arterial phase fluorescein angiogram of the lesion shown in Fig. 19-7 demonstrating early hypofluorescence of the lesion.

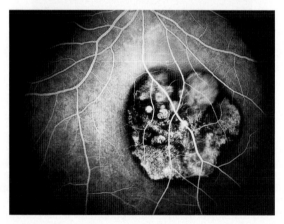

Figure 19-9. Full venous phase showing hypofluorescence of the areas of pigmentation and transmission hyperfluorescence in the areas of depigmentation.

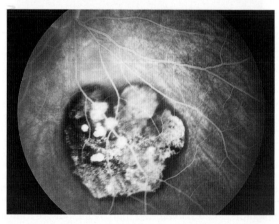

Figure 19-10. Late phases showing continued similar pattern of fluorescence.

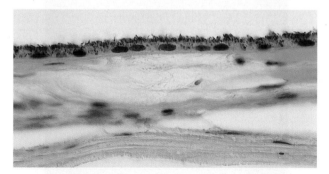

Figure 19-11. Pathology of normal retinal pigment epithelium (hematoxylin–eosin, original magnification × 100).

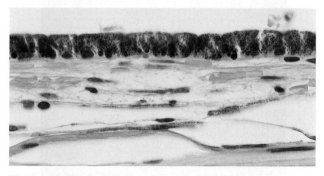

Figure 19-12. Pathology of congenital hypertrophy of the retinal pigment epithelium from the same eye shown in Fig. 19-11. Note that the retinal pigment epithelial cells are slightly taller and have more dense pigmentation as compared to normal retinal pigment epithelial cells (hematoxylin–eosin, original magnification × 100).

Solitary Congenital Hypertrophy of the Retinal Pigment Epithelium—
Larger Lesions and Growing Lesions

In some instances, solitary CHRPE can be unusually large and can be confused clinically with choroidal melanoma. In some instances, it can show photographic evidence of gradual enlargement.

Figs. 19-15 and 19-16 courtesy of Dr. John Norris. From Norris JL, Cleasby GW. An unusual case of congenital hypertrophy of the retinal pigment epithelium. *Am J Ophthalmol* 1976;94:1910–1911.

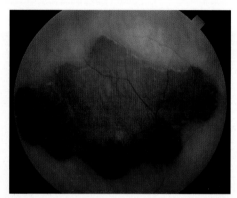

Figure 19-13. Large solitary congenital hypertrophy of the retinal pigment epithelium in a 17-year-old man. He was referred for enucleation because of suspected choroidal melanoma, but the enucleation was canceled when the lesion was diagnosed as congenital hypertrophy of the retinal pigment epithelium.

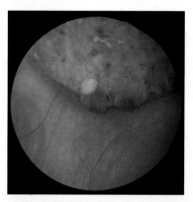

Figure 19-14. Large, peripheral congenital hypertrophy of the retinal pigment epithelium. Such peripheral lesions often give the false impression of being elevated when examined with indirect ophthalmoscopy.

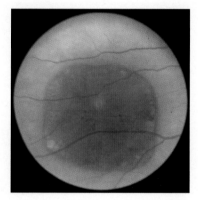

Figure 19-15. Appearance of solitary congenital hypertrophy of the retinal pigment epithelium. Note that the horizontal retinal blood vessel superior to the lesion has no underlying pigment.

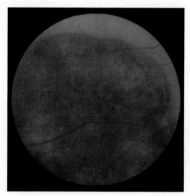

Figure 19-16. Appearance of the lesion shown in Fig. 19-15 about 13 years later demonstrating slight but definite enlargement. Note that the pigment now extends beneath the horizontal vessel.

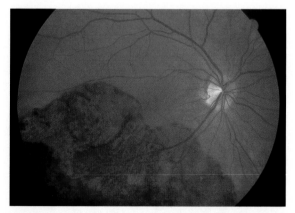

Figure 19-17. Large solitary congenital hypertrophy of the retinal pigment epithelium inferotemporal to the optic disc.

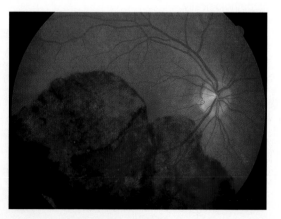

Figure 19-18. Appearance of the same lesion shown in Fig. 19-17 after 2 years. Note that it has enlarged slightly, is closer to the optic disc margin, and now crosses the horizontal blood vessel that was not involved in the earlier photograph.

Multifocal Congenital Hypertrophy of the Retinal Pigment Epithelium

Multifocal CHRPE also is known as congenital grouped pigmentation of the retinal pigment epithelium or "bear tracks." Other than being multifocal, it is similar clinically and histopathologically to solitary CHRPE. Like the solitary form, it can be deeply pigmented or nonpigmented. It often assumes a sector distribution with the small lesions near the disc and large lesions toward the peripheral fundus.

Figs. 19-21 through 19-23 from Regillo CD, Eagle RC Jr, Shields JA, Shields CL, Arbizo VV. Histopathologic findings in congenital grouped pigmentation of the retina. *Ophthalmology* 1993:100:400–405.

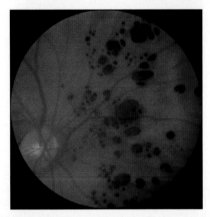

Figure 19-19. Typical multifocal congenital hypertrophy of the retinal pigment epithelium in a 12-year-old boy.

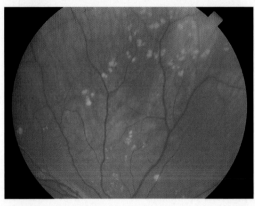

Figure 19-20. Nonpigmented congenital hypertrophy of the retinal pigment epithelium, sometimes called "polar bear tracks," in a 10-year-old girl.

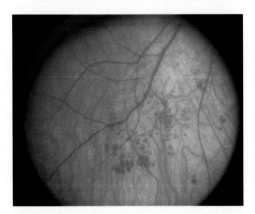

Figure 19-21. Multifocal congenital hypertrophy of the retinal pigment epithelium in a 2-year-old child with retinoblastoma. The opposite eye, which had similar lesions, was managed by enucleation, providing an opportunity to study the lesions pathologically.

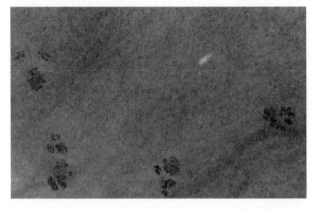

Figure 19-22. Gross photograph of the retinal pigment epithelium in the enucleated eye showing foci of hyperpigmentation.

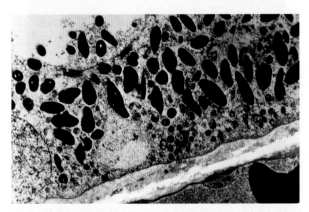

Figure 19-23. Electron microscopy of one of the lesions shown in Fig. 19-19 demonstrating the large, densely packed melanosomes in the cytoplasm of the retinal pigment epithelial cells (original magnification × 4,000).

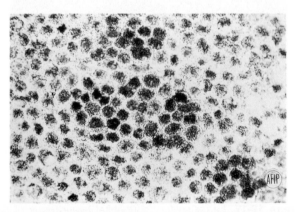

Figure 19-24. Flat preparation of the retinal pigment epithelium of another case of multifocal congenital hypertrophy of the retinal pigment epithelium (hematoxylin–eosin, original magnification × 300).

Hypertrophy and Hyperplasia of the Retinal Pigment Epithelium Associated with Familial Adenomatous Polyposis

Multifocal lesions of hypertrophy and hyperplasia of the RPE are known hallmarks of patients with familial adenomatous polyposis and Gardner's syndrome, familial conditions that predispose them to colorectal cancer. Gardner's syndrome consists of familial adenomatous polyposis with extracolonic manifestations, such as desmoid tumors, osteomas, and other benign tumors. It is unfortunate that the term CHRPE has been used to describe this fundus finding, because it has led to undue alarm that patients with the typical CHRPE also have a predisposition to colonic cancer. However, it appears that patients with typical CHRPE are not at a greater risk for colonic cancer. Depicted are various fundus lesions in patients with familial adenomatous polyposis.

Figs. 19-25 and 19-26 courtesy of Dr. Nicholas Zakov. From Romania A, Zakov N, McGannon E, et al. Congenital hypertrophy of the retinal pigment epithelium in familial adenomatous polyposis. *Ophthalmology* 1989;96:879–884.

Fig. 19-30 courtesy of Dr. James Orcutt. From Whitson WE, Orcutt JC, Walkinshaw MD. Orbital osteoma in Gardner's syndrome. *Am J Ophthalmol* 1986;101:236–241.

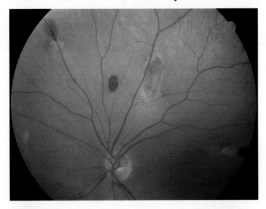

Figure 19-25. Multifocal fundus lesions.

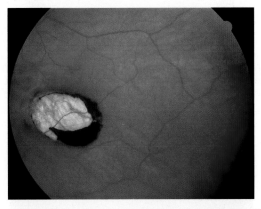

Figure 19-26. Larger lesion with partial depigmentation.

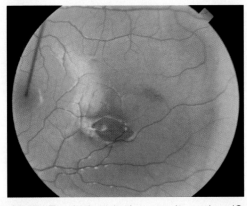

Figure 19-27. Two lesions in the macular region. (Courtesy of Dr. J. Arch McNamara.)

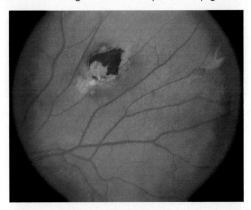

Figure 19-28. Typical fundus lesion in a patient with familial adenomatous polyposis. (Courtesy of Dr. Norman Blair.)

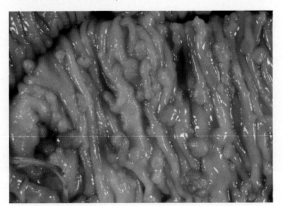

Figure 19-29. Sections of colon showing numerous polyps in a patient with typical fundus lesions. (Courtesy of Dr. James Bolling.)

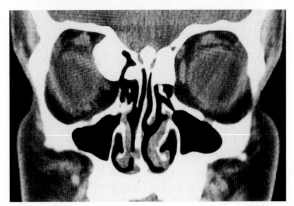

Figure 19-30. Coronal computed tomogram showing orbital osteoma as part of Gardner's syndrome.

Hyperplasia of the Retinal Pigment Epithelium

Reactive hyperplasia of the RPE can range from a small focal nodule in the macular area that is presumed to be congenital to larger more irregular forms.

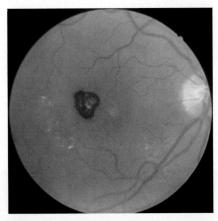

Figure 19-31. Focal foveal nodule in a child, presumably congenital hyperplasia of the retinal pigment epithelium. (Courtesy of Dr. Richard Chenoweth.)

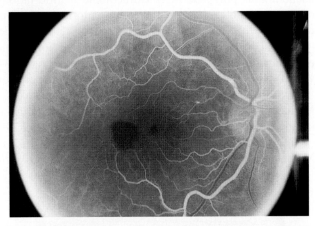

Figure 19-32. Fluorescein angiogram of the lesion shown in Fig. 19-31. Note the hypofluorescence of the lesion.

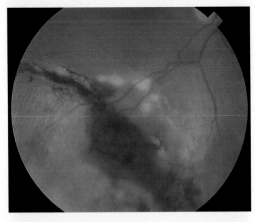

Figure 19-33. Reactive hyperplasia of the retinal pigment epithelium after ocular trauma in a 66-year-old woman.

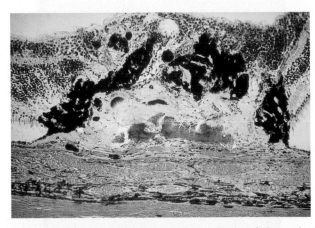

Figure 19-34. Histopathology of hyperplasia of the retinal pigment epithelium. Note that the irregular pigment proliferation has caused an elevated nodule beneath the retina that clinically can simulate a choroidal melanoma (hematoxylin–eosin × 10). (Courtesy of Armed Forces Institute of Pathology, Washington, DC.)

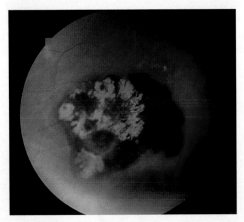

Figure 19-35. Presumed hyperplasia of the retinal pigment epithelium arising in a typical congenital hypertrophy of the retinal pigment epithelium in a 54-year-old woman. Note that a small pigmented nodule is beginning to develop at the inferior margin of the lesion.

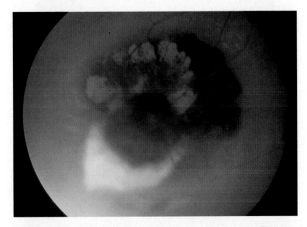

Figure 19-36. Appearance of the lesion shown in Fig. 19-35 after 2 years. Note that the nodule is larger. This is presumed to be hyperplasia, or perhaps a true adenoma, arising from congenital hypertrophy of the retinal pigment epithelium.

Hyperplasia and Migration of the Pigment Epithelium Simulating a Uveal Melanoma with Extraocular Extension

Occasionally, the RPE can undergo massive proliferation and migration, simulating a uveal melanoma. Such a case is depicted.

Figs. 19-37 through 19-42 from Shields JA, Green WR, McDonald PR. Uveal pseudomelanoma due to post-traumatic pigmentary migration. *Arch Ophthalmol* 1973;89: 519–522.

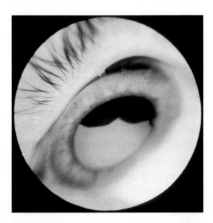

Figure 19-37. Bilobed pigmented ciliary body mass in an 11-year-old girl. The diagnosis of ciliary body "hemorrhage" was made elsewhere, and an attempt was made to drain the blood through a limbal incision.

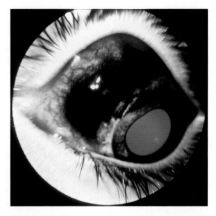

Figure 19-38. Following attempted intraocular biopsy, there was progressive migration of pigment into the epibulbar tissue. The clinical diagnosis was changed to ciliary body melanoma with extraocular extension, and an epibulbar biopsy was done.

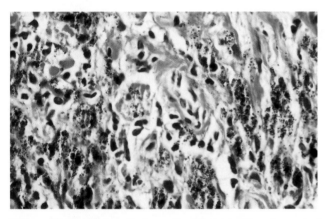

Figure 19-39. Histopathology showing peculiar pigmented lesions presumed to be migration and proliferation of the pigment epithelium, and no treatment was given (hematoxylin–eosin, original magnification × 150).

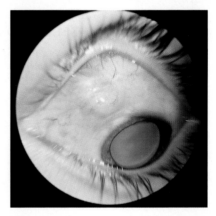

Figure 19-40. Appearance of the epibulbar area 4 years later. Note that the epibulbar pigmentation has resolved entirely.

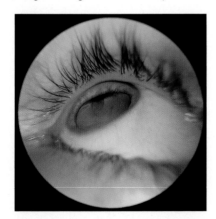

Figure 19-41. View of the ciliary body area at the same time as photograph shown in Fig. 19-40. Note that the intraocular component has decreased markedly in size.

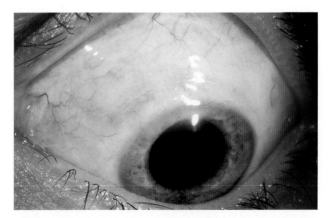

Figure 19-42. Appearance 21 years later when the patient was 32 years old. Note that the epibulbar tissues remain normal. Only a flat area of pigmentation was seen in the ora serrata region.

COMBINED HAMARTOMA OF THE RETINA AND RETINAL PIGMENT EPITHELIUM

Combined hamartoma of the retina and RPE is a fundus lesion that also has rather characteristic, but variable, clinical features (1–3). It generally is believed to be congenital and nonhereditary, and the etiology is uncertain. The most characteristic ophthalmoscopic finding is an ill-defined gray retinal mass that demonstrates abnormal retinal blood vessels, probably due to secondary retinal traction from excessive glial tissue on the surface of the lesion. It most often is located on or adjacent to the optic disc, but it occasionally can be located in the extrapapillary areas of the fundus. In either location, the abnormal, tortuous retinal vessels show characteristic straightening as they pass anterior to the lesion toward the peripheral fundus. It is generally a stable lesion, but excessive glial proliferation may lead to retinal traction and visual loss. Other complications, such as retinal exudation and vitreous hemorrhage, are rather uncommon. Somewhat similar lesions have been recognized as a component of neurofibromatosis type 2. Fluorescein angiography shows markedly abnormal retinal blood vessels in the mass and gradual late staining of the mass.

Histopathologically, the lesion is located mostly in the sensory retina or optic disc tissue and is composed of an admixture of pigment epithelial cells, proliferating blood vessels, and glial tissue. There is no highly effective method for treating combined hamartoma. Amblyopic therapy may be helpful in selected young children. Vitrectomy and membrane peeling may be helpful in cases with vitreous hemorrhage and preretinal gliosis.

SELECTED REFERENCES

1. Gass JDM. An unusual hamartoma of the pigment epithelium and retina simulating choroidal melanoma and retinoblastoma. *Trans Am Ophthalmol Soc* 1973;71:171–185.
2. Shields JA, Shields CL. *Intraocular tumors. A text and atlas.* Philadelphia: WB Saunders, 1992:43–60.
3. Schachat AP, Shields JA, Fine SL, Sanborn GE, Weingiest TA, Valenzuela RE, Brucker AJ. Combined hamartoma of the retina and retinal pigment epithelium. *Ophthalmology* 1984;91:1609–1615.

Combined Hamartoma—Juxtapapillary and Papillary Type

Most combined hamartomas are located over, or adjacent to, the optic disc. In some cases, the diagnosis must remain presumptive, and it is possible that some lesions diagnosed as combined hamartoma may be a result of ocular insults such as inflammation and trauma.

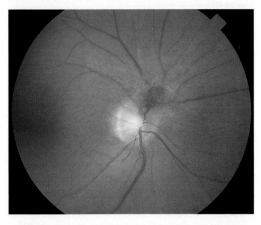

Figure 19-43. Small combined hamartoma on the superonasal margin of the optic disc in a 40-year-old man.

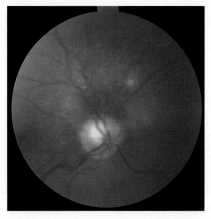

Figure 19-44. Slightly larger combined hamartoma surrounding the superior half of the optic disc in a 45-year-old man.

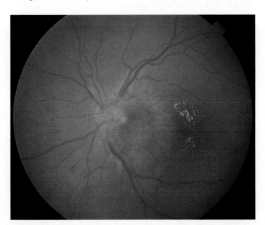

Figure 19-45. Combined hamartoma inferotemporal to the optic disc in a 32-year-old man. In this case, there is a small amount of intraretinal exudation in the foveal area.

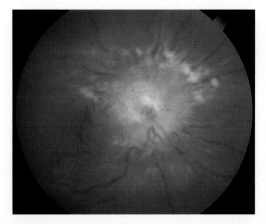

Figure 19-46. Combined hamartoma temporal to the optic disc in a 19-year-old woman. In this case, there is extensive gliosis over the disc.

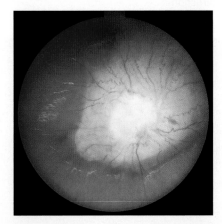

Figure 19-47. Extensive combined hamartoma over and around the optic disc. This was noted shortly after birth in a boy and has been followed for about 16 years without appreciable change.

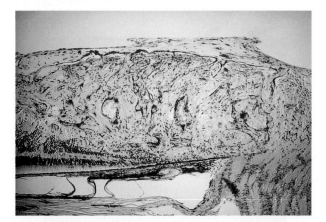

Figure 19-48. Histopathology of combined hamartoma showing thickened sensory retina adjacent to the optic disc with intraretinal pigment, excessive blood vessels, and a glial membrane of the inner surface of the lesion (hematoxylin–eosin, original magnification × 10). (Courtesy of Armed Forces Institute of Pathology, Washington, DC.)

Combined Hamartoma—Peripheral (Extrapapillary) Type

Extrapapillary combined hamartoma can be located in the posterior fundus or as peripheral as the equator. It can cause significant secondary dragging of the sensory retina.

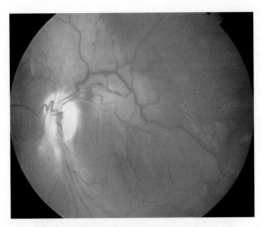

Figure 19-49. Inferior dragging of the sensory retina in a 3-year-old boy evaluated for chronic visual loss.

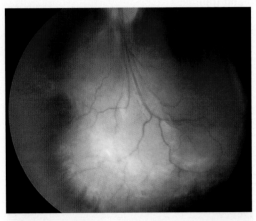

Figure 19-50. Curvilinear combined hamartoma along the inferior vascular arcade in the patient shown in Fig. 19-49. Contraction of the white glial tissue on the tumor surface accounts for the retinal dragging.

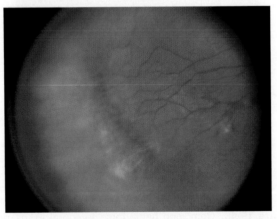

Figure 19-51. Combined hamartoma in the equator inferonasally in a 15-year-old girl. Note that in the area peripheral to the lesion (to the *left*), the retinal vessels become straightened and attenuated.

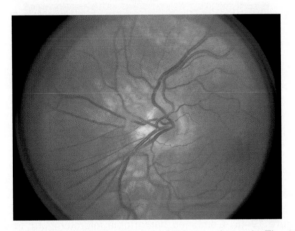

Figure 19-52. Posterior fundus of the eye shown in Fig. 19-51. Note the dragging of the inferonasal retinal blood vessels in a nasal direction.

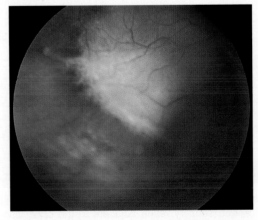

Figure 19-53. Peripheral combined hamartoma in a 6-year-old boy.

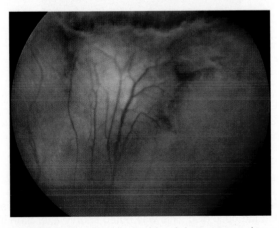

Figure 19-54. Peripheral combined hamartoma in a 30-year-old man.

Combined Hamartoma—Fluorescein Angiography

Fluorescein angiography of combined hamartoma shows rather characteristic features.

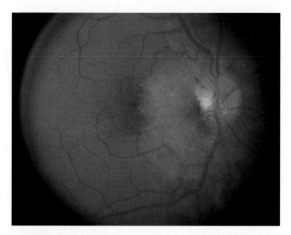

Figure 19-55. Combined hamartoma temporal to the optic disc in a 30-year-old man.

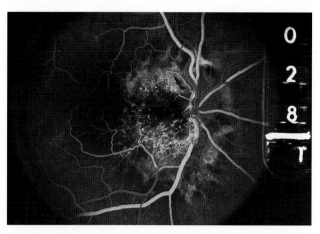

Figure 19-56. Venous-phase fluorescein angiogram of the lesion shown in Fig. 19-55 demonstrating central hypofluorescence and hyperfluorescence due to early leakage from abnormal blood vessels in the lesion.

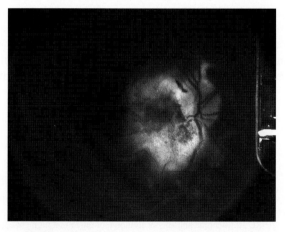

Figure 19-57. Late angiogram showing ill-defined hyperfluorescence of the lesion.

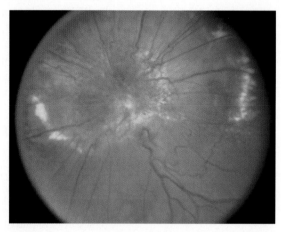

Figure 19-58. Larger combined hamartoma surrounding the optic disc.

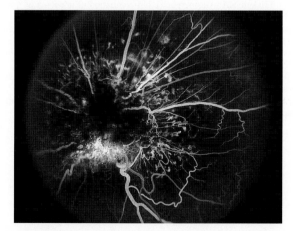

Figure 19-59. Full venous-phase fluorescein angiogram. Note that some of the blood vessels in the region of the lesion are tortuous, but the blood vessels peripheral to the lesion are straightened.

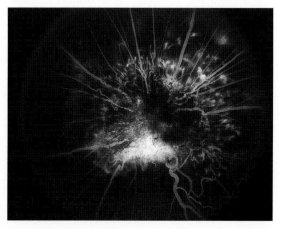

Figure 19-60. Late angiogram showing rather typical pattern of hyperfluorescence.

ADENOMA AND ADENOCARCINOMA OF THE CILIARY PIGMENT EPITHELIUM AND RETINAL PIGMENT EPITHELIUM

True tumors can develop in the pigment epithelium. Both benign adenoma and malignant adenocarcinoma are locally aggressive tumors that lack the potential to metastasize, but they can cause complications leading to visual loss (1–11). Because adenoma and adenocarcinoma are similar clinically and in their biologic behavior, they are discussed together. Adenoma of the iris pigment epithelium was covered in Chapter 3.

A neoplasm of the pigment epithelium is usually, but not always, dark brown-black in color. When it develops in the ciliary body region, it can grow slowly and produce subluxation of the lens and invasion of the anterior chamber. When it arises in the retina, it appears as a relatively stable, abruptly elevated mass. It is known to develop occasionally in an eye that has experienced trauma or inflammation. It can also arise from an area of CHRPE (3). It is not widely known that a neoplasm of the pigment epithelium can develop a feeding retinal artery and a draining retinal vein and can induce retinal exudation, exudative retinal detachment, and orbital extension (4,11).

Fluorescein angiography usually shows hypofluorescence in the filling phases and mild late staining of the lesion (6). Ultrasonography reveals high internal reflectivity with A-scan and acoustic solidity with B-scan. Histopathologically, it is composed of a proliferation of pigment epithelium cells, the pattern of which varies with the tumor location. A tumor of the ciliary body shows more microcystic features, and a tumor of the RPE reveals more cords and acini but lacks the microcystic features.

The treatment of a neoplasm of the pigment epithelium varies with the size and extent of the tumor. A tumor located in the pigment epithelium of the iris, ciliary body, or anterior retina can be sometimes managed by surgical resection. A stable lesion in the posterior segment can be observed, but progressive lesions are eventually treated by enucleation in many cases.

SELECTED REFERENCES

1. Shields JA, Shields CL. *Intraocular tumors. A text and atlas.* Philadelphia: WB Saunders, 1992:43–60.
2. Shields JA, Shields CL. *Intraocular tumors. A text and atlas.* Philadelphia: WB Saunders, 1992:137–153.
3. Shields JA, Shields CL, Mercado G, Gunduz K, Eagle RC Jr. Adenoma of the iris pigment epithelium. A report of 20 cases. The 1998 Pan-American Lecture. *Arch Ophthalmol (in press).*
4. Shields JA, Shields CL, Gunduz K, Eagle RC Jr. Adenoma of the ciliary body pigment epithelium. The 1998 Albert Ruedemann Sr. Memorial Lecture. Part 1. *Arch Ophthalmol (in press).*
5. Shields JA, Shields CL, Gunduz K, Eagle RC Jr. Adenoma and adenocarcinoma of the retinal pigment epithelium. The 1998 Albert Ruedemann Sr. Memorial Lecture. Part 2. *Arch Ophthalmol (in press).*
6. Shields JA, Sanborn GE, Augsburger JJ, Klein RM. Adenoma of the iris pigment epithelium. *Ophthalmology* 1983;90:735–739.
7. Shields CL, Shields JA, Cook GR, Von Fricken MA, Augsburger JJ. Differentiation of adenoma of the iris pigment epithelium from iris cyst and melanoma. *Am J Ophthalmol* 1985;100:678–681.
8. Lieb WE, Shields JA, Eagle RC, Kwa D, Shields CL. Cystic adenoma of the pigmented ciliary epithelium. Clinical, pathological and immunohistochemical findings. *Ophthalmology* 1990;97:1489–1493.
9. Shields JA, Eagle RC Jr, Shields CL, De Potter P. Pigmented adenoma of the optic nerve head simulating a melanocytoma. *Ophthalmology* 1992;99:1705–1708.
10. Shields JA, Eagle RC Jr, Barr CC, Shields CL, Jones DE. Adenocarcinoma of the retinal pigment epithelium arising from a juxtapapillary histoplasmosis scar. *Arch Ophthalmol* 1994;112:650–653.
11. Edelstein C, Shields CL, Shields JA, Eagle RC Jr. Presumed adenocarcinoma of the retinal pigment epithelium in a blind eye with a staphyloma. *Arch Ophthalmol* 1998;116:525–528.

Adenoma of the Iridociliary Pigment Epithelium

It may be difficult to determine clinically if a pigment epithelium tumor in the anterior chamber angle region arose primarily in the iris or the ciliary body. Microscopically, however, the iris pigment epithelium tumor is characterized by cords of pigment epithelial cells without cysts, and the ciliary pigment epithelial tumor has more microcystic features.

Figs. 19-61 and 19-62 from Shields JA, Sanborn GE, Augsburger JJ, Klein RM. Adenoma of the iris pigment epithelium. *Ophthalmology* 1983;90:735–739.

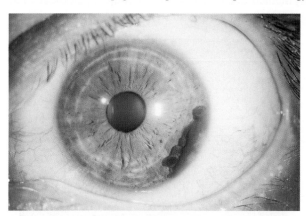

Figure 19-61. Multinodular pigmented tumor in peripheral portion of the anterior chamber seen initially in a young teenager. The lesion was followed, and it showed slow progression and induced secondary glaucoma from seeding of pigment into the trabecular meshwork.

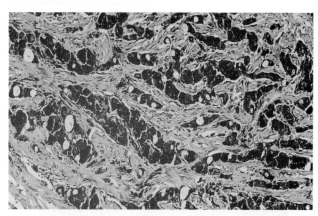

Figure 19-62. Histopathology of the tumor shown in Fig. 19-61 after removal by iridocyclectomy showing cords of proliferating pigment epithelium (hematoxylin–eosin, original magnification × 200).

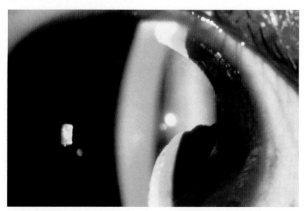

Figure 19-63. Pigmented tumor posterior to the iris as seen with the slit lamp in a 30-year-old African-American man.

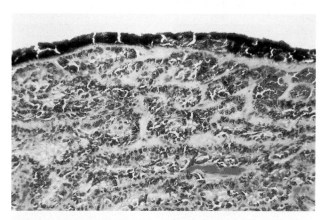

Figure 19-64. Photomicrograph of the lesion shown in Fig. 19-63 revealing cords of proliferating pigment epithelial cells. In this section, the iris pigment epithelium *(top)* is intact (hematoxylin–eosin, original magnification × 150).

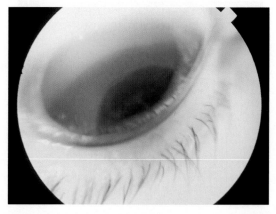

Figure 19-65. Adenoma of the cilioretinal pigment epithelium in a 73-year-old woman. Adenoma of the cilioretinal pigment epithelium was a primary diagnostic consideration, but melanoma could not be excluded.

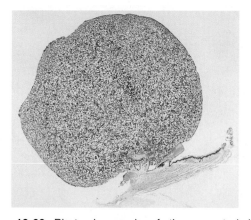

Figure 19-66. Photomicrograph of the resected lesion showing the pedunculated shape of the lesion. Numerous small cysts are present throughout the mass (hematoxylin–eosin, original magnification × 15).

Adenoma of the Cilioretinal Pigment Epithelium

Some adenomas appear to arise in the cilioretinal pigment epithelium and extend posteriorly into the RPE. Such a tumor can be removed by partial lamellar resection. A clinicopathologic correlation of such a case is shown.

Figs. 19-67 through 19-72 from Lieb WE, Shields JA, Eagle RC, Kwa D, Shields CL. Cystic adenoma of the pigmented ciliary epithelium. Clinical, pathological and immunohistochemical findings. *Ophthalmology* 1990;97:1489–1493.

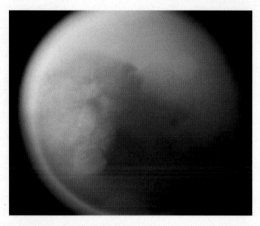

Figure 19-67. Fundus photograph of a peripheral, pigmented, hemorrhagic mass in a 52-year-old man. There is overlying vitreous hemorrhage.

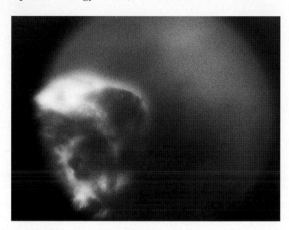

Figure 19-68. Late fluorescein angiogram showing hazy hyperfluorescence of the mass.

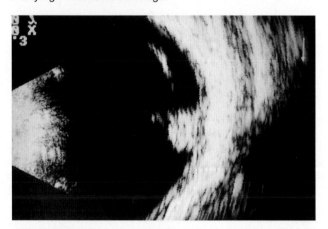

Figure 19-69. B-scan ultrasonogram showing abruptly elevated mass with acoustic solidity.

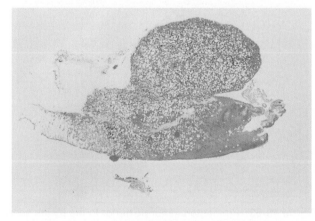

Figure 19-70. Low-magnification photomicrograph showing the mass after removal by cyclochoroidectomy.

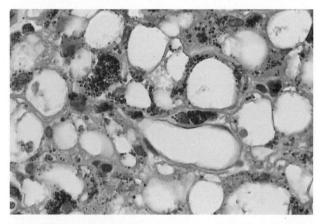

Figure 19-71. Microscopic appearance of the tumor shown in Fig. 19-70. Note the pigmented cells with numerous clear cystic spaces (hematoxylin–eosin, original magnification × 300).

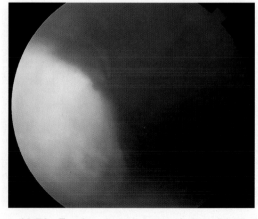

Figure 19-72. Fundus appearance of the resected area after 2 years showing clear margins without tumor recurrence.

Adenoma of the Retinal Pigment Epithelium—Fluorescein Angiography and Ultrasonography

Fluorescein angiography and ultrasonography may provide help in differentiating a neoplasm of the RPE from choroidal melanoma. With angiography, the RPE tumor is more likely to have retinal feeding and draining vessels, and it tends to be less hyperfluorescent than most melanomas. With ultrasonography, it tends to show more high internal reflectivity than melanoma.

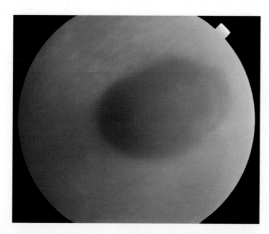

Figure 19-73. Abruptly elevated deeply pigmented oval-shaped mass near the equator of the eye in a 47-year-old woman.

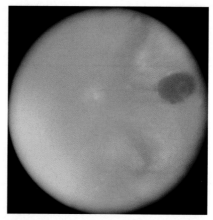

Figure 19-74. Wide-angle fundus photograph showing the full extent of the lesion.

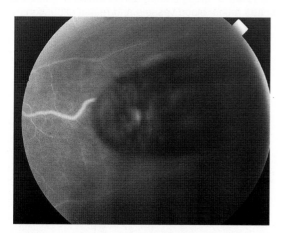

Figure 19-75. Early fluorescein angiogram showing hypofluorescence of the mass and the slightly prominent retinal feeder vessel.

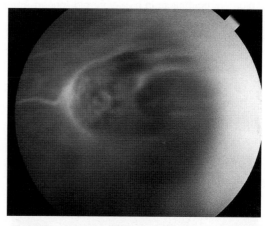

Figure 19-76. Late fluorescein angiogram showing relative hypofluorescence of the mass with marginal leakage of fluorescein.

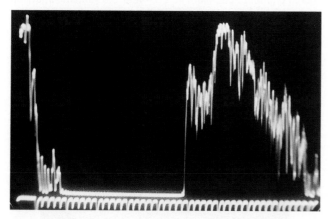

Figure 19-77. A-scan ultrasonogram showing medium to high internal reflectivity of the mass.

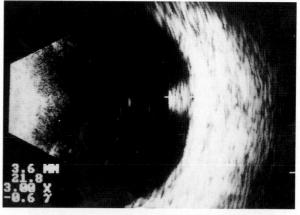

Figure 19-78. B-scan ultrasonogram showing pedunculated mass with acoustic solidity. The lesion has remained stable for 8 years, but vitreous hemorrhage has occurred.

Atypical Adenomas of the Retinal Pigment Epithelium in African-American Patients

In some patients, particularly African-Americans, an adenoma of the RPE can become highly elevated, invade the sensory retina, assume a dilated retinal feeding artery and draining vein, and produce an exudative retinal detachment. Two such cases are illustrated. Both patients declined enucleation after plaque radiotherapy failed to control the tumor, and the affected eye has become phthisical in both instances.

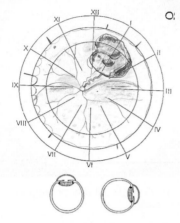

Figure 19-79. Fundus drawing of presumed adenoma of the retinal pigment epithelium in a 28-year-old African-American man.

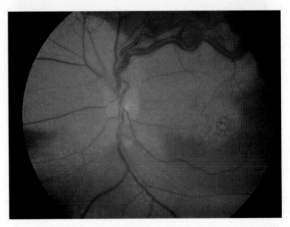

Figure 19-80. Fundus photograph of the same patient showing dilated retinal blood vessels and retinal exudation.

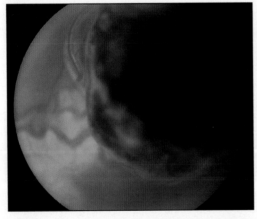

Figure 19-81. Fundus photograph of a more peripheral area showing the black pedunculated tumor.

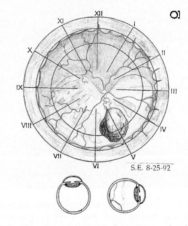

Figure 19-82. Fundus drawing of presumed adenoma of the retinal pigment epithelium in a 31-year-old African-American woman.

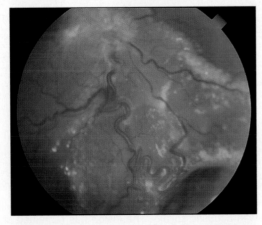

Figure 19-83. Fundus photograph of the patient shown in Fig. 19-82 showing dilated retinal blood vessels and retinal exudation.

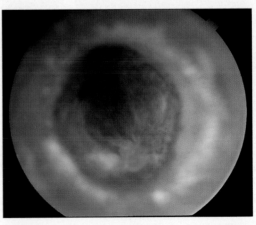

Figure 19-84. Fundus photograph of a more peripheral area of the lesion shown in Fig. 19-82 showing the black pedunculated tumor.

Juxtapapillary Adenoma of Retinal Pigment Epithelium Simulating a Melanocytoma

In some instances, an adenoma of the RPE can occur on the optic disc and clinically simulate a melanocytoma.

Figs. 19-85 through 19-90 from Shields JA, Eagle RC Jr, Shields CL, De Potter P. Pigmented adenoma of the optic nerve head simulating a melanocytoma. *Ophthalmology* 1992;99:1705–1708.

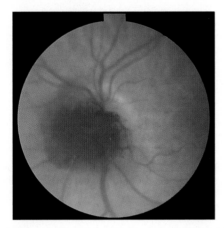

Figure 19-85. Fundus photograph of a pigmented juxtapapillary lesion in an 86-year-old woman. The lesion was believed clinically to be a melanocytoma.

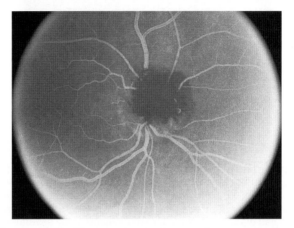

Figure 19-86. Fluorescein angiogram in venous phase showing hypofluorescence of the lesion.

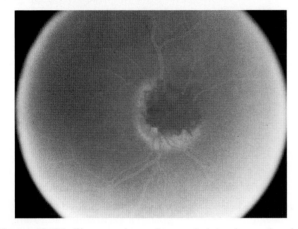

Figure 19-87. Fluorescein angiogram in late phase showing continued hypofluorescence of the lesion.

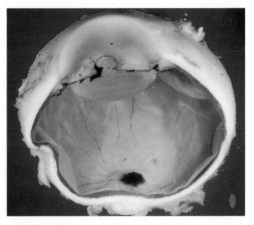

Figure 19-88. The eye was studied after the patient died of an unrelated cause. Gross photograph shows the pigmented lesion adjacent to the optic disc.

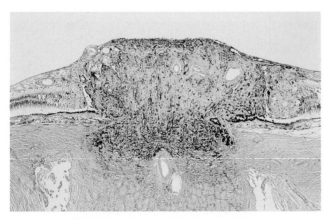

Figure 19-89. Histopathology showing epipapillary mass (hematoxylin–eosin, original magnification × 20).

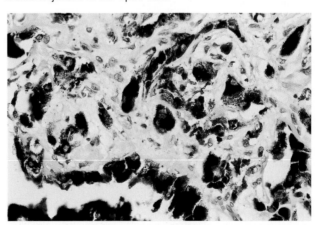

Figure 19-90. Histopathology showing cords of pigment epithelial cells with moderate connective tissue stroma (hematoxylin–eosin × 150).

Atypical Adenocarcinoma of Retinal Pigment Epithelium
Diagnosed by Fine-needle Aspiration Biopsy

Figs. 19-91 through 19-96 from Shields JA, Eagle RC Jr, Barr CC, Shields CL, Jones DE. Adenocarcinoma of the retinal pigment epithelium arising from a juxtapapillary histoplasmosis scar. *Arch Ophthalmol* 1994;112:650–653.

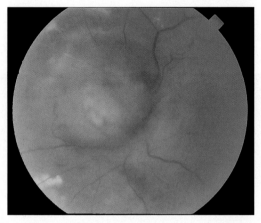

Figure 19-91. Fundus photograph of amelanotic dome-shaped tumor adjacent to the optic disc and exudative retinal detachment in a 69-year-old woman with ocular histoplasmosis syndrome. The lesion had shown progressive growth and was diagnosed as a choroidal melanoma by several retinal specialists.

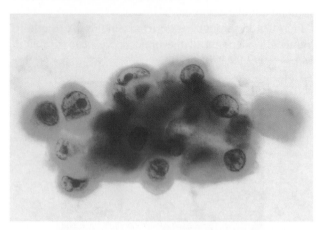

Figure 19-92. Cytology of fine-needle aspiration biopsy specimen showing cluster of tumor cells (Papanicolaou, original magnification × 250).

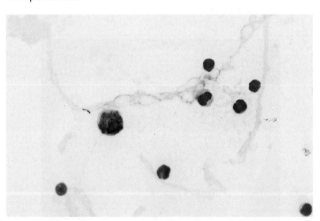

Figure 19-93. Immunohistochemical stain for cytokeratin showing immunoreactivity in the tumor cells. This suggested a malignant tumor of the pigment epithelium. Because of the progressive growth of the tumor and poor vision, the patient chose to have enucleation (CAM 52 cytokeratin, original magnification × 200).

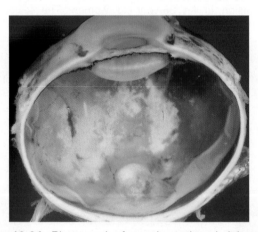

Figure 19-94. Photograph of grossly sectioned globe showing elevated mass in the posterior pole. Note the extensive yellow exudation throughout a wide area of the fundus.

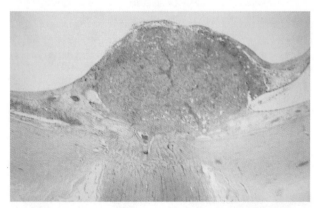

Figure 19-95. Low-magnification photomicrograph showing the tumor occupying the prepapillary region (hematoxylin–eosin, original magnification × 25).

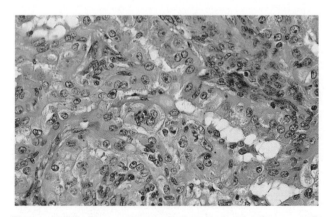

Figure 19-96. Photomicrograph showing cords of tumor cells that show moderate nuclear pleomorphism and prominent nucleoli (hematoxylin–eosin, original magnification × 200).

Aggressive Adenocarcinoma of the Retinal Pigment Epithelium

In some cases, adenocarcinoma of the RPE can become highly aggressive, fill the globe, and extend into the extraocular tissues.

Figs. 19-97 through 19-102 from Edelstein C, Shields CL, Shields JA, Eagle RC Jr. Presumed adenocarcinoma of the retinal pigment epithelium in a blind eye with a staphyloma. *Arch Ophthalmol* 1998;116:525–528.

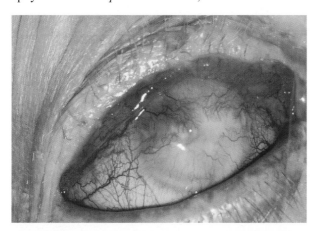

Figure 19-97. External photograph of the right eye showing pannus and complete opacification of the cornea in a 77-year-old woman. The eye had been blind for several years.

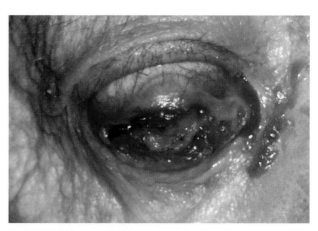

Figure 19-98. Photograph 1 year later showing proptosis of the right eye and scar tissue in the inferior part of the conjunctiva and cornea.

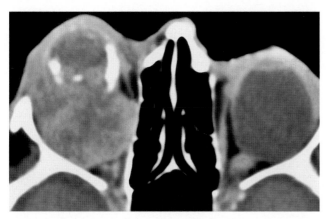

Figure 19-99. Axial computed tomographic scan demonstrating proptosis of the right globe and linear calcification along the eye wall. Massive lesion filling the orbit is contiguous with the posterior aspect of the globe.

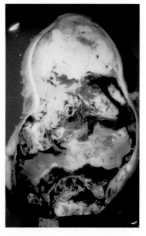

Figure 19-100. Photograph of grossly sectioned globe showing thin-walled posterior staphyloma filled with a mixture of blood and tumor tissue protruding from the posterior aspect of the eye. Light-colored necrotic tumor fills the vitreous cavity.

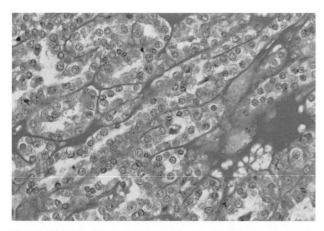

Figure 19-101. Photomicrograph showing cords of nonpigmented adenocarcinoma cells (hematoxylin–eosin, original magnification × 200).

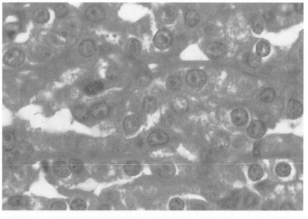

Figure 19-102. Photomicrograph showing cords of adenocarcinoma cells (hematoxylin–eosin, original magnification × 300).

CHAPTER 20

Tumors of the Nonpigmented Ciliary Epithelium

CONGENITAL NEOPLASMS OF THE NONPIGMENTED CILIARY EPITHELIUM (MEDULLOEPITHELIOMA)

The most common congenital tumor of the nonpigmented ciliary epithelium (NPCE) is medulloepithelioma, a nonhereditary, embryonal neoplasm generally diagnosed in the first decade of life (1–7) It most commonly occurs in the ciliary body and rarely in the optic nerve (8–10). It arises from the medullary epithelium, or inner layer of the optic cup, prior to its differentiation into its adult derivatives (2). An early clinical feature is a "lens coloboma" due to congenital absence of zonule in the quadrant of the tumor. Examination of the adjacent ciliary body reveals a rather typical fleshy cystic mass. A characteristic neoplastic cyclitic membrane can develop, and secondary glaucoma occurs in 60% of cases. Retinal detachment is a common complication (1–4). There is often a long delay in diagnosis and sometimes misdirected therapy (3). Fluorescein angiography shows early hyperfluorescence and gradual late staining of the mass. Ultrasonography reveals a mass pattern with acoustic solidity and high internal reflectivity (1,6).

Medulloepithelioma can be classified histopathologically into nonteratoid and teratoid types, and both can be cytologically benign or malignant. The nonteratoid type consists purely of cells that resemble ciliary epithelium and sometimes is called a diktyoma. The teratoid type demonstrates elements of heteroplasia, like cartilage, rhabdomyoblasts, and brain. Cysts found in both types contain vitreous, secreted by the epithelial cells in the tumor (2).

Although most eyes require enucleation, a small, circumscribed medulloepithelioma can be managed by iridocyclectomy. Because deaths have occurred only in patients with advanced extrascleral extension, orbital exenteration should be considered if there is extensive orbital involvement. The role of irradiation and chemotherapy for intraocular medulloepithelioma is not established.

SELECTED REFERENCES

1. Shields JA, Shields CL. *Intraocular tumors. A text and atlas.* Philadelphia: WB Saunders, 1992:461—487.
2. Broughton WI, Zimmerman LE. A clinicopathologic study of 56 cases of intraocular medulloepitheliomas. *Am J Ophthalmol* 1978;85:407–418.
3. Shields JA, Eagle RC Jr, Shields CL, De Potter P. Congenital neoplasms of the nonpigmented ciliary epithelium (medulloepithelioma). *Ophthalmology* 1996;103:1998–2006.
4. Canning CR, McCartney ACE, Hungerford J. Medulloepithelioma (diktyoma). *Br J Ophthalmol* 1988;72:764–767.
5. Hennis HL, Saunders RA, Shields JA. Malignant teratoid medulloepithelioma of the ciliary body. *J Clin Neuro-ophthalmol* 1990;10:291–292.
6. Shields JA, Eagle RC Jr, Shields CL, Marcus S. Fluorescein angiography and ultrasonography of malignant intraocular medulloepithelioma. *J Pediatr Ophthalmol Strabismus* 1996;33:193–196.
7. Shields JA, Shields CL, Schwartz RL. Malignant teratoid medulloepithelioma of the ciliary body simulating persistent hyperplastic primary vitreous. *Am J Ophthalmol* 1989;107:296–298.
8. Reese AB. Medulloepithelioma (dictyoma) of the optic nerve. *Am J Ophthalmol* 1957;44:4–6.
9. Green WR, Iliff WJ, Trotter RR. Malignant teratoid medulloepithelioma of the optic nerve. *Arch Ophthalmol* 1974;91:451–454.
10. O'Keefe M, Fulcher T, Kelly P, Lee W, Dudgeon J. Medulloepithelioma of the optic nerve head. *Arch Ophthalmol* 1997;115:1325–1327.

Ciliary Body Medulloepithelioma—Clinical and Gross Pathologic Features

Ciliary body medulloepithelioma can have a variety of clinical manifestations, depending on the size and extent of the tumor at the time of diagnosis.

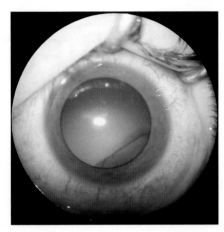

Figure 20-1. Typical lens notch or "coloboma" in a 4-year-old girl with benign nonteratoid medulloepithelioma.

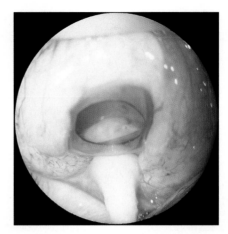

Figure 20-2. Appearance of the same eye shown in Fig. 20-1 with scleral depression showing a fleshy-white ciliary body mass.

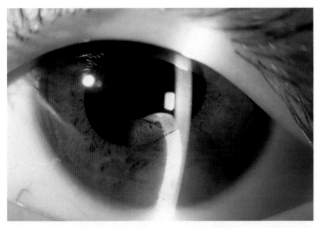

Figure 20-3. Inferior ciliary body mass in a 6-year-old boy. The tumor was found after the child underwent surgery for a congenital cataract. It initially was suspected to be a "cyst," but later examination established the diagnosis of medulloepithelioma.

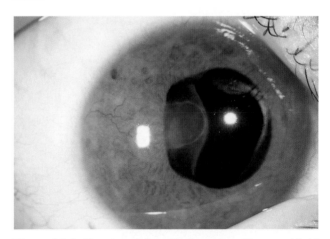

Figure 20-4. Nasal medulloepithelioma in a 10-year-old girl. Note the large clear cyst near the tumor surface.

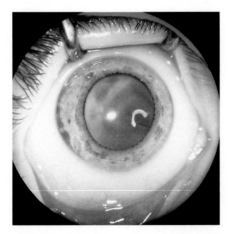

Figure 20-5. Characteristic tumor-induced cyclitic membrane secondary to ciliary body medulloepithelioma.

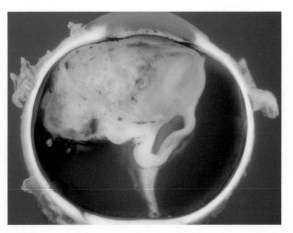

Figure 20-6. Gross pathology of the eye seen in Fig. 20-5 following enucleation. Note the irregular ciliary body mass and the secondary retinal detachment.

Ciliary Body Medulloepithelioma—Clinicopathologic Correlation

Figs. 20-7 through 20-12 from Hennis HL, Saunders RA, Shields JA. Malignant teratoid medulloepithelioma of the ciliary body. *J Clin Neuro-ophthalmol* 1990;10:291–292.

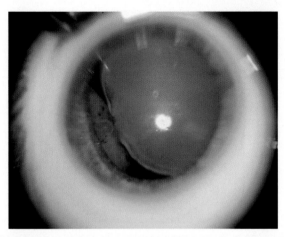

Figure 20-7. Inferotemporal medulloepithelioma in a 6-year-old boy. Note the fleshy-white lesion with a cyst near the surface.

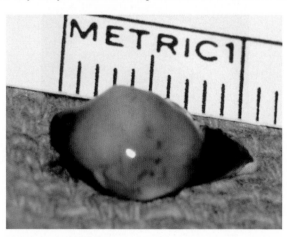

Figure 20-8. Appearance of the lesion after successful removal by iridocyclectomy.

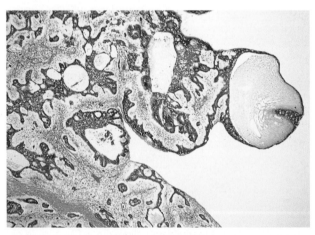

Figure 20-9. Photomicrograph of the lesion showing cyst near the surface (hematoxylin–eosin, original magnification × 40).

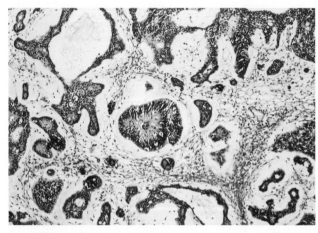

Figure 20-10. Area of tumor showing tubules and acini of proliferating epithelial cells. This pattern has been called a "diktyoma" (hematoxylin–eosin, original magnification × 150).

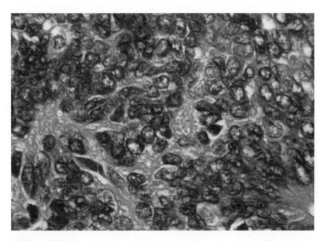

Figure 20-11. Another area of the same tumor showing closely compact cells with malignant features (hematoxylin–eosin, original magnification × 200).

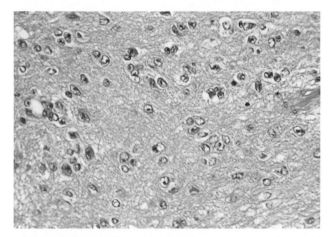

Figure 20-12. Another area of the same tumor showing tissue compatible with brain. The tumor was classified histopathologically as a malignant teratoid medulloepithelioma (hematoxylin–eosin, original magnification × 150).

Ciliary Body Medulloepithelioma—Clinicopathologic Correlation

Although most ciliary body medulloepitheliomas are difficult to demonstrate with fundus photography and ultrasonography, the case depicted here was successfully demonstrated with those techniques.

Figs. 20-13 through 20-18 from Shields JA, Eagle RC Jr, Shields CL, Marcus S. Fluorescein angiography and ultrasonography of malignant intraocular medulloepithelioma. *J Pediatr Ophthalmol Strabismus* 1996;33:193–196.

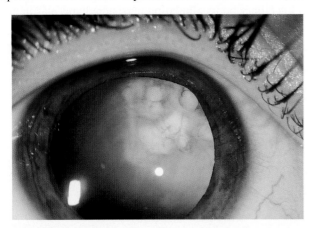

Figure 20-13. Clinical photograph of superonasal mass in the right eye of a 7-year-old girl. Note the chalky-gray–white areas in the tumor and the gray neoplastic cyclitic membrane.

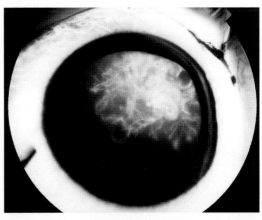

Figure 20-14. Fluorescein angiogram showing fine blood vessels that are leaking fluorescein in the tumor.

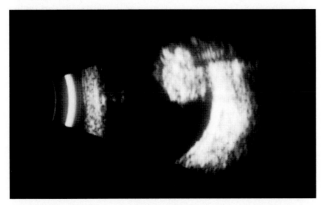

Figure 20-15. B-scan ultrasonogram showing the pedunculated mass with dense echoes. These persisted at lower sensitivities. Although the fluorescein angiogram and ultrasonogram suggested retinoblastoma, the diagnosis was made of medulloepithelioma and the eye was enucleated.

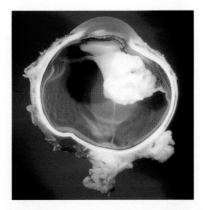

Figure 20-16. Photograph of sectioned globe showing the white ciliary body mass. Note the retrolental cyclitic membrane and the faint hyaloid blood vessel passing from the tumor toward the optic disc.

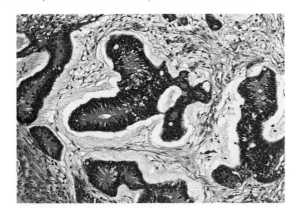

Figure 20-17. Area of tumor showing tubules and acini of proliferating epithelial cells (hematoxylin–eosin, original magnification × 150).

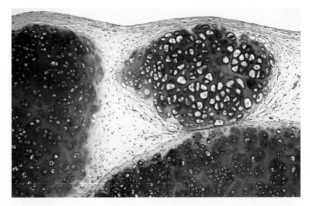

Figure 20-18. Area of tumor showing foci of hyaline cartilage (hematoxylin–eosin, original magnification × 150). It was the foci of cartilage that accounted for the chalky-gray foci seen clinically, the hypofluorescent foci seen with angiography, and the dense echoes seen ultrasonographically.

Ciliary Body Medulloepithelioma Simulating
Persistent Hyperplastic Primary Vitreous

In many instances, ciliary body medulloepithelioma can masquerade as or produce a congenital cataract or glaucoma, or it can be confused with persistent hyperplastic primary vitreous. There is a positive association of medulloepithelioma with persistent hyperplastic primary vitreous.

Figs. 20-19 through 20-24 from Shields JA, Shields CL, Schwartz RL. Malignant teratoid medulloepithelioma of the ciliary body simulating persistent hyperplastic primary vitreous. *Am J Ophthalmol* 1989;107:296–298.

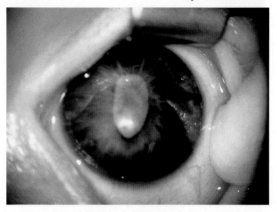

Figure 20-19. Leukocoria due to cataract in an infant.

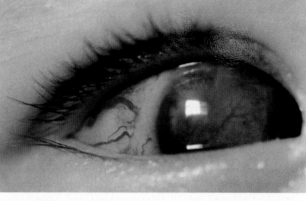

Figure 20-20. Appearance of the same eye after three operations elsewhere for presumed persistent hyperplastic primary vitreous. The anterior chamber is filled with red-yellow material, and the blind painful eye was enucleated.

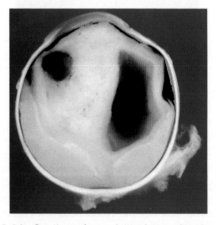

Figure 20-21. Section of enucleated eye showing irregular ciliary body mass that extends into the posterior segment and produces a retinal detachment.

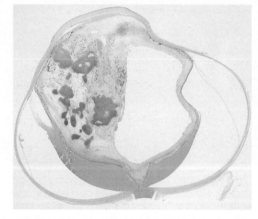

Figure 20-22. Low-magnification photomicrograph showing triangular-shaped ciliary body mass with foci of cartilage and exudative retinal detachment.

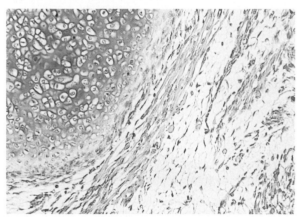

Figure 20-23. Photomicrograph of a large focus of hyaline cartilage lined with skeletal muscle (hematoxylin–eosin, original magnification × 50).

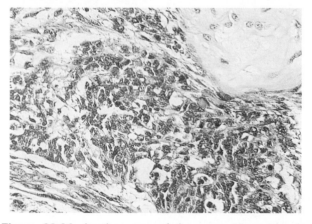

Figure 20-24. Another area of the same tumor showing atypical, closely packed epithelial cells with malignant features (hematoxylin–eosin, original magnification × 200). The final diagnosis was malignant teratoid medulloepithelioma.

Optic Nerve Medulloepithelioma—Clinicopathologic Correlation

In rare instances, medulloepithelioma can affect the optic disc and retrobulbar portion of the optic nerve. A clinicopathologic correlation of such a case is shown.

Figs. 20-25 through 20-30 courtesy of Dr. Michael O'Keefe. From O'Keefe M, Fulcher T, Kelly P, Lee W, Dudgeon J. Medulloepithelioma of the optic nerve head. *Arch Ophthalmol* 1997;115:1325–1327.

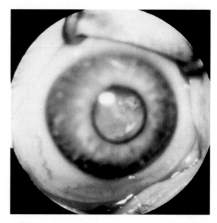

Figure 20-25. Leukocoria in a child with optic-nerve tumor.

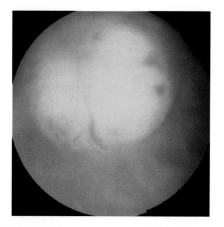

Figure 20-26. Fundus photograph of the same eye showing fluffy-white mass overlying the optic nerve.

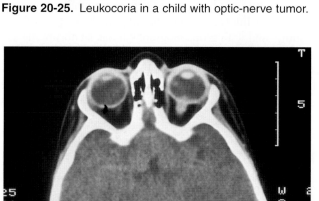

Figure 20-27. Axial computed tomogram showing mass in anterior portion of the optic nerve.

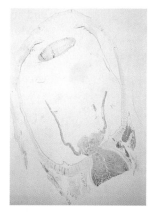

Figure 20-28. Photograph of pathology slide of enucleated eye showing basophilic mass involving the disc and retrobulbar portion of the optic nerve.

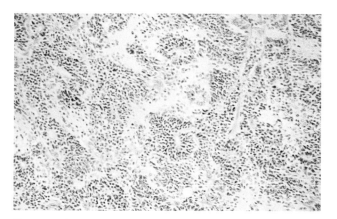

Figure 20-29. Photomicrograph showing cuboidal and columnar epithelial cells forming tubules and acini (hematoxylin–eosin, original magnification × 150).

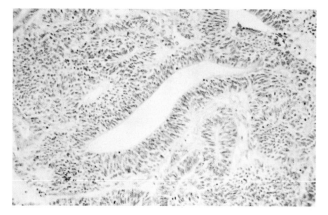

Figure 20-30. Photomicrograph of another area showing typical multilayer sheets of medullary epithelium (hematoxylin–eosin, original magnification × 200).

ACQUIRED NEOPLASMS OF THE NONPIGMENTED CILIARY EPITHELIUM (ADENOMA AND ADENOCARCINOMA)

In contrast to a congenital tumor, an acquired neoplasm of the NPCE appears in adulthood and arises from the fully differentiated ciliary epithelium (1–3). Age-related hyperplasia of the NPCE (Fuch's adenoma) is not a true neoplasm but rather a benign proliferation of the NPCE that occurs in older individuals and only rarely has clinical significance (4–6). Cytologically, a true tumor of the NPCE can be benign (adenoma) or malignant (adenocarcinoma). The clinical differentiation between adenoma and adenocarcinoma generally is not possible, and the prognosis for the two is similar (1–3).

Clinically, an acquired tumor of the NPCE usually is nonpigmented, is yellow to light tan, and has an irregular surface that directly impinges on the vitreous cavity (2–8). A few small cysts in the tumor and mild intraocular inflammatory signs often are present, and a secondary focal cataract occurs early. On rare occasions, it can show extrascleral extension (9,10).

Tumors of the NPCE have been divided into solid, papillary, and pleomorphic types (1). Most are composed of a variable combination of these three patterns (3). A consistent feature is the presence of epithelial cells that rest on prominent periodic acid–Schiff–positive basement membrane. Some tumors contain large quantities of hyaluronidase-sensitive acid mucopolysaccharide, identical to vitreous.

Awareness of this tumor and recognition of its clinical features are vitally important in making the clinical diagnosis. With fluorescein angiography, it shows progressive hyperfluorescence and late staining, and with ultrasonography it has an abrupt margin and acoustic solidity with B-scan and high internal reflectivity with A-scan.

Most reported cases of acquired neoplasms of the NPCE were managed by enucleation. However, recent studies strongly indicate that local resection is an effective treatment (3). The visual prognosis is usually good and the systemic prognosis is excellent.

SELECTED REFERENCES

1. Zimmerman LE. The remarkable polymorphism of tumors of the ciliary epithelium. The Norman McAlister Gregg Lecture. *Trans Aust Coll Ophthalmol* 1970;2:114–125.
2. Shields JA, Shields CL. *Intraocular tumors. A text and atlas.* Philadelphia: WB Saunders, 1992:461–487.
3. Shields JA, Eagle RC Jr, Shields CL, De Potter P. Acquired neoplasms of the nonpigmented ciliary epithelium (adenoma and adenocarcinoma). *Ophthalmology* 1996;103:2007–2016.
4. Iliff WJ, Green WR. The incidence and location of Fuch's adenoma. *Arch Ophthalmol* 1972;88:249–254.
5. Bronwyn-Bateman J, Foos RY. Coronal adenomas. *Arch Ophthalmol* 1979;97:2379–2384.
6. Zaidman GW, Johnson BL, Aslamon SM, et al. Fuch's adenoma affecting the peripheral iris. *Arch Ophthalmol* 1983;101:771–773.
7. Shields JA, Eagle RC Jr, Shields CL. Adenoma of the nonpigmented ciliary epithelium with smooth muscle differentiation. *Arch Ophthalmol (in press)*.
8. Shields JA, Augsburger JJ, Shah H, Wallar PH. Adenoma of the nonpigmented epithelium of the ciliary body. *Ophthalmology* 1983;90:1528–1530.
9. Rodrigues M, Hidayat A, Karesh J. Pleomorphic adenocarcinoma of ciliary epithelium simulating an epibulbar tumor. *Am J Ophthalmol* 1988;106:595–600.
10. Grossniklaus HE, Zimmerman LE, Kachmer ML. Pleomorphic adenocarcinoma of the ciliary body. *Ophthalmology* 1990;97:763–768.

Age-related Hyperplasia of the Nonpigmented Ciliary Epithelium (Fuch's Adenoma)

Age-related hyperplasia of the NPCE is a benign proliferation of epithelial cells with elaboration of basement membrane material that is more common with increasing age. It usually is not seen clinically but is discovered on pathologic examination of eyes of older individuals.

Figs. 20-35 and 20-36 courtesy of Drs. Gerald Zaidman and Bruce Johnson. From Zaidman GW, Johnson BL, Aslamon SM, et al. Fuch's adenoma affecting the peripheral iris. *Arch Ophthalmol* 1983;101:771–773.

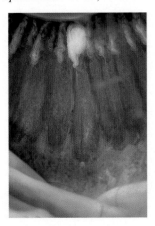

Figure 20-31. Close-up view of grossly sectioned eye enucleated for an unrelated choroidal melanoma. Note the white nodule in a ciliary process *(above)*.

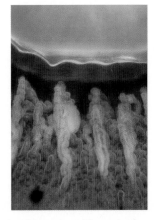

Figure 20-32. Another eye with a similar view showing a white nodule on the edge of a ciliary process.

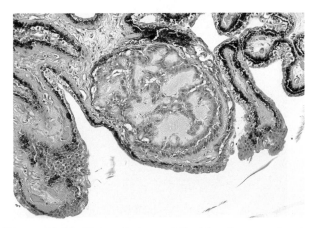

Figure 20-33. Histopathology of Fuch's adenoma showing proliferation of epithelial cells with abundant basement membrane material (hematoxylin–eosin, original magnification ×20).

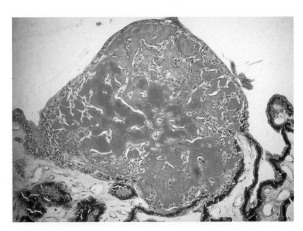

Figure 20-34. Histopathology of Fuch's adenoma showing histopathology similar to that shown in Fig. 20-33 (hematoxylin–eosin, original magnification ×20).

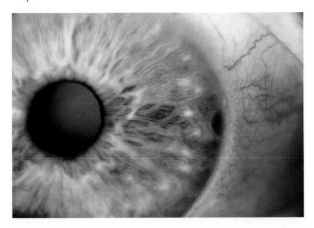

Figure 20-35. Fuch's adenoma presenting through the iris root.

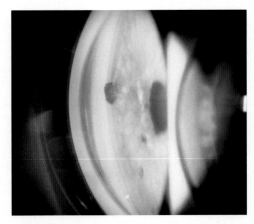

Figure 20-36. Goniophotograph showing lesion in the anterior chamber angle. The lesion was removed surgically and the diagnosis of Fuch's adenoma was established.

Adenoma of Nonpigmented Ciliary Epithelium—Clinical Features

Adenoma of the NPCE is an amelanotic ciliary body mass that can have variable clinical features. It frequently causes an adjacent cataract that can preclude a clear view of the lesion. Fluorescein angiography and ultrasonography are difficult to perform because of the hidden location of the lesion in most cases. In all cases shown here, the diagnosis was confirmed histopathologically following surgical resection.

Figs. 20-39 and 20-40 from Shields JA, Eagle RC Jr, Shields CL. Adenoma of the nonpigmented ciliary epithelium with smooth muscle differentiation. *(Arch Ophthalmol (in press).*

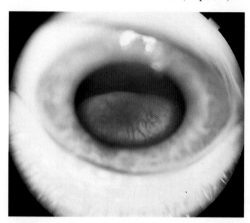

Figure 20-37. Inferior adenoma of nonpigmented ciliary epithelium in a 39-year-old man. This lesion is atypical in that it has a very smooth surface.

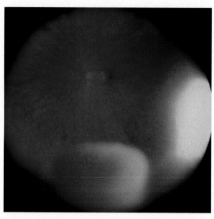

Figure 20-38. Wide-angle fundus photograph of the lesion shown in Fig. 20-37 showing that the lesions transmit light.

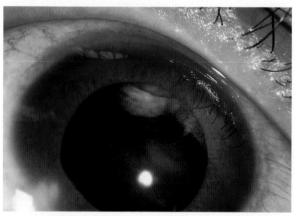

Figure 20-39. Superior adenocarcinoma of the nonpigmented ciliary epithelium in a 58-year-old African-American patient showing the margin of the lesion, an adjacent secondary cataract, and subluxation of the lens.

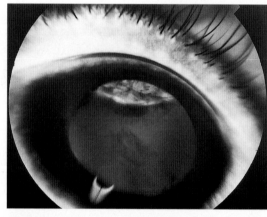

Figure 20-40. Fluorescein angiogram of the lesion shown in Fig. 20-39 demonstrating nonspecific hyperfluorescence of the lesion.

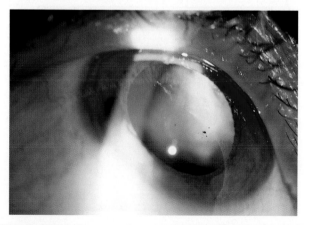

Figure 20-41. Dense cataract overlying a faintly visualized adenoma of the nonpigmented ciliary epithelium in a 45-year-old woman.

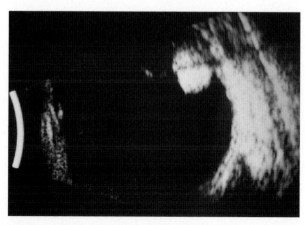

Figure 20-42. B-scan ultrasonogram of the lesion shown in Fig. 20-41. Note that the lesion has abrupt margins and is markedly pedunculated.

Adenoma of Nonpigmented Ciliary Epithelium—Clinicopathologic Correlation

Adenoma of the NPCE is sometimes a white fluffy tumor with numerous cystic spaces that contain an acid mucopolysaccharide characteristic of vitreous. The patient shown here had local resection of a large tumor with removal of a dislocated lens at the time of surgery and had excellent vision 7 years later.

Figs. 20-43 through 20-48 from Shields JA, Eagle RC Jr, Shields CL, De Potter P. Acquired neoplasms of the nonpigmented ciliary epithelium (adenoma and adenocarcinoma). *Ophthalmology* 1996;103:2007–2016.

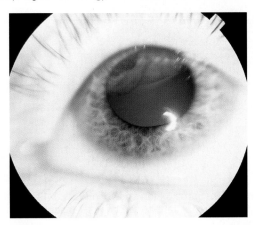

Figure 20-43. Superior ciliary body mass in a 31-year-old woman.

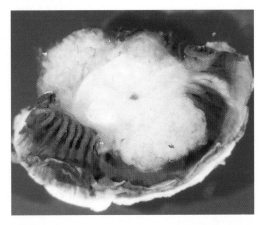

Figure 20-44. Flat view of the tumor after removal by partial lamellar iridocyclochoroidectomy.

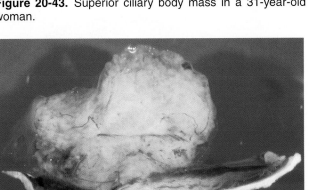

Figure 20-45. Side view of the lesion showing scleral base and friable appearance of the lesion.

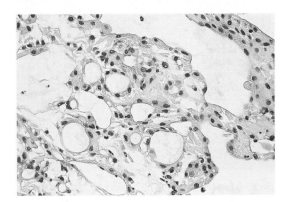

Figure 20-46. Photomicrograph showing cords of bland epithelial cells and cystic spaces (hematoxylin–eosin, original magnification × 200).

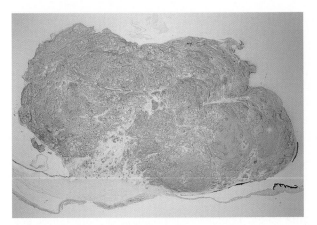

Figure 20-47. Low magnification of lesion stained for mucin showing marked positivity within the numerous cystic spaces. This was a hyaluronidase-sensitive mucopolysaccharide identical to vitreous (Alcian-blue, original magnification × 10).

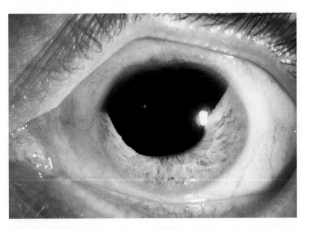

Figure 20-48. Appearance of the anterior segment several years later showing large sector iridectomy. The posterior fundus was normal. A cosmetic contact lens was fitted to cover the defect.

Adenoma of Nonpigmented Ciliary Epithelium— Clinicopathologic Correlation and Treatment

A dense cortical cataract near the lens equator is a common finding in a patient with a neoplasm of the NPCE.

Figs. 20-49 through 20-54 from Shields JA, Augsburger JJ, Shah H, Wallar PH. Adenoma of the nonpigmented epithelium of the ciliary body. *Ophthalmology* 1983; 90:1528–1530.

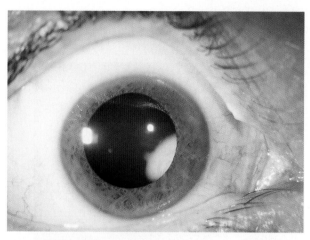

Figure 20-49. Dense cortical cataract in a 41-year-old man.

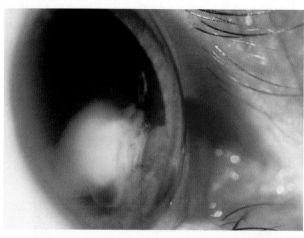

Figure 20-50. Same lesion shown in Fig. 20-49 with the eye rotated showing a light-brown mass adjacent to the lens opacity.

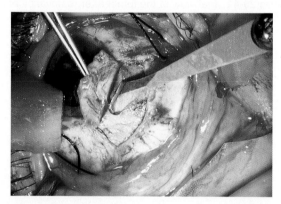

Figure 20-51. Removal of the lesion by partial lamellar iridocyclectomy.

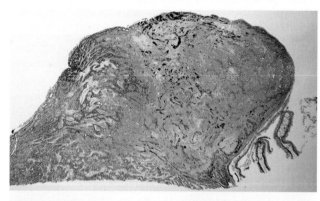

Figure 20-52. Low-magnification photomicrograph showing well-circumscribed lesion (hematoxylin–eosin, original magnification × 10).

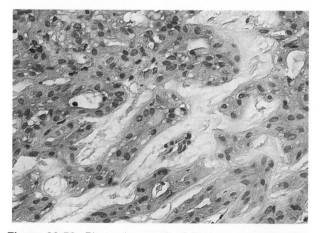

Figure 20-53. Photomicrograph of the tumor showing characteristic cords of proliferating nonpigmented ciliary epithelium (hematoxylin–eosin, original magnification × 150).

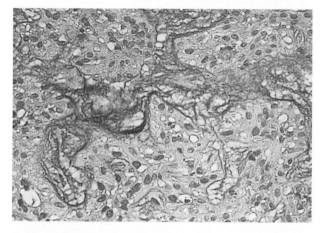

Figure 20-54. Photomicrograph showing characteristic positive staining for mucin (Alcian blue, original magnification × 150).

Adenocarcinoma of the Nonpigmented Ciliary Epithelium—Clinicopathologic Correlations

Adenocarcinoma of the NPCE can be localized in the globe, or it can exhibit extraocular extension. Even though it is cytologically malignant and may exhibit aggressive local behavior, the tumor does not have a tendency to metastasize.

Figs. 20-58 through 20-60 courtesy of Dr. Hans Grossniklaus. From Grossniklaus HE, Zimmerman LE, Kachmer ML. Pleomorphic adenocarcinoma of the ciliary body. *Ophthalmology* 1990;97:763–768.

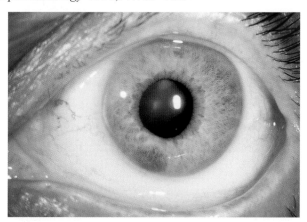

Figure 20-55. Ciliary body mass causing inferior compression of the iris stroma in a 50-year-old woman.

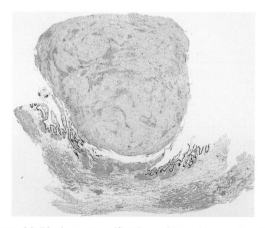

Figure 20-56. Low-magnification photomicrograph of the mass after removal by partial lamellar iridocyclectomy (hematoxylin–eosin, original magnification × 5).

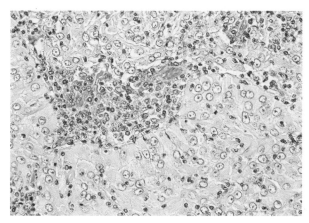

Figure 20-57. Photomicrograph showing solid pattern of abnormal epithelial cells (hematoxylin–eosin, original magnification × 150).

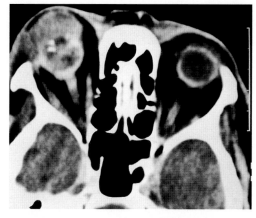

Figure 20-58. Axial computed tomogram of an aggressive adenocarcinoma that filled the entire globe and extended through the sclera in an 80-year-old man with a chronically blind eye.

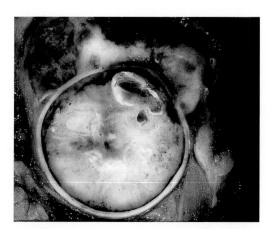

Figure 20-59. Gross appearance of sectioned specimen after orbital exenteration showing white mass filling the globe and extending through the sclera anteriorly.

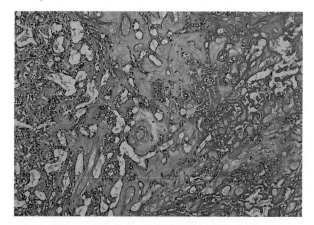

Figure 20-60. Microscopic appearance showing poorly differentiated carcinoma (hematoxylin–eosin, original magnification × 200). Special stains supported the diagnosis of adenocarcinoma of the nonpigmented ciliary epithelium.

CHAPTER 21

Intraocular Lymphoid Tumors and Leukemias

INTRAOCULAR LYMPHOID TUMORS AND LEUKEMIAS

Intraocular lymphoid tumors and leukemias include benign uveal lymphoid infiltration, malignant lymphoma, plasmacytoma, leukemia, and other rare variations (1,2). Uveal lymphoid infiltration (reactive lymphoid hyperplasia) affects mainly adults and usually is unilateral (3–5). It can occur in the iris, ciliary body, or choroid, and it simultaneously can involve the conjunctiva and orbit. In the choroid, it appears as a diffuse or circumscribed yellow thickening, often with a secondary retinal detachment. It may be difficult to differentiate from lymphoma, metastasis, or amelanotic choroidal melanoma. It is characterized by a proliferation of benign lymphocytes and plasma cells.

Intraocular lymphoma is the infiltration of the uveal tract, retina, vitreous, or optic nerve head with malignant lymphocytes. Non-Hodgkin's B-cell lymphoma (reticulum cell sarcoma) is most common, and Burkitt's lymphoma or T-cell lymphomas are less common. It can be unilateral or bilateral (1).

There are two general types of intraocular large-cell lymphoma: the retinovitreal form and the uveal form, although both can be present simultaneously. The retinovitreal form generally is associated with central nervous system lymphoma, and the uveal type generally is associated with visceral or nodal lymphoma. The retinovitreal form is characterized by signs of vitreous inflammation, simulating "uveitis." The uveal type more often presents as one or more characteristic yellow uveal or subpigment epithelial masses. Plasmacytoma in the uveal tract may be a forerunner of multiple myeloma or related conditions (6). It generally is similar to uveal lymphoid infiltration and lymphoma. Management of any of the conditions described is systemic evaluation and appropriate chemotherapy or irradiation. If chemotherapy is employed for associated systemic disease, then the ocular tumor(s) can be followed closely to ascertain the response. If there is no detectable systemic disease or if chemotherapy does not succeed in controlling the ocular disease, ocular irradiation is justified.

Most patients with ocular involvement by leukemia already have known systemic disease, although the ophthalmic findings rarely can be the initial manifestations of the disease (7). It can involve iris, ciliary body, choroid, retina, or optic nerve. Management usually is treatment of the systemic disease combined with ocular irradiation, especially if optic nerve involvement threatens the patient's vision.

SELECTED REFERENCES

1. Shields JA, Shields CL. *Intraocular tumors. A text and atlas.* Philadelphia: WB Saunders, 1992:489–512.
2. Char DH. *Clinical ocular oncology,* 2nd ed. Philadelphia: Lippincott–Raven Publishers, 1997:192–202.
3. Jakobiec FA, Sacks E, Kronish J, Weiss T, Smith M. Multifocal static creamy choroidal infiltrates. An early sign of lymphoid neoplasia. *Ophthalmology* 1987;74:397–406.
4. Grossniklaus HE, Martin DF, Avery R, Shields JA, Shields CL, Kuo I, Green RL, Rao NA. Uveal lymphoid infiltration. Report of four cases and clinicopathologic review. *Ophthalmology* 1998;105:1265–1273.
5. Ryan SJ, Zimmerman LE, King FM. Reactive lymphoid hyperplasia. An unusual form of intraocular pseudo-tumor. *Trans Am Acad Ophthalmol Otolaryngol* 1972;76:652–670.
6. Adkins JW, Shields JA, Shields CL, Eagle RC Jr, Flanagan JC, Campanella PC. Plasmacytoma of the eye and orbit. *Int Ophthalmol* 1977;20:339–343.
7. Schachat AP, Markowitz JA, Guyer DR, et al. Ophthalmic manifestations of leukemia. *Arch Ophthalmol* 1989;107:697–700.

Uveal Lymphoid Infiltration

Uveal lymphoid infiltration (benign reactive lymphoid hyperplasia) is a benign lesion in which the uveal tract is infiltrated by a combination of lymphocytes and plasma cells. Because it simultaneously can involve the conjunctiva, careful external ocular examination may suggest the diagnosis of the ocular lesion.

Figs. 21-1 and 21-2 from Shields JA, Augsburger JJ, Gonder JR, McLeod D. Localized benign lymphoid tumor of the iris. *Arch Ophthalmol* 1981;99:2147–2148.

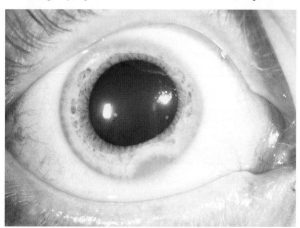

Figure 21-1. Peripheral iris involvement with localized mass in a 33-year-old woman. The lesion was excised successfully by iridocyclectomy, and it proved histopathologically to be a benign lymphoid infiltration.

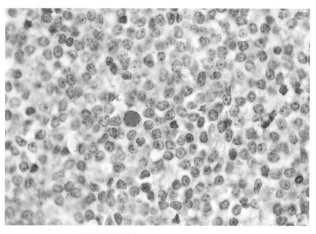

Figure 21-2. Histopathology of uveal lymphoid infiltration showing mature lymphocytes, of which one near the center of the photomicrograph has an intranuclear inclusion (Dutcher body) (periodic acid–Schiff, original magnification × 200).

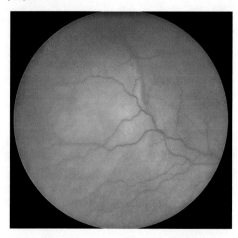

Figure 21-3. Localized choroidal involvement with uveal lymphoid infiltration near the temporal equator of the right eye in a 49-year-old man.

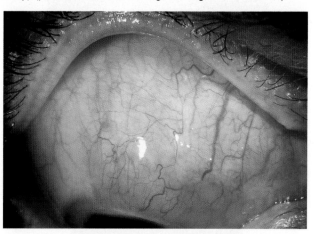

Figure 21-4. Characteristic lymphoid infiltration of the conjunctiva in the same eye shown in Fig. 21-3. A conjunctival biopsy revealed benign lymphoid infiltration.

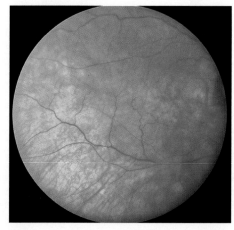

Figure 21-5. Appearance of the fundus lesion shown in Fig. 21-3 after 2,000 cGy of ocular irradiation, demonstrating excellent response.

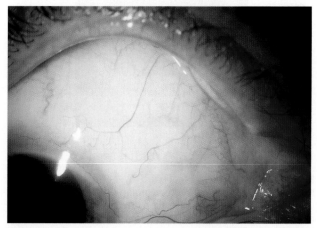

Figure 21-6. Appearance of the conjunctival lesion after the ocular irradiation showing excellent response.

Uveal Lymphoid Infiltration—Clinical and Pathologic Features

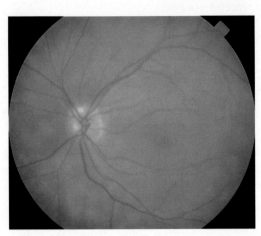

Figure 21-7. Multiple subtle yellow choroidal lesions in the left eye of a 65-year-old woman.

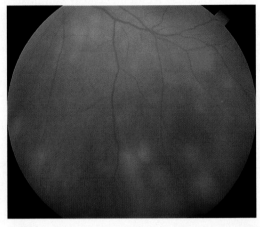

Figure 21-8. More pronounced peripheral fundus lesions in the same eye shown in Fig. 21-7. Note the similarity to the lesions seen with vitiliginous or birdshot choroidopathy.

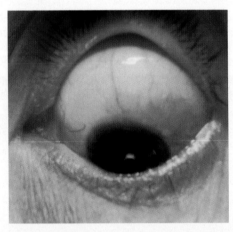

Figure 21-9. Conjunctiva of the same eye shown in Fig. 21.8. Note the salmon patch infiltration. This is seen with lymphoid infiltration but not with birdshot choroidopathy.

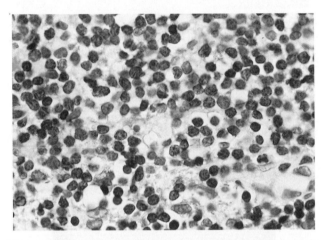

Figure 21-10. Histopathology of biopsy of the lesion shown in Fig. 21-9. The uniform small lymphocytes suggested the diagnosis of a benign to intermediate uveal lymphoid infiltration.

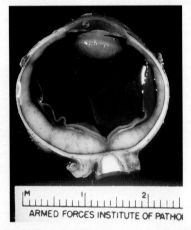

Figure 21-11. Grossly sectioned eye with uveal lymphoid infiltration. Note the marked thickening of the entire posterior uvea and the perineural infiltration adjacent to the optic nerve in the orbit. (Courtesy of Armed Forces Institute of Pathology, Washington, DC.)

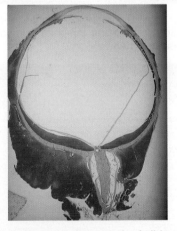

Figure 21-12. Low-power photograph of slide of an eye with uveal lymphoid infiltration. The lesion has a dark-blue color characteristic of lymphoid tumor. (Courtesy of Armed Forces Institute of Pathology, Washington, DC.)

Intraocular Lymphoma—Retinovitreal Form

The retinovitreal type of intraocular lymphoma involves primarily the retina, vitreous, and optic nerve. Although it has been known to involve only the eye, most patients have, or will develop, central nervous system lymphoma as part of the same disease process. The diagnosis generally is made by vitreous biopsy and cytology. The most common method of treatment is radiotherapy.

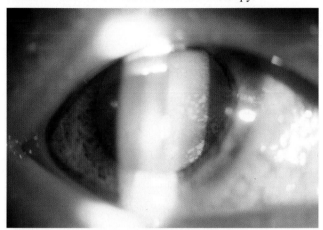

Figure 21-13. Slit-lamp view of anterior vitreous cells in a patient with the retinovitreal form of intraocular lymphoma.

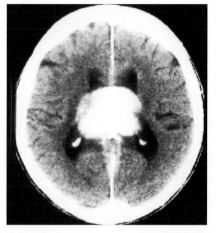

Figure 21-14. Cranial computed tomogram showing large intracranial lymphoma. Patients with suspected intraocular lymphoma should have cranial computed tomography or magnetic resonance imaging. (Courtesy of Dr. Alan Cruess.)

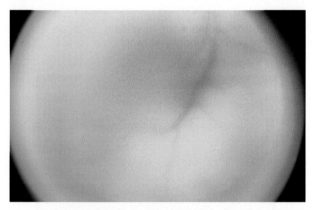

Figure 21-15. Fundus appearance of retinovitreal lymphoma showing a hazy view of yellow-white tumor tissue.

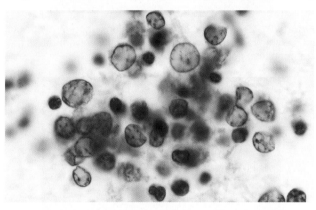

Figure 21-16. Cytology of vitreous biopsy showing malignant lymphoma cells (hematoxylin–eosin, original magnification × 300).

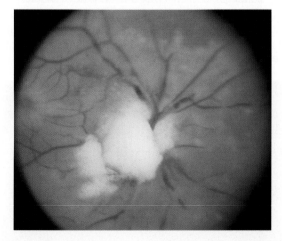

Figure 21-17. Fundus view of optic nerve involvement with non-Hodgkin's lymphoma in a 57-year-old woman. (Courtesy of Dr. W. Richard Green.)

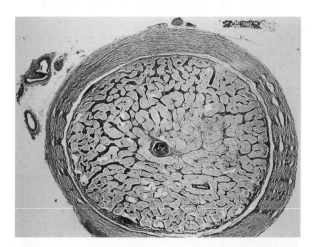

Figure 21-18. Histopathology of cross-section of the optic nerve in the patient shown in Fig. 21-17 demonstrating basophilic lymphoma cells infiltrating the pial septa (hematoxylin–eosin, original magnification × 20). (Courtesy of Dr. W. Richard Green.)

Intraocular Lymphoma—Uveal Form and Response to Chemotherapy and Radiotherapy

The uveal form of intraocular lymphoma can occur in the iris, ciliary body, choroid, or subretinal space. It can have a variety of clinical presentations, can be diagnosed by fine-needle biopsy or eye wall resection, and responds favorably to radiotherapy.

Fig. 21-19 from Leff SR, Shields JA, Augsburger JJ, et al. Unilateral eyelid, conjunctival, and choroidal tumors as initial presentation of diffuse large cell lymphoma. *Br J Ophthalmol* 1985;69:861–864.

Figs. 21-23 and 21-24 courtesy of Dr. Michael Novak. From Dean JM, Novak MA, Chan CC, Green WR. Tumor detachments of the retinal pigment epithelium in ocular/central nervous system lymphoma. *Retina* 1996;16:47–56.

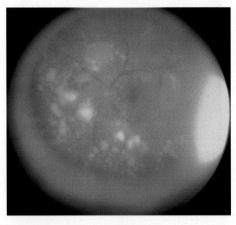

Figure 21-19. Multiple choroidal lesions in a 70-year-old man with eyelid, conjunctival, and orbital involvement as the first manifestation of systemic lymphoma.

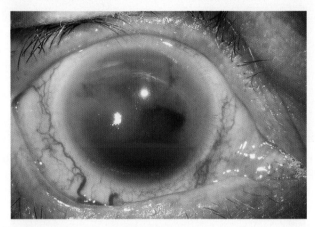

Figure 21-20. Spontaneous hyphema secondary to iris involvement in non-Hodgkin's lymphoma in a 60-year-old woman.

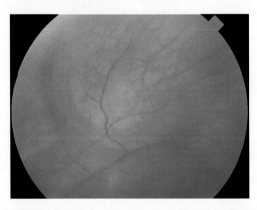

Figure 21-21. Peripheral choroidal lymphoma in a 55-year-old man. The lesion was about 3 mm thick. Biopsy of an ipsilateral conjunctival lesion confirmed lymphoma, and systemic involvement was subsequently found.

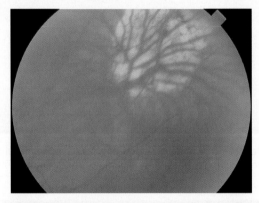

Figure 21-22. Appearance of the lesion shown in Fig. 21-21 after a course of chemotherapy. The lesion has disappeared, and atrophy of the pigment epithelium enhances visibility of underlying choroidal blood vessels.

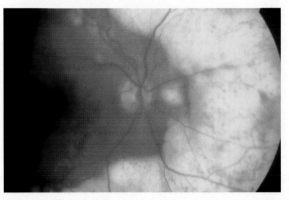

Figure 21-23. Massive subpigment epithelial deposits of lymphoma. This is a classic appearance of lymphoma, most commonly the central nervous systemic variant.

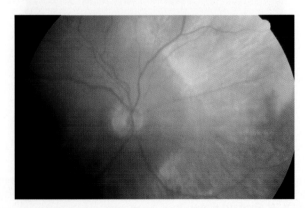

Figure 21-24. Appearance of the area shown in Fig. 21-23 after irradiation showing complete resolution of the lesion and residual retinal pigment epithelial alterations.

Intraocular Lymphoma—Aggressive Uveal Form

In some instances, lymphoma can cause massive thickening of the uveal tract and lead to a blind painful eye. A patient with massive lymphomatous infiltration of the iris and ciliary body is depicted.

Figs. 21-25 through 21-30 from Duker JS, Shields JA, Ross M. Intraocular large cell lymphoma presenting as massive thickening of the uveal tract. *Retina* 1987;7:41–45.

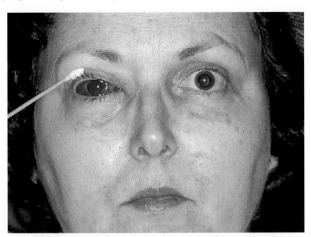

Figure 21-25. A 46-year-old woman who was noted a few weeks earlier to have an unexplained thickening of the iris. She subsequently developed a blind, painful right eye.

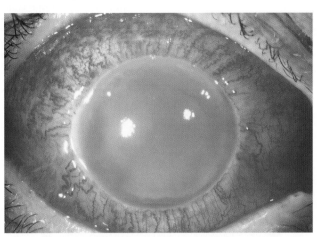

Figure 21-26. Close-up view of affected eye showing marked epibulbar injection, corneal edema, and diffuse hyphema.

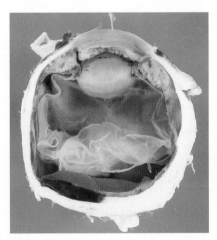

Figure 21-27. Section of enucleated eye showing marked amelanotic thickening of uvea, mostly the iris, and ciliary body.

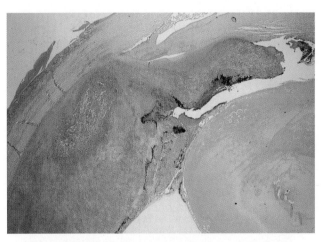

Figure 21-28. Ciliary body region. Note the thickening of the iris and ciliary body by a diffuse mass that also abuts the lens equator (hematoxylin–eosin, original magnification × 20).

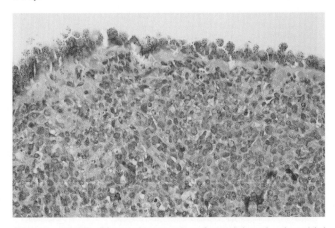

Figure 21-29. Photomicrograph of peripheral choroidal region showing replacement of the choroid by lymphoma. Note that the overlying pigment epithelium is intact (hematoxylin–eosin, original magnification × 100)

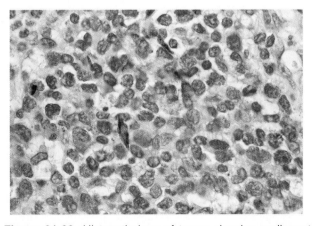

Figure 21-30. Histopathology of tumor showing malignant lymphoma cells (hematoxylin–eosin, original magnification × 200).

Aggressive Lymphoma Presenting as a Uveal and Orbital Mass

Sometimes a patient with uveal and orbital lymphoma can create diagnostic difficulty. A patient who underwent unsuccessful retinal detachment surgery where no retinal break was identified is shown. She later developed an orbital mass that aroused suspicion of uveal melanoma with extraocular extension, and the patient was referred for orbital exenteration. Lymphoma was discovered to be the cause of the retinal detachment and the orbital mass, and the patient was treated successfully with ocular radiotherapy.

Figs. 21-31 through 21-36 from Grossniklaus HE, Martin DF, Avery R, Shields JA, Shields CL, Kuo I, Green RL, Rao NA. Uveal lymphoid infiltration. Report of four cases and clinicopathologic review. *Ophthalmology* 1998;105:1265–1273.

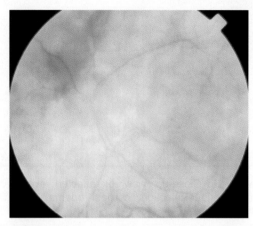

Figure 21-31. Fundus photo done elsewhere of the thickened choroid . An overlying retinal detachment prompted surgery.

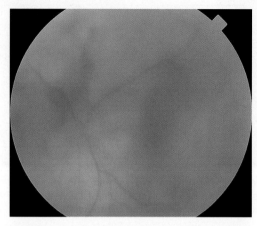

Figure 21-32. Fundus appearance several months later when larger intraocular masses became apparent.

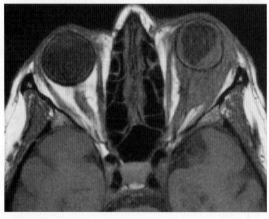

Figure 21-33. Axial magnetic resonance imaging in T1-weighted image showing continuous uveal and orbital mass.

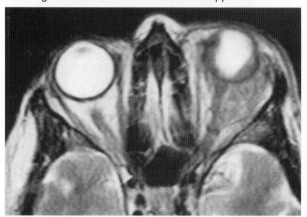

Figure 21-34. Axial magnetic resonance imaging in T2-weighted image showing the same mass.

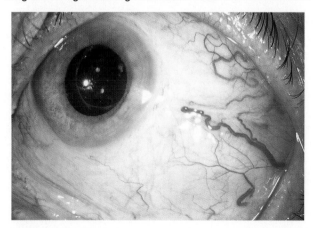

Figure 21-35. Epibulbar surface examination found at referral showing a diffuse mass in bulbar conjunctiva compatible with lymphoid infiltration.

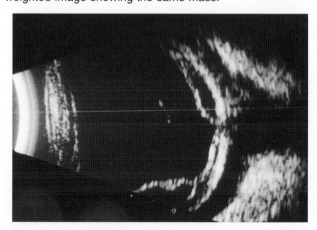

Figure 21-36. B-scan ultrasonogram showing diffuse choroidal and episcleral tumor. The extrascleral component of the lymphoma shows low internal reflectivity that extends posteriorly around the optic nerve.

Intraocular Plasmacytoma

Intraocular plasmacytoma, an uncommon neoplasm, can occur as an isolated lesion or as part of multiple myeloma. It has clinical features similar to lymphoma. A case is depicted where cytologic study of a fine-needle aspiration biopsy made the diagnosis. The tumor responded dramatically to radiotherapy.

Figs. 21-37 through 21-42 from Adkins JW, Shields JA, Shields CL, Eagle RC Jr, Flanagan JC, Campanella PC. Plasmacytoma of the eye and orbit. *Int Ophthalmol* 1977;20:339–343.

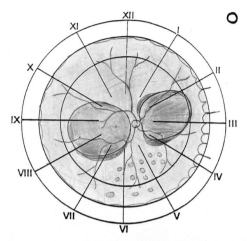

Figure 21-37. Fundus drawing showing two large choroidal masses in the right eye of a systemically healthy 77-year-old woman.

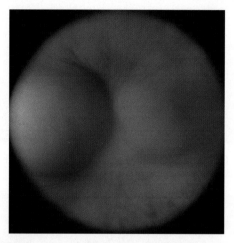

Figure 21-38. Wide-angle fundus photograph showing the two masses.

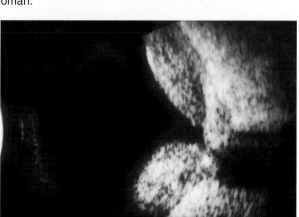

Figure 21-39. B-scan ultrasonogram showing the two masses with acoustic solidity.

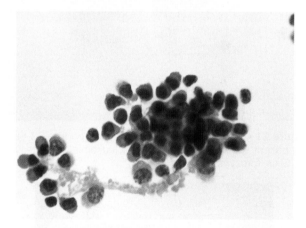

Figure 21-40. Cytology of fine-needle aspiration biopsy showing mature plasma cells.

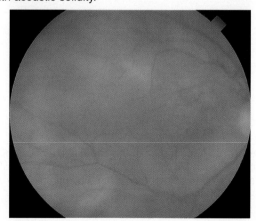

Figure 21-41. Appearance of macular area after 300 cGy of ocular irradiation showing disappearance of the macular mass.

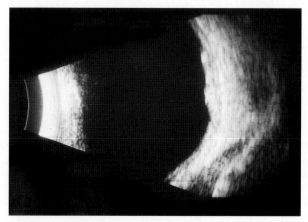

Figure 21-42. B-scan ultrasonogram after irradiation showing marked flattening of the tumors.

Intraocular and Optic Nerve Involvement with Leukemia

Intraocular findings in leukemia usually occur as retinal hemorrhages secondary to the hematologic abnormality. Occasionally, however, the iris, ciliary body, choroid, retina, and vitreous can be involved directly with leukemic infiltration.

Figs. 21-47 and 21-48 from Wallace RT, Shields JA, Shields CL, Ehya H, Ewing M. Leukemic infiltration of the optic nerve. *Arch Ophthalmol* 1991;109:1027.

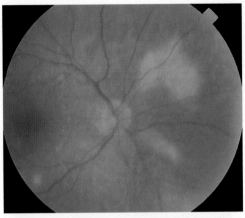

Figure 21-43. Choroidal lesions in a 72-year-old woman with leukemia.

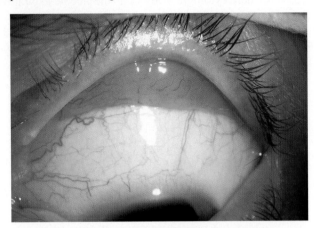

Figure 21-44. Salmon-colored leukemic infiltration in superior fornix of the same patient shown in Fig. 21-43.

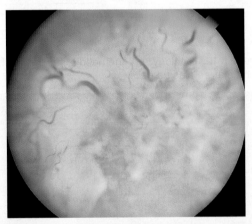

Figure 21-45. Spontaneous pseudohypopyon in a 23-year-old patient with acute lymphoblastic leukemia. (Courtesy of Dr. Elise Torczynski.)

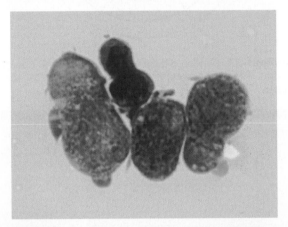

Figure 21-46. Cytology of aspiration biopsy of the anterior chamber material shown in Fig. 21-45 demonstrating leukemic blast cells (original magnification × 500).

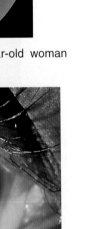

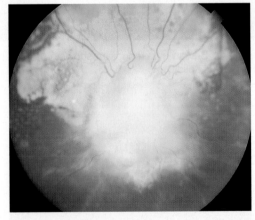

Figure 21-47. Marked involvement of the optic nerve head and surrounding fundus in a 28-year-old woman with leukemia. The differential diagnosis was leukemic infiltration or opportunistic infection. The diagnosis of leukemia was confirmed by study of a fine-needle aspiration specimen, and ocular radiation was given.

Figure 21-48. Appearance of the same eye after irradiation. Most of the leukemic infiltration has resolved, but profound optic atrophy was present and the patient had no useful vision in the affected eye.

Intraocular and Optic Nerve Involvement with Leukemia—Clinicopathologic Correlation

Leukemia has a tendency to affect the posterior fundus and to invade the optic nerve, causing profound visual loss. Such a case is illustrated.

Figs. 21-49 through 21-54 from Brown GC, Shields JA, Augsburger JJ, Serota FT, Koch P. Leukemic optic neuropathy. *Int Ophthalmol* 1991;3:111–116.

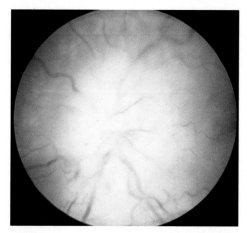

Figure 21-49. Atypical optic disc swelling in an 8-year-old boy with 20/20 vision in the affected left eye. He underwent chemotherapy for systemic relapse of previously diagnosed leukemia at this time.

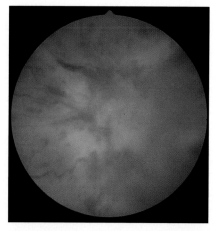

Figure 21-50. Eye shown in Fig. 21-49, 3 months later, when the patient developed rapid blindness. Radiotherapy was given without visual recovery and the child died shortly thereafter.

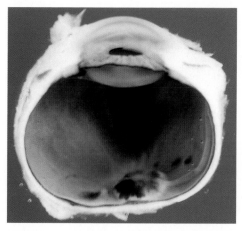

Figure 21-51. Photograph of sectioned eye obtained post-mortem. Note the hemorrhagic swelling of the optic disc and surrounding tissues.

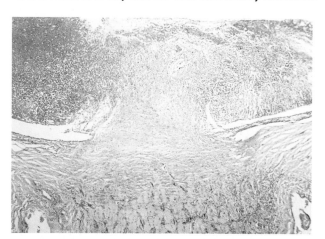

Figure 21-52. Low-power photomicrograph of the optic disc region showing massive infiltration of the retina with minimal involvement of the adjacent choroid (hematoxylin–eosin, original magnification × 25).

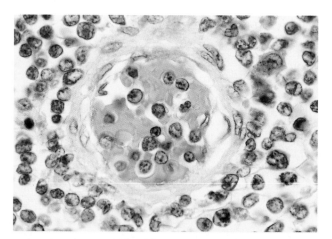

Figure 21-53. Photomicrograph of the involved retina showing intravascular and extravascular infiltration of leukemic blast cells (hematoxylin–eosin, original magnification × 200).

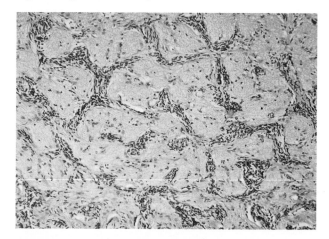

Figure 21-54. Cross-section of the optic nerve showing infiltration of the pial septae with leukemic blast cells (hematoxylin–eosin, original magnification × 100).

CHAPTER 22

Surgical Management of Intraocular Tumors

SURGICAL MANAGEMENT OF INTRAOCULAR TUMORS

Surgical management of intraocular tumors has been mentioned in several parts of this atlas, but specific steps have not been illustrated. Techniques to be briefly illustrated here include fine-needle aspiration biopsy, application of radioactive plaque, iridocyclectomy, cyclochoroidectomy, choroidectomy, enucleation, and orbital exenteration. Laser photocoagulation and cryotherapy also are discussed elsewhere (1,2).

Intraocular fine-needle aspiration biopsy is a method of diagnosing selected lesions that defy an accurate diagnosis using less invasive diagnostic modalities (3). It is a rather difficult procedure that requires the cooperation of an experienced ocular oncologist and cytopathologist (3). It should be reserved for selected cases in which an accurate diagnosis will influence the therapeutic choice. It is performed by passing a fine needle into the suspicious tissue and obtaining cells for special preparation and cytologic analysis. Although false results sometimes occur, it is an accurate diagnostic procedure in most cases (3).

Selected iris tumors can be removed by partial iridectomy. Selected ciliary body or choroidal tumors can be removed by techniques of partial lamellar sclerouvectomy. It is used mainly for melanoma, leiomyoma, and tumors of the pigment epithelium or nonpigmented ciliary epithelium (4,5). Enucleation is indicated for advanced malignant tumors such as retinoblastoma and uveal melanoma that cannot be managed safely by other methods (2). A gentle technique should be employed in all cases, and the method may vary depending on whether the tumor is a melanoma (2) or a retinoblastoma (6). Orbital exenteration, particularly the eyelid-sparing technique, is reserved for some advanced tumors, particularly uveal melanoma with extraocular extension (7,8).

The techniques employed are discussed in more detail in the references cited.

SELECTED REFERENCES

1. Shields JA, Shields CL. *Intraocular tumors. A text and atlas.* Philadelphia: WB Saunders, 1992:11–23.
2. Shields JA, Shields CL. *Intraocular tumors. A text and atlas.* Philadelphia: WB Saunders, 1992:25–43.
3. Shields JA, Shields CL, Ehya H, Eagle RC Jr, De Potter P. Fine needle aspiration biopsy of suspected intraocular tumors. The 1992 Urwick Lecture. *Ophthalmology* 1993;100:1677–1684.
4. Shields JA, Shields CL. Surgical approach to lamellar sclerouvectomy for posterior uveal melanomas. The 1986 Schoenberg Lecture. *Ophthal Surg* 1988;19:774–780.
5. Shields JA, Shields CL, Shah P, Sivalingam V. Partial lamellar sclerouvectomy for ciliary body and choroidal tumors. *Ophthalmology* 1991;98:971–983.
6. Shields JA, Shields CL, De Potter P. Enucleation technique for children with retinoblastoma. *J Pediatr Ophthalmol Strabismus* 1992;29:213–215.
7. Shields JA, Shields CL, Suvarnamani C, Tantasira M, Shah P. Orbital exenteration with eyelid sparing: indications, technique and results. *Ophthalmic Surg* 1991;22:292–297.
8. Shields JA, Shields CL. Massive orbital extension of posterior uveal melanoma. *J Ophthal Plast Reconstr Surg* 1991;7:238–251.

Fine-needle Aspiration Biopsy—Instruments and Technique

The instruments, techniques, limitations, complications, and results for fine-needle aspiration biopsy of suspected intraocular tumors and inflammations are reported in more detail in the references cited and are only illustrated briefly here.

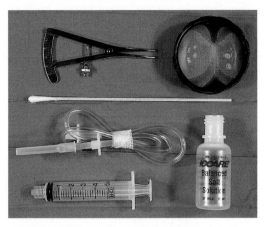

Figure 22-1. Instruments used for intraocular fine-needle aspiration biopsy.

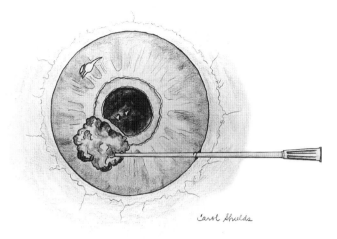

Figure 22-2. Limbal, transaqueous approach for iris lesions, front view. The surgical microscope generally is used for this technique.

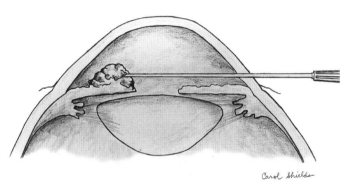

Figure 22-3. Limbal, transaqueous approach for iris lesions, side view.

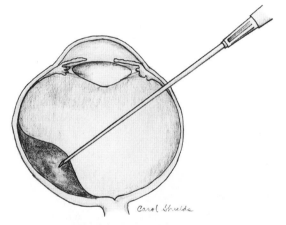

Figure 22-4. Pars plana, transvitreal approach for ciliary body and choroidal lesions. Indirect ophthalmoscopy usually is used for needle guidance. The technique requires considerable experience.

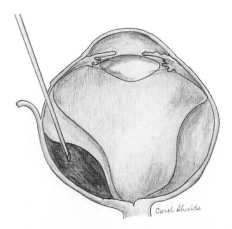

Figure 22-5. Method used for choroidal mass overlying bullous retinal detachment. An equatorial sclerotomy is performed, the choroid is cauterized, and the needle is passed obliquely through the subretinal space.

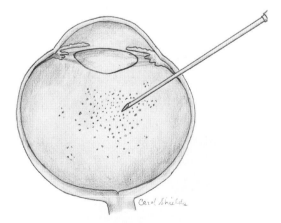

Figure 22-6. Pars plana approach for fine-needle aspiration biopsy of free cells in the vitreous cavity. This technique is most appropriate to diagnose vitreous lymphoma or to differentiate conditions such as vitreous melanoma cells from blood cells. Standard vitrectomy techniques also can be used to make the diagnosis of lymphoma.

Application of Radioactive Plaque

Brachytherapy, using a radioactive plaque sutured to the sclera over the base of the intraocular tumors, is used most often for selected malignant tumors such as uveal melanoma, retinoblastoma, and uveal metastasis. It can be used under special circumstances for circumscribed choroidal hemangioma, retinal vascular tumors, and perhaps other intraocular lesions. The use of radioactive plaques for these tumors is illustrated in the specific chapters in this atlas.

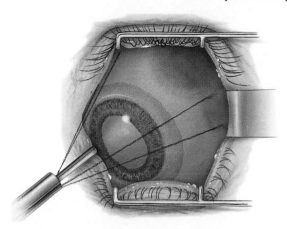

Figure 22-7. Transscleral transillumination is performed after a conjunctival peritomy. Note the shadow of the tumor.

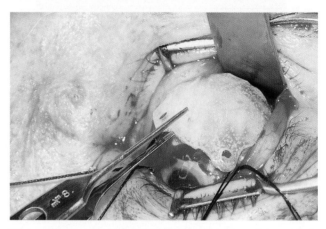

Figure 22-8. A dummy plaque without radioactive seeds is placed for suture alignment.

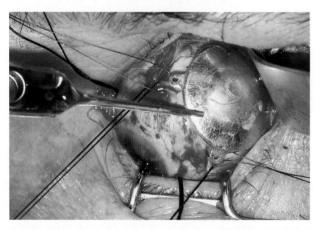

Figure 22-9. The dummy plaque has been removed and a radioactive iodine-125 plaque is inserted.

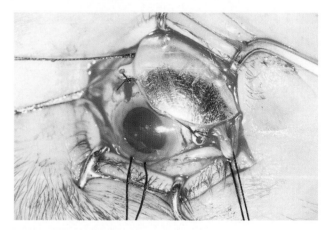

Figure 22-10. The radioactive plaque is sutured into the proper position.

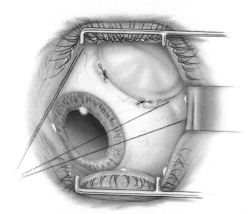

Figure 22-11. Drawing showing gold-shielded plaque sutured to the sclera.

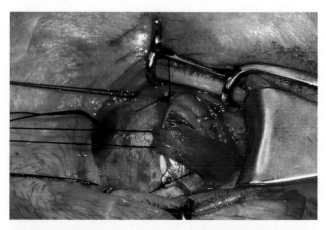

Figure 22-12. There are a number of special considerations in plaque application for intraocular tumors. In this case, the plaque is placed under the lateral rectus muscle because of the tumor location near the equator temporally.

Removal of Iris Tumor by Partial Iridectomy

Partial iridectomy is used mostly for resectable iris melanoma but it can be used to resect other benign and malignant tumors under certain circumstances.

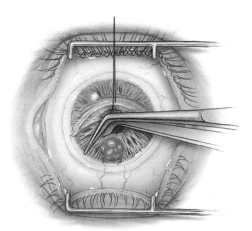

Figure 22-13. A limbal incision has allowed entrance into the anterior chamber. The cornea is retracted with a suture and the iris is being cut radially about 3 mm from the tumor.

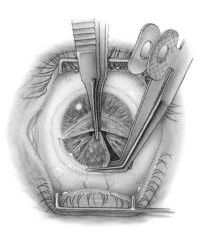

Figure 22-14. Both radial cuts have been made and a basal iris cut is being made outside the tumor margin, allowing tumor removal.

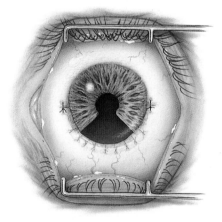

Figure 22-15. The sector iridectomy has been completed and the limbal wound has been closed with interrupted 10-0 nylon sutures.

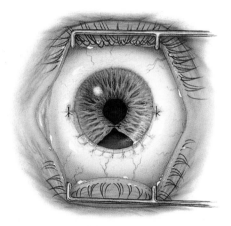

Figure 22-16. In cases in which the sector iridectomy is not too large, the iris defect can be repaired with a permanent intraocular suture (iridoplasty), creating a more round pupil.

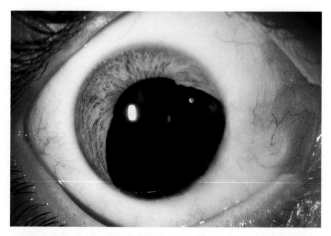

Figure 22-17. Postoperative photograph of sector defect too large to close with iridoplasty.

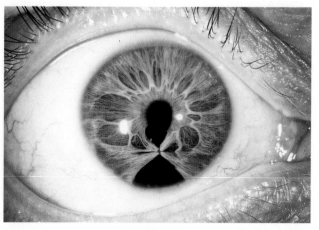

Figure 22-18. Postoperative photograph of smaller sector defect closed with iridoplasty.

Removal of Iridociliary Tumor by Partial Lamellar Iridocyclectomy

This technique is useful for uveal melanoma, leiomyoma, epithelial tumors of the ciliary body, and other selected lesions. It is a difficult surgical method that requires considerable experience.

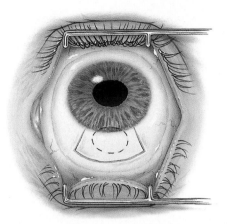

Figure 22-19. The *dotted line* depicts the margins of the tumor as determined with transillumination. The *solid line* shows the extent of the limbus-based scleral flap to be developed.

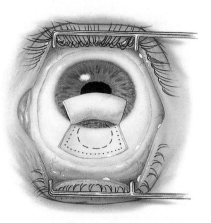

Figure 22-20. A scleral limbus-based flap of 80% thickness has been developed. The *dotted line* represents diathermy marks approximately 3 mm from the tumor margin.

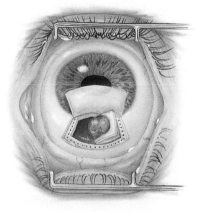

Figure 22-21. The inner scleral fibers have been incised and the tumor is exposed.

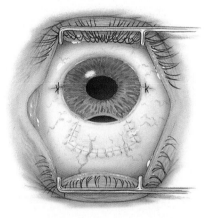

Figure 22-22. The tumor has been removed, a peripheral iridectomy has been performed, and the scleral wound has been closed with 9-0 interrupted nylon sutures.

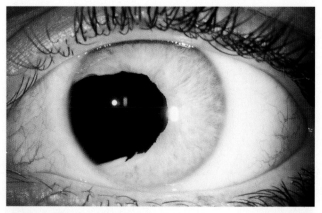

Figure 22-23. Postoperative photograph of sector defect after tumor removal by iridocyclectomy.

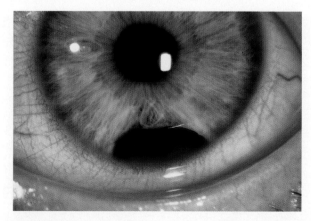

Figure 22-24. Postoperative photograph of peripheral iris defect after tumor removal by iridocyclectomy. In this case, a full-sector iridectomy was not necessary, so a peripheral iridectomy was performed.

Removal of Peripheral Choroidal Tumor by Partial Lamellar Cyclochoroidectomy

This technique is used for more posteriorly located tumors including melanoma, leiomyoma, neurilemoma, and larger tumors of the ciliary body epithelia. It is a very difficult surgical method that requires considerable experience.

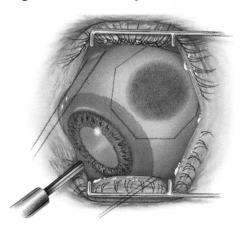

Figure 22-25. A conjunctival peritomy has been performed, the rectus muscles isolated with traction sutures, and the shadow of the tumor, seen with transillumination, will be marked with a sterile pen. The *solid line* depicts the size of the posteriorly hinged scleral flap that will be developed.

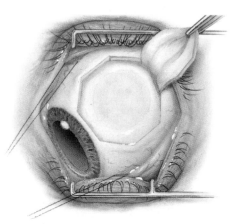

Figure 22-26. The dissected scleral flap has been reflected posteriorly, revealing the inner scleral bed.

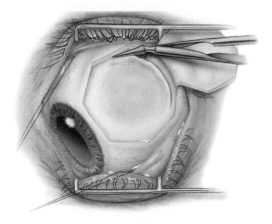

Figure 22-27. A circular incision is being made through the inner scleral bed about 4 mm outside the tumor margin as determined with transillumination.

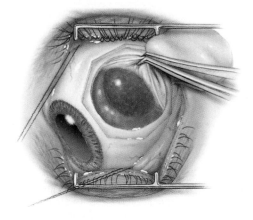

Figure 22-28. The inner scleral bed has been incised, revealing the tumor.

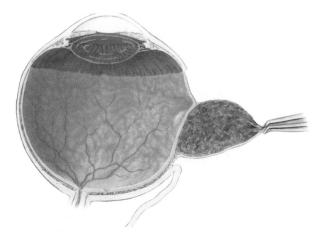

Figure 22-29. Side view of tumor being removed, leaving intact the sensory retina and vitreous.

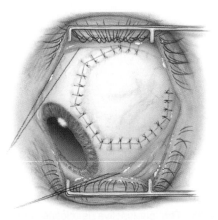

Figure 22-30. The tumor has been removed and the scleral flap sutured into its original position with 8-0 interrupted nylon sutures.

Enucleation

In ocular oncology, enucleation is performed mostly for advanced cases of uveal melanoma and retinoblastoma in which there is little hope for useful vision in the affected eye. It occasionally is warranted for uveal metastases that have produced a blind painful eye. It also is performed for uveal melanomas and retinoblastomas that have not been controlled following conservative methods of treatment. In cases of intraocular tumor, a minimal manipulation enucleation should be performed. In cases of retinoblastoma, it is important to obtain a long section of optic nerve along with the intact globe.

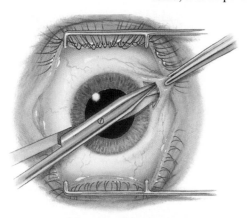

Figure 22-31. A conjunctival incision is made and a peritomy will be performed at the limbus for 360 degrees.

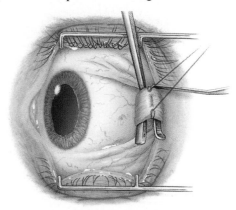

Figure 22-32. The rectus muscles are hooked, tagged with absorbable sutures, and cut near their insertions. The oblique muscles also are cut at their insertions.

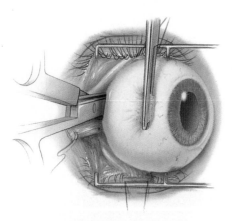

Figure 22-33. A hemostat is placed on the medial rectus muscle stump, the enucleation scissors are passed along the medial wall of the orbit, and the optic nerve is cut.

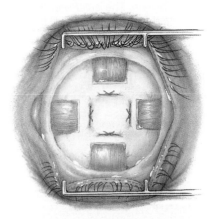

Figure 22-34. After hemostasis is achieved, the orbital implant is placed in the socket and the rectus muscles are attached to the implant. Although there are a variety of orbital implants, the authors most recently have used a hydroxyapatite or medpore motility implant lined with eye-bank sclera.

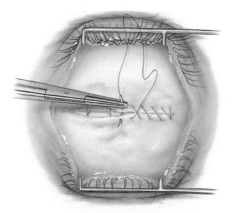

Figure 22-35. The conjunctiva is closed with a running absorbable suture. A conformer is inserted and a pressure patch applied.

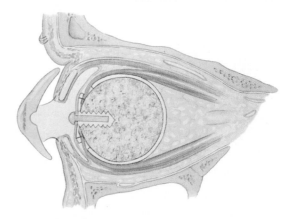

Figure 22-36. Side view showing vascularization of the hydroxyapatite implant 6 months after surgery. Also depicted is the peg that integrates the implant to the overlying prosthesis to provide better ocular motility.

Orbital Exenteration

Orbital exenteration most often is employed for malignant orbital tumors or for eyelid or conjunctival tumors that secondarily have invaded the orbit. With regard to intraocular tumors, it is used most often for massive orbital extension of uveal melanoma, retinoblastoma, and rarely other tumors. Because most intraocular tumors do not extend to affect the eyelids, an eyelid-sparing exenteration can be done in the majority of cases.

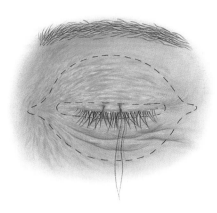

Figure 22-37. A suture is used to close the eyelids and a skin incision is made either just outside the cilia *(inner dotted line)* or in the midportion of the eyelid *(outer dotted line).*

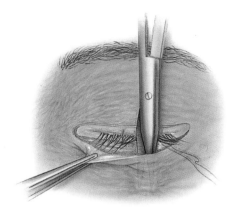

Figure 22-38. The skin and orbicularis muscle are undermined superiorly and inferiorly to the bony orbital rim.

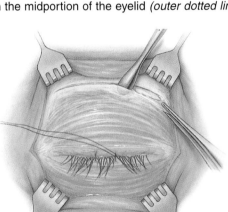

Figure 22-39. The periosteum is incised about 3 mm outside the orbital rim and a periosteal elevator is used to separate the periosteum from the bone into the orbit for 360 degrees.

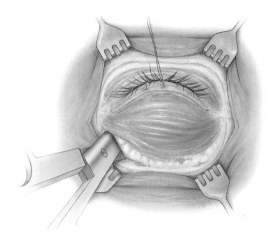

Figure 22-40. The enucleation scissors are inserted outside the orbital periosteum on the medial side and the optic nerve is cut near the orbital apex.

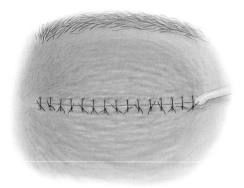

Figure 22-41. After hemostasis is achieved in the orbital cavity, interrupted 5-0 nylon sutures are used to suture the upper to the lower eyelid flap and a surgical drain is inserted.

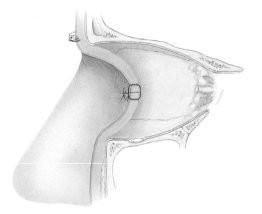

Figure 22-42. Side view postoperatively showing the bare orbital cavity with the eyelids sutured together over the defect.

Subject Index

Figures are noted with a page number first succeeded by the notation for the specific figure in italic numerals: for example, figure 1-27 on page 3 is shown as 3:*1-27.*